HEALTH CARE FOR CHILDREN

HEALTH CARE FOR CHILDREN

What's Right, What's Wrong, What's Next

Ruth E. K. Stein, M.D.
Editor

Phyllis Brooks
Associate Editor

United Hospital Fund of New York

Printed in the United States of America.

Library of Congress Cataloging-in-Publication Data

Health care for children : what's right, what's wrong, what's next /
   edited by Ruth E. K. Stein
      p.   cm.
   Includes bibliographical references and index.
   ISBN 1-881277-31-3
   1. Child health services—United States.   2. Children—Health and
hygiene—United States.   I. Stein, Ruth E. K.
   [DNLM: 1. Child Health Services—United States.   2. Child welfare—
United States.   3. Managed Care Programs—United States.   4. Health
Services Accessibility—United States.   WA 320 H4335 1997]
RJ102.H386   1997
362.1'982'000973—dc21
DNLM/DLC
for Library of Congress   97-12033
                                                                      CIP

For information, write, Publications Program, United Hospital Fund, Empire State Building, 350 Fifth Avenue, 23rd Floor, New York, NY 10118-2399.

Contents

Foreword

In recent years, public policy has more often been challenged for doing harm than praised for doing good. It is rare indeed that we pause to consider policy's power to crystallize a nation's present values and future aspirations, even rarer that we celebrate its victories.

But there are victories. In health care, one of the most impressive is the Medicare program. As recently as the early 1960s, elderly people in this nation lived in fear that a serious illness might bankrupt them. Health insurance was expensive, unreliable, and often inadequate; the dual results were high rates of poverty and poor health among the elderly.

Then in 1965, we as a society determined that we were not willing to tolerate this situation and enacted sweeping measures to combat it. In the 32 years since the passage of Medicare, there have been dramatic changes. All the elderly in the United States have access to some basic level of care. Disparities in health status among high-income and low-income older Americans have been virtually eliminated. Moreover, the poverty rate among the elderly has been significantly reduced, reflecting the extent to which earlier rates had been driven by health care costs. This is not to say, of course, that we have addressed all the health care needs of the elderly or that we have solved the problem of poverty among older Americans. Nor is it to imply that the Medicare program is without both short- and long-term challenges. Nonetheless, the story of Medicare is an instructive and inspirational one, an example of how we as a society can make a major commitment to improve conditions for a certain sector of our society and keep that commitment, with impressive results.

Contrast this story of success with our society's commitment to the health of children. Children are among the most vulnerable of our people, because they are so entirely dependent on others for care and nurture. Yet efforts to protect and support children have been fitful at best. In this century, the zeal to improve children's living conditions and health had its high point more than 60 years ago when laws were passed barring child labor and a national Children's Bureau with responsibility for children's health was created.

The record since then has been much spottier. The gains that have been made have often targeted segments of the child population, with the result being a dizzying array of programs, services, and funding mechanisms. The Children's Bureau was dismantled in 1969, its responsibilities parcelled out among various other agencies. As recently as the 1980s, we set out to expand coverage for children, using Medicaid as a vehicle. Gains were made, which in the first instance were reasonably impressive. But subsequent turmoil in the organization and financing of health care services threatens to erode that hard-won ground. The number of children without health insurance now stands at 10 million, and recent changes in the federal welfare program will decrease the number of children eligible for Medicaid and other social services. All these developments are bound to have an impact on children, some of them by affecting children's access to health care services, others by increasing the number of children in poverty, itself linked to health status.

All of this is cause for grave concern. Yet we as a nation have not managed to focus in a sustained way on children and their health care and other needs. A vigorous commitment is required, along with a serious examination of the health status of children and the ways in which they get care, and a thoughtful analysis of what would be needed to build a more rational and equitable system of care for them.

That, of course, is where this book comes in. With contributions from leading experts in the fields of pediatrics, public health, and health policy, it lays out the components of a rationalized system of care for children, one that would provide better and more consistent access to care for all of them. It makes the argument for a uniform standard of care for all children, as well as sustained investment in public health and pediatric research and education. It also reminds us that the United States stands alone in its failure to guarantee universal access to care for its children.

The question of children's health and access to health services generally is one that has occupied us over the years at the United Hospital Fund. The Fund was the lead sponsor of a 1989 child health policy retreat, which resulted in a series of recommendations, some of which were reflected in New York State's subsequent Child Health Plus legislation. Children are at the center of much of our work around Medicaid, access to care, and primary care development. Most recently, they were the focus of our 1996 conference "Child Health in a Managed Care Environment: Balancing Personal and Community Health Needs," which linked the Fund once again with Ruth E. K. Stein, MD, who has spent the last two years as a scholar in residence at the Fund and who had edited *Caring for Children with Chronic Illness* (Springer/United Hospital Fund 1989). In addition to providing the impetus for and organizing the conference, Dr. Stein—together with the Fund's ace editor, Phyllis Brooks—shaped and developed this book. We believe the book makes an important contribution to the literature, reflecting Dr. Stein's unique perspective, which blends the clinician's view of the individual child with the policy analyst's vision of the child population. The eloquence with which she espouses the cause of children, particularly those whom poverty or poor health renders especially vulnerable; the clarity with which she describes the problems of the current system; and her hopes for a more equitable system have guided and inspired us all.

There is no minimizing the problems that Dr. Stein and the other authors lay out here, nor the ambitious scope of the solutions proposed, but we must not forget how much is at stake. As we look ahead, let us remember that investing in children is one of the few ways we have of really making a difference.

James R. Tallon, Jr.
President
United Hospital Fund

Acknowledgments

This kind of volume is not possible without many different kinds of contributions from many different people. I am grateful to the authors who contributed their expertise and wisdom, helping to build a compelling argument on behalf of children. It is all the more powerful because it reflects the variety of their approaches and perspectives.

Several staff members at the United Hospital Fund helped shape and strengthen the book by reading and reacting to various drafts, including David A. Gould, Deborah E. Halper, Kathryn Haslanger, Avery Hudson, Sally Rogers, and Anthony Tassi. A special thanks to Phyllis Brooks for her exceptionally thoughtful editorial input. This book as a whole and every chapter in it have benefited from her unique skill and singular gift for language.

I would also like to express my gratitude to the United Hospital Fund and its president, James R. Tallon, Jr. I have had the privilege of being a scholar-in-residence at the Fund for the last two years, first to plan and develop a child health conference and then to work on this book. The Fund offered an oasis for reflection, which was particularly welcome for someone otherwise immersed in a busy urban health care facility.

Finally, on behalf of the Fund, I express a debt of gratitude to the funders who supported the publication of this volume, the William T. Grant Foundation, the Foundation for Child Development, and the David and Lucile Packard Foundation's Center for the Future of Children, as well as to United Way of New York City, which provides core support for the United Hospital Fund's myriad activities.

REKS

1

Changing the Lens: Why Focus on Children's Health?

Ruth E. K. Stein

CHILDREN ARE SOCIETY'S most precious resource. Caring for children—helping them to grow into healthy and productive members of society—is a significant responsibility, because both the long-term well-being of individual children and the collective vitality of society depend upon it. This responsibility is unique in that it must be fulfilled by one generation on behalf of the next. Children themselves do not vote; they have no direct political strength or voice in the policy decisions that affect them. Instead, society as a whole must make the commitment to care for them, demonstrating in the process its willingness to invest in the general good and the future.

How then does the United States care for, nurture, and protect its children? Others have described in detail the successes and failures of the U.S. educational and social welfare systems, but there has been far less discussion of the impact of health care practices and policy on the well-being of the next generation. This book seeks to fill that gap. It takes a look at just how healthy U.S. children are, both in comparison to each other and to children in other nations, and describes how they currently get health care, including, increasingly, through managed care arrangements. It outlines needed improvements in children's health services and assesses the prospects for such reforms in an era of shrinking budgets for health care delivery and social welfare programs and wavering commitment to the role of government in assuring access to basic human services for the most vulnerable members of society. What are the implications for children of current policy directions, and how can the interests of children and ultimately of society be protected?

Children in Our Society

One in every four people in the United States is under 18 years of age (Figure 1.1). While it is clear that the health status of U.S. children is considerably better than it was a few decades ago, it is equally apparent that their health lags significantly behind that of children in most western and industrialized nations. There are large segments of the nation in which child health status compares unfavorably with third-world nations. In part this reflects the fact that problems of child health are integrally related to poverty, and that there are substantial differentials in mortality and morbidity between those who are raised in middle-class environments and those who are poor.

Children constitute 38 percent of the nation's poor, and the proportion of U.S. children in all racial and ethnic groups living in poverty is growing (Figure 1.2). One in every five children lives below the federal poverty line, and one in ten lives in extreme poverty (less than 50 percent of the federal poverty level) (U.S. Bureau of the Census, 1995). An astounding 43 percent of black children and 41 percent of children of Hispanic descent live below the poverty line (CPS, 1994). The rates are even higher among children raised in female-headed households; approximately two-thirds of both black and Hispanic children living with a single mother are poor (Saluter, 1994).

Despite the need that these figures suggest, the United States finds itself alone among the nations of the western world in having failed to guarantee universal health care coverage to children and adolescents. Ten million, al-

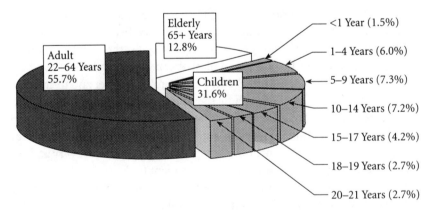

Figure 1.1
Population by age group, United States, 1995. (From HRSA, 1996.)

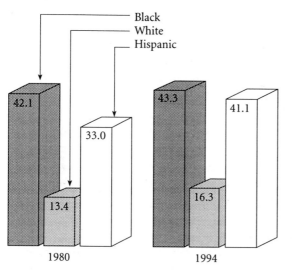

Figure 1.2
Children living in poverty, United States, 1980 and 1994. (From HRSA, 1996.)

most 14 percent, of U.S. children are uninsured (EBRI, 1996), and as many as one-quarter of all uninsured persons are children (U.S. Bureau of the Census, 1995). An even greater proportion, 35 percent, of children are uninsured for at least part of the year. Almost two-thirds of uninsured children live in families in which the head of household is employed year-round (EBRI, 1996).

Exacerbating the high rates of poverty and uninsurance among U.S. children is the lack of a solid public health or primary care infrastructure. Many of the services routinely available in other countries are unavailable to U.S. children. A child born in the United States has no guarantee of being provided basic health care services, no certainty of receiving immunizations against preventable infectious diseases, and no promise of being screened for avoidable health conditions. It is not certain that anyone will monitor the adequacy of the child's growth and development, nor is there any assurance that new parents will receive health education or assistance with common issues in child rearing. The universal home visitor programs that exist in other nations to teach young families to parent and to make the home safe for children have not been widely adopted here, despite repeated demonstrations that such interventions improve child rearing and decrease child abuse and neglect. When children in the United States are ill, their families have inconsistent access to care for them, and many find themselves unable to pay for services and medicines. Those children unfortunate enough to have chronic health conditions often have no choice but to rely on a bewildering patchwork of underfunded and uncoordinated systems with inconsistent eligibility requirements and enormous amounts of red tape.

The consequences of children's poor physical and emotional health are far-reaching. Because children are at the beginning of the life cycle, early problems may result in long-term costs for care and services, not to mention losses in productivity for both parents and, eventually, the grown children themselves. A child who is well and is able to grow normally, one who is nurtured and helped, is far more likely to become self-sufficient and to contribute to the community than one whose growth, development, and learning are stunted.

Furthermore, children learn from adults in their communities; they emulate their behavior and values. In a society that does not prioritize caring for each other, they may learn to be selfish and egocentric, to take but not to give back to others. A child, particularly one who is disadvantaged and who is reared in an uncaring environment, is far more likely to be in poorer health and to develop physical and mental health problems. Our failure to improve the situation for children contributes to substantially higher rates of adult physical and social morbidity, including high rates of substance abuse, crime, violence, and sustained poverty.

Toward a System of Health Care for Children

In short the United States has failed in its commitment to children, too often putting short-sighted economic considerations ahead of long-term goals. The current focus on how changes in welfare will affect children may paradoxically provide an opportunity for a more global reassessment of the ways in which we as a nation care for children and build the policies and services that would assure that all children have a chance to grow into healthy and productive members of society.

The first step in designing a system of care for children is recognizing the significant ways in which children's health care needs differ from adults'.

- Children are inherently dependent on their adult caretakers to protect and nurture them; they cannot be expected to act independently in securing health care.
- Children's rate of development and of biological, cognitive, and emotional change exceeds that at any other stage of life, making them uniquely vulnerable to a host of social, environmental, and develop-

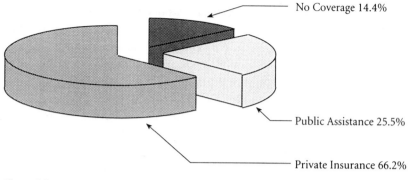

No Coverage 14.4%

Public Assistance 25.5%

Private Insurance 66.2%

Figure 1.3
Health insurance coverage for children, United States, 1994. Note that details may add to more than 100 percent because individuals may receive coverage from more than one source. (From HRSA, 1996.)

mental risks. As a result, their health status may be much more dramatically affected than adults' by social and economic factors, including environmental pollutants, violence, and poor nutrition.

- As infectious diseases have been brought under check, the predominant morbidity experienced by children increasingly is in the environmental, developmental, behavioral, and emotional spheres.
- While children are more likely to experience chronic conditions than is generally appreciated, the substantial majority do not have chronic health conditions. Those who do have chronic conditions are more likely to have relatively rare conditions.
- Because they are at the beginning of the life cycle, the patterns of health-related behavior that children develop form the basis of lifelong habits, which may have an impact much later in life and may contribute to or protect against long-term morbidity.

What does all this mean for the design of a health care system for children? First and foremost, it means that children are not just small adults whose care needs can be met by a system designed for grown-ups or by health care practitioners trained to treat adults. Children require a system and professionals that are able to address their particular needs.

- Preventive care, health education, and care of acute illness should form the cornerstone of a health care system for children, not the acute episodic care and chronic disease management that are the focus of the adult system.

- Care for children requires personnel who are knowledgeable about the unique manifestations of their disorders and who are intimately familiar with the dynamic nature of childhood behavior and physiology. They must be well versed in the wide range of developmental trajectories and the special forms of illness that children manifest.
- Health care services must be coordinated with social welfare and educational services. This is true for both those children who are healthy and those who have chronic disorders.
- All children benefit from the protection provided by good standards of community health, including environmental protection, "herd immunity" afforded by high rates of immunization against infectious diseases, and safety education.
- Finally, the schemes used to evaluate the efficacy and cost-effectiveness of child health services must recognize that the time frame for children's health outcomes is inevitably a long-term one and that poor child health has an impact not only on health care budgets but on many other sectors of the economy.

Taken together, these characteristics suggest that *medical necessity* must be defined differently for children and for adults. Medical necessity is the standard set forth in statute, regulations, and health insurance contracts that defines the scope of required services. The need for a child-specific definition of medical necessity was first developed by Jameson and Wehr (1994), who suggested that one must consider both children's present medical needs and their long-term developmental needs in deciding what services should be covered or provided. They also stress the great diversity of relatively rare childhood conditions that require access to specialized pediatric care. A child-specific standard, therefore, includes treatments or interventions that may be necessary now because of the high probability that they will prevent a future impairment. It sometimes has assured the provision of a broader and more inclusive package of health and related services to children than to adults, thus buffering children who needed services that were beyond their own family's ability to provide them.

This future orientation is reflected in the Medicaid program's standards for Early and Periodic Screening, Diagnosis and Treatment (EPSDT). Medicaid includes, as a fundamental part of the health care package for children, many services designed to prevent future impairments or conditions, including screening and early intervention services. It also includes enabling or wraparound services such as transportation and outreach. EPSDT has been the cornerstone of much of the past policy that has led to improvements in health care delivery for children, especially among those at highest medical and social risk. Current changes in the health care system threaten to erode this fundamental and hard-won concept, however.

The Role of Medicaid

As the foregoing discussion implies, Medicaid is central to any discussion of children's health care. Medicaid is not specifically designed for children, yet 58.5 percent of all those eligible for Medicaid are children (CPS, 1994), and 23.5 percent of all children are covered by Medicaid (EBRI, 1995). In many communities, the rates are even higher. In New York City and many other metropolitan areas, for example, more than 50 percent of births are paid for by Medicaid (City of New York, Department of Health, 1993). In the country as a whole, 39 percent of all births are paid for by Medicaid. Yet despite these high percentages, children account for only 16 percent of Medicaid expenditures. The average annual cost for each child enrolled in Medicaid is only $646 (Nather, 1997).

The number of children who rely on Medicaid for coverage has grown in recent years. More than half a million children have joined the Medicaid rolls each year as a result of the loss of private health insurance and the deliberate expansion of Medicaid coverage to children above the poverty line by the Omnibus Budget Reconciliation Acts of the late 1980s; between 1992 and 1993 the number increased by 900,000 (EBRI, 1995; Newacheck et al., 1995).

Because Medicaid is a means-tested program, and not like Medicare an entitlement, it is subject to all of the problems of programs for the poor. Moreover, eligibility is constantly fluctuating. Four percent of children on Medicaid lose their eligibility each month. Thus, Medicaid is hardly an ideal mechanism for financing the continuous care that children require.

Even more troubling are current discussions about the need to reduce Medicaid spending and to transfer responsibility for the program from the federal government to individual states. Either of these changes is likely to increase the proportion of uninsured children and reduce the package of services available to those who receive Medicaid benefits as a result of stretching limited appropriations to cover larger numbers of beneficiaries. It is also likely to make advocacy on behalf of children more difficult, as the locus of decision making about children's issues is further fragmented and diffused and as the battles over the distribution of shrinking funds are fought locally.

The Impact of Managed Care on Children's Health

Managed care in a wide variety of forms is being broadly implemented in both the private and the public sectors, based in large measure on the evidence that it can save money and slow the rate of growth in health care expenditures.

As of 1994, 16.7 million children were enrolled in managed care organizations (AAHP, 1994), and the numbers continue to grow dramatically. By 1995, 34 states were enrolling children in Medicaid in fully capitated plans in at least some geographic areas (Fox and McManus, 1996). However, there are few data demonstrating the impact or effectiveness of managed care for children, especially for the most vulnerable children and adolescents, such as those living in poverty and those who are disabled.

In principle, managed care offers an opportunity to do much that is good. It can increase the emphasis on primary and preventive care and improve the coordination of services. It seeks to develop links between individual physicians and individual children. Having a doctor who knows the child may reduce unnecessary and expensive visits to emergency rooms, where laboratory and diagnostic tests often substitute for the clinician's knowledge of how the child's appearance and examination differ from usual. In addition, managed care generally pays for health care maintenance for children, an otherwise expensive and often uncovered element of care for most families with young children outside the public sector.

Managed care, with its emphasis on continuity, care coordination, and flexibility, holds particular promise for hard-to-serve and vulnerable populations, those for whom continuity is most important and whose families face the most financial barriers to care. However, managed care's capitated rates do not, for the most part, differentiate among those with intensive and those with routine health care needs; managed care organizations thus have financial incentives to avoid enrolling the most socially disadvantaged and medically complex children, and to place restrictions on access to all but the most basic services.

Another issue is the relationship between managed care and the public health services and infrastructure that are so important to children's health. Managed care changes the way personal health care services are financed and organized, and it is sometimes viewed as the solution to all health problems; in some states, funds have been diverted from public health agencies to managed care plans. However, it is not clear that plans are able or willing to assume the full range of public health responsibilities. It is vital that the public health infrastructure be maintained and that the relationship between managed care and public health be closely monitored.

Overview of the Book

In the pages that follow, a number of experts have come together to share their understanding and analyses of these issues and to provide the insight necessary to improve the way we address children's health care needs.

To lay the groundwork and to demonstrate why we need to provide better health care for children, the first portion of the book asks how well we are currently doing. Chapter 2 reviews the health status of the entire child population and of large subgroups of U.S. children. Chapter 3 looks at the influence of social and environmental factors and health care services on children's health status. Next, chapter 4 assesses the issue of access to care using the most recent national data to point to some of the most glaring inequities in the availability and use of child health services.

The second part of the volume addresses how children get care. Chapter 5's historical perspective on the evolution of child health policy and pediatrics in the United States is followed by an analysis in chapter 6 of the current organization of health care services; it illustrates the extent to which current services are neither comprehensive nor consistent. Chapter 7 focuses on the changing role and pressures on the individual child health practitioner as the overall system evolves and reflects on how alterations in the financing of medical education and technological advances are likely to shape the future of health care. The final chapter in the section, chapter 8, reviews the important tensions that underlie, and in some cases paradoxically strengthen, current services and that must be taken into account in designing a more cohesive system of care.

The third section of the book focuses on managed care. Chapter 9 describes the challenges of defining and measuring the quality of health care delivered to children through managed care arrangements. Chapters 10 and 11 follow with analyses of some of the best practices of managed care organizations, along with some frank assessment of the incentives that may limit the extension of these practices.

The final section of the book presents a framework for considering and designing a new system of health care for children. First, chapter 12 lays out the moral and ethical arguments for ensuring all children access to health care. Chapter 13 discusses some of the recent efforts by child health advocates, highlighting the ways in which child advocacy has changed as decision making around child health issues has moved outside the traditional legislative mechanisms. Using a discussion of vulnerable children as a starting point, chapter 14 defines the financial, procedural, and conceptual barriers that must be overcome in order to provide an adequate system of care for children and argues for a "three-dimensionally" integrated system, in which care is coordinated vertically (primary and specialty care), horizontally (health care services and social welfare and education services), and longitudinally (over time). Chapter 15 discusses how the role of public health departments is evolving with the growth of managed care and stresses the need for a strong public health function in assuring and evaluating health care. This chapter is followed by one that outlines several innovative and promising collaborations that have been developed within the constraints of the changing paradigms. Finally the book ends with a health policy agenda in chapter 17 that sets out the choices and suggests changes that are needed to improve the situation for children. These are predicated on the strong belief that there is a great deal of work to do in maximizing the ways we invest in our children. In the final analysis, children and our nation's future depend on how well we face these challenges.

References

[AAHP] American Association of Health Plans. 1994. National Directory of HMOs. AAHP.

City of New York, Department of Health. 1993. Summary of vital statistics. New York: Office of Vital Statistics and Epidemiology.

[CPS] Current Population Survey. 1994. Washington: U.S. Department of Commerce, Bureau of the Census.

[EBRI] Employee Benefits Research Institute. 1995. Issue report 158. Washington: EBRI.

[EBRI] Employee Benefits Research Institute. 1996. Sources of health insurance and characteristics of the uninsured: Analysis of the March 1995 Current Population Survey. Issue brief no. 170. Washington: EBRI.

Fox H, McManus M. 1996. Impacts of state Medicaid waiver programs on children: Results from Hawaii, Oregon, Rhode Island, and Tennessee. Policy Center.

[HRSA] Health Resources and Services Administration, Maternal and Child Health Bureau, U.S. Department of Health and Human Services, Public Health Service. 1994. Child Health USA. Washington: U.S. Government Printing Office.

[HRSA] Health Resources and Services Administration, Maternal and Child Health Bureau, U.S. Department of Health and Human Services, Public Health Service. 1996. Child Health USA. Washington: U.S. Government Printing Office.

Jameson EJ, Wehr E. 1994. Drafting national health care reform legislation to protect the health interests of children. Stanford Law and Policy Review 5(1):152–76.

Nather D. 1997. Special report on children's health: Consensus on need for legislation weakened by range of possible options. BNA's Health Report 5:202–4.

Newacheck PW, Hughes, DC, Cisternas, M. 1995. Children and health insurance: An overview of recent trends. Health Affairs 14(1):244–54.

Saluter A. 1994. Marital status and living arrangements. Current population reports (series P-20-484). Washington: Bureau of the Census.

U.S. Bureau of the Census. 1995. Statistical abstract of the United States: 1995. Washington: U.S. Bureau of the Census.

I

HOW HEALTHY ARE AMERICA'S CHILDREN?

One theme emerges unambiguously from the following chapters, that efforts in the United States to preserve recent advances in child health and achieve further improvements will require addressing the needs of an increasingly ethnically and economically diverse child population. In the United States of the 1990s, a third of the children are nonwhite, a fifth of them live in poverty, and a tenth are uninsured—and more than half of American children fall into one or more of these risk groups. Childhood poverty, if anything, is growing and deepening, and the number of uninsured children will likely grow even larger in coming years. Even the rapid growth in Medicaid coverage since 1989 has failed to compensate entirely for the simultaneous deterioration of employment-related health benefits.

Children in the United States lack the guaranteed access to health services that is characteristic of all other industrialized countries, and they must rely on a health system that lacks a strong primary care infrastructure. A few health problems seem actually to have worsened in recent years, among them child abuse and neglect, asthma and other chronic respiratory conditions, AIDS, limitation of activity, and overweight. Children in the United States are far more likely than children in other industrialized nations to die from injuries, and they are less likely to be up to date on their immunizations. The United States also has higher rates of unintended pregnancies, abortions, teenage pregnancies, and infant mortality than many industrialized countries.

Still, in recent decades mortality from all causes except for violent deaths has fallen; several childhood diseases have virtually disappeared; and anemia, lead poisoning, and dental caries have declined. Several measures—such as low birthweight, preterm delivery, shortness, and thinness—appear stable. Local, state, and federal health policies—changes in legislation, enforcement of regulations, and health promotion efforts—indubitably have contributed to these advances. Improvement in environmental conditions, including safe water supplies, pasteurized milk, pure food, and elimination of lead from gasoline and paint, has reduced mortality and morbidity. And children from lower-class families who receive Medicaid to pay for health services are far more likely to receive care for their acute and chronic illnesses than are those who have no such coverage. However, the continued absence of a direct federal role creates conditions for increased inequities in the provision of health services across economic, ethnic, and regional boundaries.

2

Recent Trends in the Health of U.S. Children

Lorraine V. Klerman and Janet D. Perloff

IN MANY WAYS the health status of children in the United States has improved considerably over the last few decades, although in some respects it shows no progress and in others, it is worsening. Also troublesome are the disparities among racial/ethnic and socioeconomic groups within this country and this country's continued low ranking on some health measures in comparison to other industrialized nations.

This chapter will first review the measures most often used to assess health. It will then describe recent trends in children's health status. Finally, it will consider the extent to which the observed trends can be ascribed to medical care.

Measures of Children's Health Status

Most child health experts believe that the U.S. system of health care for children is adequate or good for middle- and upper-income children, but inadequate for poor and near-poor children, particularly those with impairments or chronic illnesses. Usually such judgments are based on utilization of health care services, such as the number of well-child visits relative to the standards of the American Academy of Pediatrics; the number of immunizations relative to the standards of the Centers for Disease Control and Prevention (CDC); or even the adequacy of health insurance

The preparation of this chapter was made possible, in part, by the Maternal and Child Health Bureau, U.S. Department of Health and Human Services (grant MCJ 9040).

coverage, whether obtained through parent's employment, individual purchase, or a public system such as Medicaid.

Such judgments assume, generally, that more care is better care or, at least, that care that does not meet professionally established standards is inadequate. While these assumptions may be true, the evidence to validate them is not powerful, except in the case of immunizations. In order to use health care utilization or insurance status as indicators of children's health status, researchers first need to demonstrate that those who meet the standards for health care use or who have health insurance are healthier than those who do not meet those standards or who are not insured, even after taking into consideration genetic makeup; physical environment; demographic characteristics such as age and gender; socioeconomic factors such as income and education; and similar factors. There are such studies, but not as many as are needed either to improve the present system of child health care or to design a better one (Budetti et al., 1995; Wagner et al., 1989).

Criteria

Among the reasons that it is difficult to show the effectiveness of health care are the limited number of easily available measures of the health status of children and the problems involved in linking these measures to health care. In chapter 3, Starfield notes that documenting population health levels is particularly difficult for children, who are not old enough to have developed the well-defined illnesses associated with the aging process. She urges that health systems be evaluated on the basis not only of their ability to reduce mortality and prevent disease, but also of their capacity to minimize symptoms and disability and decrease vulnerability to threats to health. Several groups have attempted to develop lists of measures that could be used to monitor children's health status (Miller et al., 1989; Walker and Richmond, 1984), most importantly the U.S. Public Health Service (1991) in *Healthy People 2000: National Health Promotion and Disease Prevention Objectives*.

Most policy analysts agree that in order to be used to evaluate or improve a system of health care for children, measures of child health status must be:

- related to a disease, condition, or cause of death whose incidence or prevalence is relatively high and that could be prevented or greatly reduced through known and available interventions;

- capable of being measured reasonably precisely and consistently across time and geographic boundaries;
- easy to obtain from data sources that are both complete and valid (i.e., they must measure the phenomena accurately);
- based on a population or, if based on a sample, chosen in such a way as to eliminate bias;
- collected on an ongoing basis so that trends can be charted and made available quickly and periodically, preferably through governmental or journal publication; and
- able to be linked to other information, such as poverty level or maternal education, which will assist in interpreting the findings.

A recent listing of measures of child health status can be found in *Trends in the Well-Being of America's Children and Youth: 1996*, which was extensively used in this review (Office of the Assistant Secretary for Planning and Evaluation, 1996). It provides three types of measures in its health section:

- mortality (infant, child, and youth mortality, and adolescent deaths from motor vehicle injuries, homicides, and suicides);
- health conditions (healthy births [defined by Apgar score, birthweight, gestational age, and adequacy of prenatal care], low and very low birthweight, general and chronic health conditions, overweight in adolescents, abuse and neglect, and suicidal adolescents); and
- health care (health insurance coverage, adequacy of prenatal care, and immunizations).

The list of health status measures generated by a federally funded project to develop a model data set for maternal and child health is similarly brief (M. Peoples-Sheps, personal communication):

- perinatal morbidity (condition at birth, congenital anomalies, and prenatal exposure);
- disease and injury morbidity (communicable diseases, sexually transmitted diseases, nutritional deficiencies, dental diseases, chronic diseases, and injuries);
- physical and psychosocial functioning (behavioral/emotional disorders, sensory impairments, and other); and
- mortality (total and cause-specific).

Clearly the experts have difficulty in generating extensive lists of health status measures that meet these criteria.

Sources

The measures that come closest to meeting the criteria cited above are those items found on birth and death certificates. They are reasonably valid, although some studies have found inaccuracies. They are collected on all children and provide information about more than just health conditions. And they are collected continuously and published annually by the National Center for Health Statistics (NCHS), state governments, and others.

Birth certificates provide information on birthweight; gestational age at birth, from which it can be determined whether the birth is preterm and whether the infant is small, normal, or large for its gestational age; and the presence of congenital anomalies. But birth certificates are of limited use in evaluating the system of child health care, because they reflect only preconception and prenatal care. The information on birth certificates is more useful for planning purposes when it is linked to the death certificates of infants (children under the age of one). Most states prepare such linked data sets in order to gain insight, relatively rapidly, into how preconception and prenatal factors affect infant mortality. A national data set linking births and infant deaths is prepared by the NCHS, but its publication lags behind the publication of birth and death data. The 1991 data were released late in 1996.

While death certificates provide information about the cause of death, as well as the infant's or child's age at the time of death, they are of limited use in measuring the health status of the child population because, fortunately, relatively few children die and those who die usually do so in the first year of life. Some additional information can be obtained when the Supplementary Classification of External Causes of Injury and Poisoning, also known as E codes, is used to "classify the environmental events, circumstances, intentionality, and conditions that cause injury, poisoning and other adverse effects." E codes can provide relatively complete data on fatal injuries sustained by children and adolescents. Because E codes are not yet widely incorporated into hospital discharge and other data systems, however, information about children's *nonfatal* injuries is much less complete (Smith et al., 1994).

Other measures of children's health status can be divided into those that examine health and those that examine the absence of health. There are many more of the latter, including the presence of chronic conditions and the limitation of activities due to these conditions; episodes of acute or chronic illness; injuries; and other items. The best-known sources of these data are the surveys of the NCHS. The National Health Interview Survey (NHIS), a continuous sample survey, collects data on all the items listed above at two-week intervals over the course of the year. The NHIS, however, does not focus exclusively or even predominantly on children's health, although in some years the NHIS has added questions about children's health and risk behaviors to its basic survey. These surveys have been a rich source of child health measures. The NHIS publishes its findings once a year in a summary form, *Current Estimates from the National Health Interview Survey.* The tapes from these surveys are available for analysis and more detailed reports are published frequently by independent researchers as well as the NCHS. These data, while based on large, representative samples, are obtained by adult report, so their validity is dependent on respondents' honesty and knowledge of their own and other family members' health.

The NCHS's National Health and Nutrition Examination Survey (NHANES) collects information not only by interview, but also by physical and psychological examinations. Thus, some NHANES data are based on actual clinical measures of health status and, in those areas, may be more valid than the NHIS. And, as indicated by its name, the NHANES also provides nutritional data. Unfortunately, because of its high cost, the NHANES is conducted infrequently and on a much smaller sample than the NHIS. An additional problem is that the NHIS and NHANES are available only for the nation or by large regions: the data are not available for most states, counties, or cities. Thus, states, counties, and cities that want information about the health status of children in their areas must either conduct their own surveys, which are very expensive, or resort to synthetic estimates.

The NCHS conducts other surveys that provide information on children's health status. These include the National Hospital Discharge Study, which indicates the health reasons for hospitalization, and the National Ambulatory Medical Care Survey and Hospital Ambulatory Medical Care Survey, which indicate the health reasons for ambulatory care visits to physicians' offices and to hospital ambulatory care and emergency departments. Like the NHIS, these surveys yield national and regional estimates, but cannot be used to describe the health status of children in smaller jurisdictions. Unlike the NHIS, which is a population-based survey, these three surveys are facility-based and capture the health problems only of health care users.

In addition, the CDC conduct or help states conduct several surveys including the Pediatric Nutrition Surveillance System, which monitors the general health and nutritional characteristics of low-income children enrolled in clinics served by publicly funded health and nutrition programs in most states, and the school-based surveys conducted in conjunction with the Youth Risk Behavior Surveillance System. Other studies of children's health have been commissioned by the federal government or undertaken by smaller governmental units, universities, and other groups.

Researchers and program planners are increasingly interested in measures of children's *health* rather than of its absence. Perhaps the easiest to obtain and most widely used measure is reported health status. In the NHIS, the respondent, usually the mother, is asked, for each of her children living at home, whether she believes that the child's health is excellent, very good, good, fair, or poor.

Multiple-Item Measures

Many researchers are working on more complex and sensitive measures of health based on a combination of items that together may reveal more than the individual measures just described. For its landmark study of the impact of health insurance on the receipt of care and on health status, the RAND Corporation administered questionnaires to parent proxies, usually mothers, from which scales were developed to measure mental health, social health, general health perceptions, and parental satisfaction with child development (Eisen et al., 1979). Stein and Jessop (1990) have developed a functional status measure that assesses how well children perform daily activities. Starfield and colleagues have published an Adolescent Child Health and Illness Profile (CHIP-AE) that measures six domains: discomfort (physical, emotional, limitation of activity); satisfaction (with health, self-esteem); disorders; achievement (school behavior, academic performance, work performance); resilience (family involvement, problem-solving, physical activity, home safety and health); and risks (individual with and without sex-related items, threats to achievement, peer influences). The information on the profile can be collected by a self-administered questionnaire. Clearly the profile includes many items that are not usually considered to measure "health" status (Starfield et al., 1995). Unfortunately, few of the multiple item measures have been administered to large populations. Most are still used exclusively as research instruments.

The increasing attention being paid to the effectiveness of treatment is creating new interest in ways of measuring health including clinical status; physical, mental, and social/role functioning and well-being; and general health perceptions and satisfaction (Stewart and Ware, 1992). While still focused primarily on adults, whose care is usually more expensive, the techniques are beginning to be used with children as well.

Trends in Child Health Status

Analyses of *trends* in children's health status are further limited because few measures, other than mortality and some perinatal measures, have been collected over a long enough period of time to allow for a study of trends. The review that follows will show, however, that by most indicators the health status of U.S. children has improved in this century. Mortality from all causes is down, except for violent deaths among adolescents; several childhood diseases have virtually disappeared; and anemia, lead poisoning, and dental caries have declined. Several measures appear stable, such as low birthweight, preterm delivery, shortness, and thinness. But a few health problems may actually have worsened, such as child abuse and neglect, asthma, limitation of activity, and overweight, although some of these upward trends may be due to improved reporting or to changes in definitions. And AIDS, a disease unknown 15 years ago, is being diagnosed in infants and adolescents.

Mortality

Infant mortality has decreased steadily in recent years, reaching a low of 7.5 deaths per 1,000 live births in 1995 (preliminary) (Rosenberg et al., 1996). Infant mortality was 29.2 in 1950, 26.0 in 1960, 20.0 in 1970, 12.6 in 1980, and 10.6 in 1985 (National Center for Health Statistics, 1996). The largest percentage declines between 1979 and 1994 were in deaths due to respiratory distress syndrome (due to the use of surfactant, a new therapy), followed by intrauterine hypoxia and birth asphyxia, and pneumonia and influenza (Singh et al., 1996). The recent decline in the Sudden Infant Death Syndrome (SIDS) is probably a result of the American Academy of Pediatrics' educational campaign about SIDS risk factors. The lack of any significant downward trend in infant deaths due to preterm deliveries and low birthweight is troubling. The percentage of low birthweight infants actually increased from a low of 6.8 percent in 1985 to 7.3 percent in 1994.

Mortality among children aged 1 to 4, 5 to 9, and 10 to 14 years, expressed as deaths per 100,000 children in the age group, has also decreased.

Among those aged 15 to 19 years, the general trend is downward, but there were some intermediate increases (Table 2.1) (Office of the Assistant Secretary for Planning and Evaluation, 1996).

Injuries are the most frequent cause of death to children over the age of one and the seventh most frequent cause of death to infants (Singh et al., 1996). Comparing rates of traumatic death in children under 20 years of age in 1978 and 1991, Rivera and Grossman (1996) found that deaths from all injuries decreased by 26.5 percent, from 40.2 per 100,000 to 29.6 per 100,000. Unintentional deaths decreased by 38.9 percent, but intentional deaths (deaths from child abuse or neglect) actually increased by 47.1 percent. The largest decreases in rates were for poisoning due to gases and vapors and for motorcyclist and pedestrian injuries. Deaths due to homicide and suicide rose, largely due to increases in firearm deaths for these causes.

The National Committee to Prevent Child Abuse reported that between 1985 and 1995, intentional deaths increased by almost 50 percent, from 810 to 1,215 per year. Reported cases per year also rose, from 2.1 million to 3.1 million in the same period (National Center on Child Abuse Prevention Research, 1996). Some of this increase may be due to heightened awareness of the problem, leading to increased reporting.

Measures of Poor Health or Injury

This century has witnessed dramatic declines in the serious communicable diseases of childhood—diphtheria, measles, pertussis, and poliomyelitis—due almost entirely to the development and widespread use of vaccines. But the last decades have seen the appearance of HIV infection and AIDS as diseases of infants, young children, and adolescents. As of September

Table 2.1
Childhood Mortality (Deaths per 100,000 Children)
United States
1960 and 1992

Age (years)	1960	1992
1–4	109	44
5–9	49	20
10–14	44	25
15–19	92	84

Source: Office of the Assistant Secretary for Planning and Evaluation, 1996.

1996, 7,472 cases of AIDS among children under age 13 had been reported. From 1988 to 1993, CDC estimated that between 6,000 and 7,000 children were born each year to HIV-infected women and that between 1,000 and 2,000 of the children born each year were infected. As a result of clinical trials showing the effectiveness of zidovudine (ZDV) therapy in preventing the transmission of HIV from mother to fetus, the Public Health Service issued recommendations in 1994 for routine ZDV treatment and in 1995 it recommended routine HIV counseling and voluntary testing for all pregnant women. The CDC is now reporting a 27 percent decline in perinatally acquired AIDS cases from an estimated peak of 905 in 1992 to 663 in 1995 (CDC, 1996). As of December 31, 1995, 2,354 cases of AIDS had been reported in adolescents 13 to 19 years of age. Of these, 405 were first reported in 1995 (Maternal and Child Health Bureau, 1996).

According to NHIS estimates, the most prevalent chronic health conditions in children under 18 years of age are respiratory conditions, particularly asthma and chronic sinusitis. The rates of several chronic health conditions have increased in the last few decades. The incidence of asthma, the condition with the highest prevalence, increased from 40 per 1,000 children under 18 years of age in 1982 to 72 per 1,000 in 1993. Increases were also reported for hay fever and allergic rhinitis without asthma, chronic bronchitis, chronic sinusitis, serious acne, and migraine headaches (Office of the Assistant Secretary for Planning and Evaluation, 1996).

Measuring the prevalence of specific chronic conditions, such as asthma, is somewhat easier than measuring the overall prevalence of childhood chronic conditions and disabilities. This is due, in part, to differences in definitions among studies. Some studies, such as the NHIS, use a "condition list." Estimates of the prevalence of chronic conditions based on such a list depend on which conditions are defined as chronic (Perrin et al., 1993). Dissatisfaction with this approach, particularly as it applies to children, has led to measurements based on the impact of acute and chronic conditions on children's lives. Such measures include school absences due to illness or injury, number of days spent in bed, and limitations in school, play, or recreational activities, all of which are used in the NHIS (Newacheck and Stoddard, 1994; Newacheck and Taylor, 1992).

For example, the percentage of children under 18 reported as having a limitation of activity increased from 1.8 percent in 1960 to 3.8 in 1981 and to 6.7 percent in 1994. This change may be partially due to increased reporting as benefits became available for children with certain conditions under the Supplementary Security Income program for Disabled Children (SSI-DC) (Adams and Marano, 1995; Newacheck et al., 1986). Another approach to the measurement of chronic conditions is that of the Current Population Survey, which asks whether a child has a disability, as well as whether the child is limited in "usual kind of activities" (McNeil, 1993). Some multiple-item health status measures also examine the impact of acute and chronic conditions on children.

Most indicators of nutritional status show improvement. According to the Pediatric Nutrition Surveillance System, the prevalence of childhood anemia declined nearly 5 percent for most racial and ethnic groups between 1980 and 1991. Over the same period, the rates of shortness (low height-for-age) and thinness (low weight-for-height) remained stable, except for Asian children, predominantly those of Southeast Asian refugee background, whose rates of shortness in 1980 were higher than those of other groups. The rates for this group have declined over time, however, and by 1991 they were similar to those for other racial/ethnic groups (Yip et al., 1992). However, overweight among adolescents is increasing. In the 1976–1980 NHANES, 15 percent of 12- to 19-year-olds were overweight, while in the 1988–1991 survey 21 percent were (Office of the Assistant Secretary for Planning and Evaluation, 1996).

NHANES has also shown that the incidence of lead poisoning (defined as more than 25 micrograms per deciliter of blood) among children 1 to 5 years of age decreased from 9.3 percent in the 1976–1980 survey to only 0.5 percent in the 1988–1991 survey. The proportion of children with more than 10 micrograms of lead per deciliter of blood (the goal the CDC [1991] established for all lead poisoning prevention activities) fell from 88.2 percent in the earlier survey to 8.9 percent in the later one (Maternal and Child Health Bureau, 1996).

Fluoridation of the water supply, along with increased use of dental sealants and other measures, has led to a marked decrease in dental caries among children. The 1989–1991 NHANES found that 62.1 percent of children 2 to 9 years of age were caries-free in their primary dentition and 54.7 percent of children 5 to 17 years of age were caries-free in their permanent dentition (Kaste et al., 1996).

Measures of Health
The percentage of children under 5 years of age reported to be in excellent or very good health remained fairly constant, at approximately 80 percent, between 1982 and 1993. For those 5 to 17 years of age, there was a slight in-

crease, from 76 percent in 1982 to 79 percent in 1993 (Office of the Assistant Secretary for Planning and Evaluation, 1996).

Health Status Differentials among U.S. Children

This overview of the health status of U.S. children obscures important differentials in health status among certain populations, however. National data indicate that the health of children in low-income families, children in racial and ethnic minority groups, children in large cities, and, to a lesser extent, children in rural areas compares unfavorably with that of children without these characteristics.

Children in Low-Income Families

By almost any measure, children in low-income families experience poorer health than their higher income counterparts. As Starfield notes in chapter 3, low-income children are consistently found to experience higher rates of illness, and low income has been found to be associated with three- to fourfold increases in the severity of illness in childhood. Rates of underimmunization are highest among low-income children (Wood et al., 1995); elevated blood lead levels are more prevalent among low-income children 1 to 5 years of age (CDC, 1994); and various indicators of inadequate nutrition—including hunger, chronic undernutrition, and iron deficiency anemia—are all disproportionately high among low-income children (Geltman et al., 1996). Reports of children being in fair or poor health, days of school lost due to acute and chronic conditions for children under 18 years of age, and the percentage of children with activity limitations all increase as family income decreases (Adams and Marano, 1995). The varied and complex reasons for the compromised health of low-income children include poor housing and hazardous neighborhoods, poor nutrition, inadequate preventive care, and poor access to care (Fossett and Perloff, 1995; Perloff, 1992; Starfield, 1992).

Although, as noted previously, the health of this nation's children has improved in many respects, the rate of improvement has probably been hindered by growing and deepening childhood poverty. The proportion of children living below 200 percent of the poverty line hovered around 43 percent between 1975 and 1993. The proportion of those living below 100 percent of the poverty line increased from a low of 14.0 percent in 1969 to a high of 22.7 in 1993 and declined only to 20.8 percent by 1995. Of even greater concern in relation to children's health status is the doubling, from

5 percent to 10 percent, in the proportion of children living in extreme poverty, that is, in families with incomes below 50 percent of the poverty line. Increases in extreme poverty have been especially pronounced for black children, rising from 14 percent in 1975 to 26 percent in 1993. The chances of being extremely poor increases to 72 percent for black and Hispanic children under the age of 6 who are living in female-headed households (Baugher and Lamison-White, 1996; Office of the Assistant Secretary for Planning and Evaluation, 1996).

Racial and Ethnic Minority Children

There are substantial differences in children's health status by racial and ethnic group. These differences are particularly pronounced between white, non-Hispanic children and children of color. Some proportion of the observed differences is no doubt attributable to the far greater likelihood of poverty and near-poverty among black and Hispanic children: 27 percent of white children under age 18 lived under 150 percent of the poverty level in 1993 as compared with 61 percent of black and 60 percent of Hispanic children (Office of the Assistant Secretary for Planning and Evaluation, 1996).

Just as the nation's overall infant mortality rate fell rapidly over the past several decades, the rate also fell by race and Hispanic origin. Between 1960 and 1992, the infant mortality rate decreased 69 percent among whites, 62 percent among blacks, 68 percent among Asians, and 77 percent among Native Americans (Office of the Assistant Secretary for Planning and Evaluation, 1996). In 1994, however, large disparities could still be observed in infant mortality rates across racial and ethnic subgroups. The infant mortality rate for blacks in 1994 was more than twice that for whites, and the rate for Puerto Ricans (8.7) was higher than that for all Hispanics (6.5) (Singh et al., 1996).

As noted in the previous section, deaths in children older than 1 year are not common, but they are found disproportionately among black children. In recent decades the mortality rate for black children has consistently been two times higher than that for white children. A notable exception to this pattern is found among 15- to 19-year-olds. For this group, the disparity among races in the mortality rate closed between 1970 and 1980, but it increased again between 1985 and 1992, a period during which the white rate remained stable. As a result, the death rate among black 15- to 19-year-olds is once again twice that of white children of the same age (Office of the Assistant Secretary for Planning and Evaluation, 1996).

While childhood deaths from injuries are decreasing overall, black children are at considerably higher risk for some types of violent death. Relative to their white counterparts, black male teenagers are at substantially elevated risk for homicide deaths. For this group, the homicide rate has increased dramatically, from 46.6 per 100,000 in 1985 to 134.6 per 100,000 in 1991. In contrast, over the past 20 years the rate of youth motor vehicle accident deaths has been consistently lower among black teenagers (Office of the Assistant Secretary for Planning and Evaluation, 1996).

Some general measures of morbidity indicate less substantial differentials in the health status of black and white children. Since 1982, the likelihood that black children would be reported as being in very good or excellent health has increased considerably, and as a result, racial disparities in this measure of children's health status have narrowed. In 1993, 71 percent of black children and 82 percent of white children under 5 years of age were reported to be in good or excellent health; for black and white children ages 5 through 17 the respective rates were 70 percent and 81 percent (Office of the Assistant Secretary for Planning and Evaluation, 1996).

Children of minority groups are at higher risk for specific acute and chronic health problems, probably because of their greater likelihood of being poor. Minority children are more likely to be underimmunized and they disproportionately experienced the recent epidemics of vaccine-preventable diseases (Wood et al., 1995). Minority children also are overrepresented among children with HIV and AIDS. Although Hispanic children constitute only 12 percent of the U.S. child population, they account for 24 percent of childhood AIDS cases, with a large proportion of these cases concentrated among Puerto Rican children (Mendoza, 1994). The rate of asthma is also particularly high among minority children. This chronic condition is associated with the highest average number of restricted activity and bed disability days among children (Halfon and Newacheck, 1993).

The different measures of chronic conditions and disabilities, discussed earlier in this chapter, produce different estimates across racial and ethnic groups. Data from the 1988 NHIS Child Health Supplement indicated that both single and multiple chronic conditions were more prevalent among white children than among black children (Newacheck, 1992; Newacheck, 1994). The 1991–1992 Current Population Survey, however, found that the percentage of children reported as having a disability was similar among whites and blacks from birth to 14 years, but slightly higher among black as compared to white 15- to 17-year-olds. The percentage of children reported as having a severe disability was similar among whites and blacks from birth to 14 years, but twice as high among black as opposed to white 15- to 17-year-olds. Hispanic children had the lowest rates of disability at all ages (McNeil, 1993). Additional research is needed to understand the reasons for these differences by racial and ethnic groups and to determine whether chronic conditions and disabilities impact these groups differently.

Children in Large Cities

The health of children living in large cities compares unfavorably with that of children living elsewhere. Large cities have high rates of poverty and of poor female-headed households with children. In 1990, 13 percent of all people and 18 percent of children residing in the nation's 100 largest cities were poor. These poverty rates are strongly implicated in the elevated rates of childhood mortality and morbidity found in those cities. Many of the income-linked health problems of children and youth are disproportionately found among the residents of large cities (Fossett and Perloff, 1995).

A recent analysis of urban social health revealed that the percentage increase in children under 5 years of age was larger in the nation's 100 largest cities, except the 25 largest, than nationally; the percentage increase in poverty rates was greater in the nation's 100 largest cities, except for the 51st to 75th, than nationally; and the increases in births was far larger in the nation's 75 largest cities than nationally. The rate of decline in infant mortality in the nation's 25 largest cities between 1980 and 1989 was substantially less than the national decline (-17.9 percent as compared to -22.2 percent). The rate of births to teenage women in these cities was also markedly higher than nationally (Andrulis et al., 1995).

Moreover, over time poor city residents become concentrated, that is, increasingly, they live in parts of the cities where a substantial proportion of the population is poor. This concentration of poor people in poor neighborhoods increased between 1970 and 1990. In 1970, in the nation's 100 largest cities, 55 percent of the poor resided in census tracts where 20 percent or more of the residents were poor; by 1990 the proportion had risen to 69 percent. The concentration of the poor within large cities has been particularly pronounced for minorities. In 1990 only about one of five poor black or Hispanic people resided outside the tracts where at least 20 percent of the population was poor. Poor white families in many cities are more dispersed spatially and are more likely to reside in less depressed areas where access to employment and services is better (Fossett and Perloff, 1995).

As poor people living in cities, and especially as poor minority group members, have become increasingly concentrated in depressed communities (sometimes called inner-city neighborhoods), many income-linked health problems have become concentrated in the same areas. Infant mortality, various forms of violent death, low weight births, vaccine-preventable illnesses, sexually transmitted diseases, maternal substance abuse, AIDS, intended and unintended injuries, asthma, and other income-linked health problems experienced disproportionately by the residents of inner-city neighborhoods (Fossett and Perloff, 1995; Fossett et al., 1992).

One study found that despite efforts to boost immunization coverage following the 1989–1991 measles outbreak, immunization rates among Hispanic and black preschoolers living in Los Angeles's poor, inner-city neighborhoods were low. Only 42 percent of the Hispanic children and 26 percent of the black children were up-to-date in their immunizations at 2 years of age, well below the federal target of 90 percent for preschool children. These rates suggest that inner-city minority children remain very vulnerable to vaccine-preventable diseases (Wood et al., 1995). Similarly, Pertowski notes that while all children are at risk for lead exposure, young children living in the deteriorated housing found in inner cities are at the highest risk (Pertowski, 1994).

Rural Children

In 1990, 23 percent of children lived outside metropolitan areas, and more than half of those, 15 percent, lived in rural areas (Office of the Assistant Secretary for Planning and Evaluation, 1996). Children living in non-metropolitan areas are known to experience special barriers to health care access that result in patterns of use that are different from those of children in metropolitan areas. The 1988 NHIS on child health indicated, for example, that children living outside metropolitan statistical areas (MSAs) were more likely to have received no medical care in the prior two years and to have higher rates of short-stay hospitalizations. But the survey did not indicate that children living outside MSAs were in poorer health than their metropolitan area counterparts. Children in MSAs and children in non-MSAs had similar levels of reported health status, of most conditions, and of morbidity as evidenced by rates of bed days (Coiro et al., 1994). The major differences in health resulted from rural children's greater likelihood of injuries as occupants of motor vehicles and of death from injuries, including those caused by farm machinery, firearms, falling objects, and drowning (Children's Safety Network, 1996; Rivera, 1985).

Comparisons with Other Industrialized Countries

A somewhat different perspective on the health of U.S. children can be gained by comparing it with the health of those living in other industrialized nations. The potential for international comparisons is limited, however, because few nations routinely collect similar health status measures and because those data that are available focus almost exclusively on mortality. Nonetheless, the data point to several areas in which the health status of this nation's children is worse than that of their counterparts in other industrialized nations (Harvey, 1990).

The United Nations considers 80 countries to have "complete" vital statistics including infant mortality. Data from these countries show that in 1994, the United States, with an infant mortality rate of 8.0, ranked 21st among countries with populations greater than 2.5 million (Guyer et al., 1996). While infant mortality has declined in this country over the past decade, the rates in other countries have also declined, and in some instances their declines have been more rapid.

Cross-national comparisons of childhood mortality indicate that mortality from natural causes declined across all industrialized countries between 1960 and 1985. By 1985, most of the leading natural causes of death in childhood occurred at about the same rate in all industrialized nations. Children in this nation, however, are far more likely than their counterparts in other industrialized nations to die from injuries both unintentional and intentional. Excess injury deaths in this country, relative to other developed nations, occur predominantly in children aged 1 to 4 and 15 to 19 years. The observed excess death rates due to unintentional injuries are primarily caused by automobiles, fires, and drowning, while the excess death rates due to intentional injuries are primarily due to homicide (Fingerhut, 1989; Fingerhut and Kleinman, 1990; Williams and Kotch, 1990).

U.S. children are also less likely to be up-to-date on their immunizations than children in many European nations (Williams, 1990). And this nation has a higher rate of unintended pregnancies, abortions (Brown and Eisenberg, 1995), and teenage pregnancies (Jones et al., 1986) than many industrialized countries.

Implications for Child Health Care

This review suggests several areas of concern for those who would design an improved health system for this nation's children.

Social and Demographic Trends

Increased attention must be paid to the social and demographic trends with implications for children's health, particularly the persistent and, in some instances, widening gaps in health status between low-income and upper-income children and among children of different racial and ethnic groups. Additional research will be needed in order to achieve a fuller understanding of the causes of some of these disparities and to develop policies aimed more explicitly at mitigating them.

Moreover, the number of children who are poor and extremely poor may increase due to the passage of welfare reform legislation. The Personal Responsibility and Work Opportunity Reconciliation Act of 1996 terminates income support for most legal as well as illegal immigrants and significantly curtails income support for many families now receiving cash assistance, including many families with children with disabilities. Given the strong relationship between income and child health, as well as the Act's health-care-related restrictions, the Act must be seen as posing a serious threat to the health and well-being of children (Rosenbaum and Darnell, 1996). Reducing income support for low-income families may increase homelessness and the number of families living in inadequate and unsafe housing, as well as worsen the nutritional status and overall health and development among children (Geltman et al., 1996).

Efforts to preserve recent gains and achieve further improvements in children's health will require addressing the needs of an increasingly racially and ethnically diverse child population. Unless there is improvement in the social and economic circumstances of blacks and Hispanics, their health problems, particularly those problems associated most closely with poverty, may grow in importance as the proportion of these groups in the population increases. In addition, health services will need to be rendered in ways that are culturally appropriate.

Managed Care

The increasing number of children cared for under various forms of managed care suggests the need for safeguards to ensure that managed care does not inadvertently reduce children's use of needed services and bring about deterioration in their health status. For some groups of children, access may improve over the fee-for-service system and improvements in health status may also be evident. It is less clear that improvements in access or health outcomes will result for disadvantaged children, especially poor children, minority group children, children living in large cities and rural underserved communities, and children who are uninsured. Sick children, especially those with chronic illnesses, may be especially vulnerable to adverse health outcomes under managed care (Ware et al., 1996). In the long term, if the current transformation of the health care system is successful, integrated managed care systems may evolve to a point where further gains in profitability and competitiveness can be achieved only by providing the enrolled population with adequate preventive and primary care services (Shortell et al., 1995). At that point, enrolled children may benefit from managed care and their health status may improve demonstrably.

Data Needs

These analyses underscore the need for improvements in the data used to gauge health status. Multiple-item measures of health, rather than death and disability measures, are badly needed. Even data to monitor morbidity are extremely limited in terms of the measures used, the frequency with which data are collected, the speed with which these data are made available for planning and research, and the populations on which these data are based. Presently, data sources produce either national and regional estimates for a limited set of morbidity indicators (such as those produced by the NHIS and its supplements), or state and local data sets that are not population-based and characterize only the experience of health care users (these data sets include state hospital discharge databases, state Medicaid claims databases, or the new encounter databases being developed by states moving heavily into Medicaid managed care).

As we move toward integrated community-oriented health care delivery systems, the need for data with which to characterize the health of communities will increase dramatically. In order to meet children's needs, health plans will need high quality data on the risk status and health status of enrolled children. Current data sources and measures will not allow health plans to develop strategies for more fully meeting the health care needs of enrolled children. States and health plans will need considerable support in their efforts to conduct state-of-the-art health needs assessments for children enrolled in health plans (Newacheck et al., 1996).

The Importance, and Limitations, of Medical Care

The current system of medical care for children can be credited with some, but not all, of the favorable trends described in this chapter. The most dramatic trend in child health status in the last half century may be the decline in infant mortality. Some of this must be attributed to the preconception and prenatal health care system and much to the new technologies and pharmaceuticals now available in hospital neonatal intensive care units for the treatment of low birthweight or otherwise compromised infants. Immunizations have lowered mortality and disability. And medical innovations have saved the lives of many victims of injury and reduced the disability days of children with serious handicaps.

But changes in legislation, enforcement of regulations, and health promotion efforts have also helped raise the health status of children. Improvement in environmental conditions, including safe water supplies, pasteurized milk, pure food, and elimination of lead from gasoline and paint, have reduced mortality and morbidity. The reduction in the rate of injuries is largely due to regulations (e.g., those pertaining to automobile restraints and health education activities) and the reduction in dental caries to water fluoridation. The federal food supplementation programs, such as school lunches, the Women, Infants and Children (WIC) program, and food stamps, are largely responsible for the improvements in nutritional indicators.

While new medical discoveries, such as the cause of preterm labor, and greater access to medical care, particularly for the poor, will undoubtedly further reduce mortality and disability, those designing an improved health system for this nation's children should not limit their efforts to the medical care system. Efforts to improve the economic status of low-income families, to reduce unintended and teenage pregnancies, to improve housing and other environmental conditions, to reduce violence, and to improve the health-related behaviors of parents and children—adolescents especially—have the potential for making significant improvements in the health status of U.S. children (Klerman, 1996).

References

Adams PF, Marano MA. 1995. Current estimates from the national health interview survey, 1994. National Center for Health Statistics, Vital and Health Statistics 10(193).

Andrulis DP, Ginsberg C, Shaw-Taylor Y, Martin V. 1995 Dec. Urban social health. A chart book profiling the nation's one hundred largest cities. Washington: National Public Health and Hospital Institute.

Baugher E, Lamison-White L. 1996. US Bureau of the Census, current population reports, Series P60-194, poverty in the United States: 1995. Washington: U.S. Government Printing Office.

Brown SS, Eisenberg L. 1995. The best intentions: Unintended pregnancy and the well-being of children and families. Washington: National Academy Press.

Budetti PP, Solloway MR, Green HL. 1995. The role of outcomes, effectiveness, and cost-effectiveness research in child health supervision. In: Solloway MR, Budetti PP, editors. Child health supervision. Analytical studies in the financing, delivery, and cost-effectiveness of preventive and health promotion services for infants, children, and adolescents. Arlington, VA: National Center for Education in Maternal and Child Health.

[CDC] Centers for Disease Control. 1991. Preventing lead poisoning in young children. Atlanta, GA: U.S. Department of Health and Human Services.

[CDC] Centers for Disease Control. 1994 Aug. 5. Blood lead levels: United States, 1988–1991. Morbidity and Mortality Weekly Report 43:545–8.

[CDC] Centers for Disease Control. 1996 Nov. 22. AIDS Among Children— United States, 1996. Morbidity and Mortality Weekly Report 45: 1005–10.

Children's Safety Network Rural Injury Prevention Resource Center. 1996 Sept. Childhood agricultural injury. Fact Sheet No. 2F.

Coiro MJ, Zill N, Bloom B. 1994. Health of our nation's children. National Center for Health Statistics, Vital and Health Statistics 10(191).

Eisen M, Ware JE, Donald CA, Brook RH. 1979. Measuring components of children's health status. Medical Care 17:902–21.

Fingerhut L. 1989. Trends and current status in childhood mortality, United States, 1900–85. National Center for Health Statistics, Vital and Health Statistics 3(26).

Fingerhut LA, Kleinman JC. 1990. International and interstate comparisons of homicide among young males. Journal of the American Medical Association 263:3292–5.

Fossett JW, Perloff JD. 1995 Dec. The "new" health reform and access to care: The problem of the inner city. Washington: Kaiser Commission on the Future of Medicaid.

Fossett JW, Perloff JD, Klekte PR, Peterson JA. 1992. Medicaid and access to child health care in Chicago. Journal of Health Politics, Policy and Law 17:273–98.

Geltman PL, Meyers AF, Greenberg J, Zuckerman B. 1996 Spring. Commentary: Welfare reform and children's health. Health Policy and Child Health. Washington: Center for Health Policy Research, George Washington University Medical Center.

Guyer B, Strobino DM, Ventura SJ, MacDorman M, Martin JA. 1996. Annual summary of vital statistics—1995. Pediatrics 98:1007–19.

Halfon N, Newacheck PW. 1993. Childhood asthma and poverty: Differential impacts and utilization of health services. Pediatrics 91:56–61.

Harvey B. 1990. Presidential address. Pediatrics 86(suppl.):1025–7.

Jones EF, Forrest JD, Goldman N, Henshaw S, Lincoln R, Rosoff JI, Westoff CF, Wulf D. 1986. Teenage pregnancy in industrialized countries. New Haven, CT: Yale University Press.

Kaste LM, Selwitz RH, Oldakowski RJ, Brunelle JA, Winn DM, Brown LJ. 1996. Coronal caries in the primary and permanent dentition of children and adolescents 1–17 years of age: United States, 1988–1991. Journal of Dental Research 75(special issue):631–41.

Klerman LV. 1996. Child health: What public policies can improve it? In: Zigler EF, Kagan SL, Hall NW, editors. Children, families, and government: Preparing for the twenty-first century, pp. 188–206. Cambridge, MA: Cambridge University Press.

Maternal and Child Health Bureau. 1996 Sept. Child Health, USA '95. Washington: U.S. Government Printing Office.

McNeil JM. 1993. Americans with disabilities: 1991–92. Current Population Reports, no. P70-33.

Mendoza FS. 1994. The health of Latino children in the United States. Future of Children 4(3):43–72.

Miller CA, Fine A, Adams-Taylor S. 1989. Monitoring children's health: Key indicators. 2d ed. Washington: American Public Health Association.

National Center on Child Abuse Prevention Research. 1996 April. Current trends in child abuse reporting and fatalities: The results of the 1995 annual fifty state survey. Chicago: National Committee to Prevent Child Abuse.

National Center for Health Statistics. 1996. Health, United States, 1995. Hyattsville, MD: Public Health Services.

Newacheck PW, Stoddard JJ. 1994. Prevalence and impact of multiple childhood chronic illnesses. Journal of Pediatrics 124:40–148.

Newacheck PW, Taylor WR. 1992. Childhood chronic illness: Prevalence, severity and impact. American Journal of Public Health 82:364–71.

Newacheck PW, Budetti PP, Halfon N. 1986. Trends in activity-limiting chronic conditions among children. American Journal of Public Health 76:178–84.

Newacheck PW, Stein REK, Walker DK, Gortmaker SL, Kuhlthau K, Perrin JM. 1996. Monitoring and evaluating managed care for children with chronic illnesses and disabilities. Pediatrics 98:952–8.

Office of the Assistant Secretary for Planning and Evaluation. 1996. Trends in the well-being of children and youth: 1996. Washington: U.S. Department of Health and Human Services.

Perloff JD. 1992. Health care resources for children and pregnant women. Future of Children 2(2):80–94.

Perrin EC, Newacheck P, Pless B, Drotar D, Gortmaker SL, Leventhal J, Perrin J, Stein RK, Walker DW, Wertzman M. 1993. Issues involved in the definition and classification of chronic health conditions. Pediatrics 91:787–930.

Pertowski CA. 1994. Lead poisoning. In: Wilcox LS, Marks JS, editors. From data to action: CDC's public health surveillance for women, infants, and children. Washington: U.S. Department of Health and Human Services.

Rivera FP. 1985. Fatal and nonfatal farm injuries to children and adolescents in the United States. Pediatrics 76:567–73.

Rivera FP, Grossman DC. 1996. Prevention of traumatic deaths to children in the United States: How far have we come and where do we need to go? Pediatrics 97:791–7.

Rosenbaum S, Darnell J. 1996 Aug. An analysis of the Medicaid and health-related provisions of the Personal Responsibility and Work Opportunity Reconciliation Act of 1996. Health Policy and Child Health 3(3):1–12.

Rosenberg HM, Ventura SJ, Maurer JD, Heuser RL, Freedman MA. 1996 Oct. 4. Births and deaths: United States, 1995. Monthly Vital Statistics Report 45(suppl. 2).

Shortell SM, Gillies RR, Devers KJ. 1995. Reinventing the American hospital. Milbank Quarterly 73:131–60.

Singh GK, Kochanek KD, MacDorman MF. 1996 Sept. 30. Advance report of final mortality statistics, 1994. Monthly Vital Statistics Report 45(suppl.).

Smith SM, Sniezek JE, Luallen JJ, McClain PW, Froehlke RG, Graitcer PL, Rodriguez JG. 1994. Injury and child abuse. In: Wilcox LS, Marks JS, editors. From data to action: CDC's public health surveillance for women, infants, and children. Washington: U.S. Department of Health and Human Services.

Starfield B. 1992. Child and adolescent health status measures. Future of Children 2(2):25–39.

Starfield B, Riley AW, Green BF, Ensminger ME, Ryan SA, Kelleher K, Kim-Harris S, Johnston D, Vogel K. 1995. The adolescent child health and illness profile: A population-based measure of health. Medical Care 33:553–6.

Stein RE, Jessop DJ. 1990. Functional status II (R): A measure of child health status. Medical Care 28:1041–55.

Stewart AL, Ware Jr. JE, editors. 1992. Measuring functioning and well-being: The medical outcomes study approach. Durham, NC: Duke University Press.

U.S. Public Health Service. 1991. Healthy people 2000: National health promotion and disease prevention objectives. Washington: U.S. Department of Heath and Human Services.

Wagner JL, Herdman RC, Alberts DW. 1989. Well child care: How much is enough? Health Affairs 8:147–57.

Walker DK, Richmond JB, editors. 1984. Monitoring child health in the United States: Selected issues and policies. Cambridge, MA: Harvard University Press.

Ware JE, Bayliss MS, Rogers WH, Kosinski M, Tarlov AR. 1996. Differences in 4-year health outcome for elderly and poor, chronically ill patients treated in HMO and fee-for-service systems. Journal of the American Medical Association 276:1039–47.

Williams BC. 1990. Immunization coverage among preschool children: The United States and selected European countries. Pediatrics 86(suppl.): 1052–6.

Williams BC, Kotch JB. 1990. Excess injury mortality among children in the United States: Comparison of recent international statistics. Pediatrics 86(suppl.)1067–73.

Wood D, Donald-Sherbourne C, Halfon N, Tucker MB, Ortiz V, Hamlin JS, Duan N, Mazel RM, Grabowsky M, Brunell P, Freeman H. 1995. Factors related to immunization status among inner-city Latino and African-American preschoolers. Pediatrics 96:295–301.

Yip R, Parvanta I, Scanlon K, Borland EW, Russell CM, Trowbridge FL. 1992 Nov. 27. Pediatric nutrition surveillance system—United States, 1980–1991. Morbidity and Mortality Weekly Report 41(SS-7):1–24.

3

Social, Economic, and Medical Care Determinants of Children's Health

Barbara Starfield

CHILDREN ARE BOTH more vulnerable and more resilient than adults. Their greater rates of development and growth, and wide fluctuations in hormonal levels and biochemical composition, widen the range of opportunity for both adverse and salutary effects. Greater plasticity also makes for an expanded range of possibility in manifestations of ill health.

This chapter examines the social, environmental, and medical and health system factors that promote or inhibit children's health. These three factors—along with genetic and biological and behavioral factors—act in combination to heighten susceptibility and reduce tolerance. Single causes of disease are the exception rather than the rule. Even single gene abnormalities had antecedent events that resulted in a mutation; diseases "caused" by multiple gene abnormalities generally depend on some environmental event for their expression. Thus, social and environmental factors, along with genetic and biological factors, behavioral factors, and medical care and health systems, must be seen as potent codeterminants of disease and its severity.

The factors leading to disease may be categorized as cues, correlates, and counteractants. A cue is the determinant without which a condition will not occur: the tuberculosis bacillus is the cue for tuberculosis; asbestos is the most common cue for mesothelioma. Correlates are those factors that predispose to the disease. Sometimes other diseases are the correlates: AIDS is a correlate to tuberculosis. Often social conditions are correlate determinants: poor living conditions and inadequate income are major ones.

Counteractants are those conditions that reduce the threat to disease posed by cues and correlates. Good nutrition, good housing, and exposure to good medical care are important counteractants to disease. It is not likely that the relative magnitude of these factors will ever be quantified, however, since their relative impact is likely to vary from condition to condition and from individual to individual.

Physical and Environmental Factors

Physical factors in the environment have effects on health that are specific to the particular developmental stage of the child. These impacts have been well described by Bearer (1995); the following summarizes her exposition. Impacts prior to birth occur through exposures of germ cells (ovum and sperm) of mother and father to toxins in the environment. For example, ingestion of cooking oils contaminated with certain chemicals by women who subsequently become pregnant is associated with abnormal physical characteristics in the future infant, even without any abnormality being manifested in the mother. Women with lead poisoning, even if asymptomatic themselves, may produce infants with frank congenital lead poisoning.

In the early months of life before infants are mobile, sustained exposures to harm occur because of an inability to move from the noxious agent. For example, without caretakers' vigilance to the potential dangers of overexposure to the sun, infants may suffer serious burns.

After the early months of life, infants and toddlers are exposed to a range of possible insults as a result of their particular developmental capacities. During the months in which they crawl, they are vulnerable to exposure to substances on the ground or floor; chemicals found on these surfaces are much more likely to have adverse effects on infants than on those at older ages. Such chemicals include substances found in carpets (such as volatile organic chemicals) and pesticides falling to the ground from aerial spraying or from the use of household canisters.

Toddlers are at increased risk of certain environmental exposures merely because of their short stature. Since heavy chemicals, heavy metals, and particulate matter fall with gravity to lower heights, youngsters are more vulnerable to their ill effects than their older counterparts in the same general environment. For example, mercury poisoning occurred in a child living in a house recently renovated with latex house paint when no other individuals in the house were similarly affected (Centers for Disease Control, 1990). The developmental stage of oral exploration further heightens the vulnerability of infants to these toxins. As a result, infants are much more susceptible to lead poisoning than adults living in the same environment. Furthermore, air pollution is a much more serious problem for children than for adults because of their more rapid breathing. Similarly, children take in more food per body weight than adults and are therefore more subject to harm from contaminated food and drink. Children drinking lead-contaminated tap water are more likely to become lead poisoned than older individuals who drink the same amount of the same water.

Different stages of cell growth, multiplication, and differentiation result in unique predisposition to harm among children and youth. Since the brain and lung continue to develop into adolescence, the vulnerability of these organs is extended throughout the entire period of growth and development. As a result, standards for exposure need to be targeted to the age of the individual; an acceptable level of exposure for an adult will be highly toxic for a child or adolescent. This is why legal and regulatory limits on contaminants must take children into consideration; standards for water quality, radon testing, and permissible levels of pesticide residues need to consider the special vulnerability of children.

Social and Economic Factors

Low social class, with its links to poverty, is an important correlate of disease. Children from lower class families are more likely to become ill and to suffer greater consequences from their illnesses. With the exception of uncorrected myopia and allergy,* diseases are at least two to three times more common among lower class infants and children as among upper income infants and children (Starfield, 1989a). Moreover, lower class children are

---

*However, even myopia, when measured with the child's normal corrective lenses, is more common among lower class children, since they have less access to medical services that ameliorate the functional disability stemming from nearsightedness. Thus, only allergy is more common among upper class children. One hypothesis for this anomaly is that it is an artifact caused by greater likelihood of diagnosis resulting from greater use of medical services (and especially specialist services) by upper class children. However, skin testing carried out by the 1976–1980 National Health and Nutrition Examination Survey found that the higher the family income of the child, the greater the skin-test reactivity (Gergen and Turkeltaub, 1986). Skin tests were performed for house dust, alternaria, cat, dog, ragweed, oak, rye grass, and Bermuda grass. Individuals living at or above the poverty level had greater reactivity to all but dog allergens and statistically significant greater reactivity to all other except house dust and cat allergens. A reasonable hypothesis and some evidence suggest that greater reactivity has to do with higher frequency of nonurban area of residence among upper class children—a social correlate of illness.

less likely to have access to all types of needed services. Families of these children are less likely to have private insurance coverage for health services, and without governmental assistance are less likely to receive both preventive services and needed illness care. They are more likely to be deprived of a regular source of health care (Kogan et al., 1995) and, as a result, are more likely to receive less effective care (Starfield, 1992).

This correlation between socioeconomic status and disease is not surprising when one considers that socioeconomic status affects such factors as area of residence, and type of housing and food available. For example, a study in Denmark (Lissau and Sorensen, 1992) showed the critical importance of area of residence on the occurrence of obesity by identifying 9- and 10-year-old school children in 1974 and examining them ten years later. Although genetic factors appear to play an important role in the genesis of obesity—obese children are much more likely to have obese parents than other children—the authors were able to show that genetics is at most only a correlate. After controlling for initial obesity (and hence the effect of parental obesity, which should have been fully expressed in the weight status of the children at the time of the initial study), for mother's and father's educational level, and for parental occupational status, area of residence during childhood remained an important predictor of adult obesity. Whether this is a result of poor income associated with area of residence, reinforcements of poor eating habits within these areas, or targeted advertising and marketing of unhealthy foods in these areas remains to be determined.

The powerful effect of area of residence also was shown in a study in Sydney, Australia, where children living in commercial areas (i.e., business districts) stood out from others in their dislike of other children and feelings of loneliness, worry, fear, anger, and unhappiness, even after controlling for the effect of family composition, social class, and culture (Homel and Burns, 1989).

The disparity in health status between low-income and high-income children widens when measured not by the occurrence of disease but by its manifestations. Low-income children die at greater rates than high-income children, and they have greater disability than high-income children, even with the same diseases. The higher death rates among poor children from both injuries and medical conditions were graphically shown several years ago by Nersesian et al. (1985) in Maine; a study in North Carolina (Nelson, 1992) extended these findings by showing that the disparity in mortality rates between poor and nonpoor children was greatest at ages 1 to 4 years, that white and nonwhite children did not differ once social status was taken into account, and that the effect of lower class was greater among whites than among nonwhites.

Analysis of data from the National Health Interview Survey (NHIS) explored the relationships among various aspects of social disadvantage and various manifestations of health. The NHIS involves a random sample of U.S. households; it measures health status and use of health services as reported by respondents for themselves and other household members. In this analysis, the relationship between family income and health characteristics was examined separately for black and white children. The health characteristics reflected the severity and impact of disease: days spent in bed due to illness, days lost from school due to illness, school failure, behavioral problems, and the mother's perception of her child's health as poor. These adverse effects were associated with low family income in both black and white children, but in different ways. For white children, low income alone increased the risk of one or more adverse effects by approximately twofold; for black children, low income had an indirect effect by increasing the likelihood that a child had a chronic illness or the mother reported herself to be in poor health, both of which generally increased the risk of the adverse impacts by four to eight times (McGauhey and Starfield, 1993).

In all of these studies it is apparent that low income increases the likelihood that health conditions will have an adverse impact by at least three- to fourfold, and that the effect is particularly evident among white children (Starfield, 1989b). In black children, other social characteristics, which are also associated with low income, act as more direct influences.

Low-income children in the United States are far more disadvantaged than their peers in all but 2 of 18 other western industrialized nations (Australia, Canada, Israel, and 14 western European countries) included in a recent study, while children at the high end of the income distribution are better off than comparable children in these other countries. Children at the bottom end of the income distribution have far lower incomes if they live in the United States than if they live in these other countries (except for Ireland and Israel), even after the contribution of social welfare programs (such as food stamps and earned income credits) is included in family income. In fact, the gap between family income in the lowest 10 percent of households and that in the highest 10 percent of households is greater in the United States than in any of the other countries (Rainwater and Smeeding, 1995).

This situation is associated with overall poorer health levels of U.S. children when compared with children in other comparably industrialized countries (Starfield, 1993). Infant mortality is higher in the United States than in more than 20 other countries; the United States ranks worst among 11 countries for neonatal mortality rates and proportion of infants born at low birthweight; and it ranks eighth on postneonatal mortality rates, and sixth and ninth respectively for female and male life expectancy at age 1 year. It ranks last or next to last (depending on the age and sex group) among seven countries with comparable data on injury death rates, and in the low half of the seven countries for rates of death due to medical causes. It also ranks last for receipt of most preventive immunizations among the nine countries with comparable data available. Children in two countries (Netherlands and Canada) that conduct surveys comparable to the NHIS have lower prevalence of disability resulting from acute illness, fewer days spent in bed from acute illness, and fewer days of activity restriction because of chronic illness than is the case in the United States (Starfield, 1991). U.S. adults, except for the very elderly, also are in worse health than adults in many of these other countries, but the disparities are not as great as they are among children (Starfield, 1993). Social inequities are generally reflected in health inequities, but the relationship is far from perfect: some countries with substantial social inequities achieve better health outcomes than would be expected because they have implemented health policies that counteract the effect of social disadvantage.

Medical Care and Health System Factors

Medical care and health systems are important determinants of children's health. Properly constituted, they can improve health, prevent disease from occurring or progressing, and reduce the impact of diseases that are themselves irreversible. Improperly constituted, medical care and health systems can cause disease. Thus, health services can act as a cue, correlate, or counteractant, both in the genesis of disease as well as in its severity and impact.

Health services act as a cue in iatrogenic disease. The dangers of medical interventions have been well catalogued and far exceed the rate of filing of malpractice suits (Brennan et al., 1991). Health services also can act as a correlate by increasing the likelihood of disease or its impact. Complications of surgery and anesthesia, and medication side effects that complicate the expression of disease fall into this category.

The conventional role of health care, however, is as a counteractant.

Health services reduce the occurrence of disease by preventing it from occurring (e.g., through immunizations), by detecting it early and dealing with it before it is manifested (e.g., through screening and consequent intervention), and by treating it so that its effects are eliminated or reduced (Starfield, 1985). Most conventional medical care falls into the last category, that is, the management of the manifestations of disease.

Children in the United States are at a special disadvantage when compared with children in many other comparably industrialized nations. Not only do they lack the guaranteed access to health services that is characteristic of all other industrialized countries, they must rely on a health system that lacks a strong primary care infrastructure. Health systems with a strong primary care infrastructure distribute health services more equitably across their populations (Starfield, 1992) and reduce barriers to care that especially impede access by the socially disadvantaged.

One manifestation of impaired access is the occurrence of hospitalizations that could have been avoided had good primary care been available. In the United States, several studies have shown marked differences in such hospitalization rates in areas differing in mean income and in the availability of primary care resources (Billings et al., 1993; Parchman and Culler, 1994; Weissman et al., 1992). In countries with a strong primary health care infrastructure, such differences do not exist. For example, a study in Spain showed that neither socioeconomic characteristics (illiteracy, unemployment, income) nor primary care characteristics of children's area of residence (type of physician and facilities for primary care) affected the probability of being admitted to the hospital for treatment of a condition that should have been preventable with good primary care, and the rate of admission for these "ambulatory care sensitive" conditions was lower in Spain than in the United States. Thus, the provision of universal financial access to care (see discussion of health policy below) and the availability of a consistent and accountable primary care provider as in Spain are associated with lower hospitalization rates for conditions that are preventable with good primary care (Casanova and Starfield, 1995). Countries with a strong primary care base also achieve better health outcomes with lower costs than the United States does. As noted above, the younger the age group, the greater the relative disadvantage in health outcomes of poor primary care infrastructure.

As this discussion implies, health policy is an important determinant of child health status, insofar as it influences the types of care available, the allocation of resources, the shape of the service system, and the financing of care. Health policy also plays a major role in converting the product of scientific discovery into effective medical services. For example, although an efficacious vaccine against measles existed for many years, its effectiveness in preventing measles depended on a commitment of public funds to distribute it (Blendon and Rogers, 1983). Increases in the incidence of infectious diseases preventable by immunization in the late 1980s, which resulted from declining insurance coverage and increasing requirements for copayment for services, were reversed by the National Immunization Program, which made vaccines available to states.

The history of neonatal mortality shows a similar impact of health policy. Although neonatal mortality had been decreasing for many decades, the decline accelerated after the formalization and governmental support of family planning programs in the early 1960s; the rate of decline accelerated again from 1968 to 1973, when an increasing number of states legalized abortion. Had there been a renewed interest in promoting contraception (as in many countries in Europe), this decline would probably have occurred even in the absence of increasingly available abortions.

Health policy has also had an impact in the case of postneonatal mortality, which decreased dramatically after the social interventions implemented by the New Deal in the mid-1930s. Marked declines were also noted in the early 1940s as a result of governmental programs for the families of servicemen. The 1950s was a decade of stagnation, with increases in postneonatal mortality in many places, probably because health services failed to accommodate the needs of populations moving from rural to urban areas. A notable decline occurred in the late 1960s and early 1970s as a result of increased accessibility of health services following the implementation of the Medicaid legislation in the mid-1960s. Postneonatal mortality again plateaued in the late 1970s and is still well above the level experienced by comparable countries, undoubtedly as a result of the absence of a universal entitlement to health services and consequent reduced access by those unable to afford care.

The impact of health policy is quite dramatically demonstrated in comparisons of children in families who receive Medicaid with those in families who do not. Compared to lower class children in families that receive Medicaid, those in families that do not receive Medicaid are less likely to receive care for their acute illnesses, including conditions such as earache, recurrent ear infections, and pharyngitis. Similarly, children with disabilities caused by chronic conditions who are in low-income families that do not receive Medicaid have only half the number of visits of those in families who do receive Medicaid, or who are in higher income families (Newacheck et al., 1995). Thus, governmental policy is critical in assuring that the most vulnerable children receive the services they need.

Public health policy also plays a major role in preventing adverse impact due to environmental conditions. The U.S. Constitution reserves no public health functions for the federal government. Thus, whatever actions the federal government takes to prevent disease or promote health are restricted to activities that are indirect: research, investigation, and encouragement (including financial inducements) of states and localities to provide needed services. Notwithstanding that much of ill health in childhood is a direct result of environmental insult, children are at the mercy of decisions made by a myriad of decentralized agencies, many of which make their policy in response to powerful and often nonlocal interests that lack a commitment to improving the quality of the local environment. Furthermore, many states and localities lack personnel or programs with jurisdiction over the environment. In 12 states and territories, there are no staff responsible for food- or water-borne disease surveillance and 24 other states have fewer than one staff person per million citizens performing such functions (National Health Policy Forum, 1996). This leaves millions of the country's children at the mercy of industrial and agricultural interests that expose them to a wide variety of infectious and toxic agents to which they are especially susceptible.

Although it is commonly assumed that the poor health levels of the U.S. population are due to social inequities or to poor health behaviors within the population, neither explanation holds. Social disparities have not been eliminated in any country. Moreover, many western industrialized nations have very large immigrant populations of different culture and class than the predominant population of the country. Some have native subpopulations as deprived as the most disadvantaged subpopulations in the United States. Rates of poor health behaviors (such as smoking, drinking, and promiscuity) are, in reality, higher in many of these other countries than in the United States. High levels of teen and young adult violence certainly inflate the U.S. death rate, but cannot explain differences for health problems not influenced by violence. These realities have relevance for health care reform: countries with more centrally organized services that focus on planning and deploying physician manpower according to needs rather than professional discretion achieve better health of their populations, especially with regard to the common diseases that are so powerfully influenced by social disadvantage (Starfield, 1994).

Interaction among Social, Environmental, Biological, and Medical Care Factors

As stated at the outset, disease is most often the product of the interaction of multiple factors. The interaction among socioenvironmental, biological, and medical care factors is graphically demonstrated in the case of low birthweight. Low birthweight is a major challenge since it is so highly related to both mortality and the subsequent health of survivors. Many studies have shown the powerful impact of social class on low birthweight, and much of the difference in low birthweight between white and black populations can be explained by the effect of social class. In fact, when low-income blacks and whites are compared, there is no difference in the frequency of low birthweight. The persistence of a racial disparity in higher income individuals, with black low birthweight rates persistently higher than white low birthweight rates, has been harder to understand. Part of the effect is a result of a clustering of non-low-income black women at the lower end of the spectrum of higher incomes. However, longitudinal studies among non-low-income individuals show the existence of another factor: a history of low income earlier in life. Higher income black women whose formative years were spent in poverty have a higher likelihood of having a low birthweight infant (Starfield et al., 1991).

By far the most salient determinant of a low birthweight infant, however, is a prior low birthweight infant to the same woman (Table 3.1). Even though prior low birthweight is a very powerful determinant of current low

Table 3.1
Risk of Low Birthweight among Offspring, According to Whether Mother Was Reared in Poverty
United States

Early poverty, prior low birthweight sibling	39%
Nonpoor, prior low birthweight sibling	27
Early poverty, prior normal birthweight sibling	7
Nonpoor, prior normal birthweight sibling	3

Source: Adapted from Starfield et al., 1991.

birthweight (the risk of low birthweight is more than seven times higher—31 percent vs. 4 percent—if the prior birth to a mother was low birthweight rather than normal birthweight), the effect is much greater among women who lived in poverty earlier in life. Presumably they are at high risk of poor physiological status upon entering pregnancy. Given this early predisposition, interventions to reduce the occurrence of low birthweight (such as nutritional enhancement in pregnancy) will operate as counteractants to modify but probably not eliminate the impact of prior poor physiological status. This is the likely explanation for the relatively small impact of enhanced prenatal care on the occurrence of low birthweight. More fundamental approaches to dealing with the social factors that act as correlates of low birthweight will be needed to reduce its occurrence substantially.

Monitoring Children's Health

Documenting the health of populations is a difficult task. Many health conditions are impossible to specify with precision. The challenge is particularly problematic in the case of children, who are still too young to manifest well-defined illnesses associated with deterioration in physiologic or anatomic status, yet who suffer from symptoms of a variety of acute, ill-defined ailments and experience disability and dysfunction from these as well as chronic illnesses. The measure of a health system is its ability not only to reduce mortality and prevent disease, but to reduce symptoms and disability, and to decrease vulnerability to and enhance resilience against threats to health. These aspects of health are increasingly recognized as important goals of health services (McDowell and Newell, 1996; Stewart and Ware, 1992).

The science of health status measurement for children lags far behind that for adults, but the gaps are rapidly being filled. One instrument, known as the Functional Status Measure II(R) (Stein and Jessop, 1990), is specifically designed to evaluate the impact of illness on the functioning of children; it quantitatively documents the degree to which children can perform the daily activities of healthy children. Another tool recently developed for youths aged 11 to 17 years, and under development for younger children, assesses domains related to discomfort, disorders, satisfaction with health status, achievement of social expectations (developmental status appropriate for age), vulnerability, and resilience (Starfield et al., 1995). These tools meet psychometric criteria for adequacy; they also document the relatively poorer health status of youths at social disadvantage.

Summary and Implications

This analysis suggests several directions for policy regarding children. First, there is a need for social and environmental as well as health services policies that are supportive of children. Planning, monitoring, and assurance of the maintenance of standards will require national direction, although implementation may be at the state or local levels. Second, good health depends on more than access to health services, although access is a necessary prerequisite. Health services should be targeted to population needs and should be evaluated according to the extent to which they succeed in meeting these needs. The current organization of the U.S. health care system, with its heavy focus on highly technological medicine, is not conducive to meeting the needs of the people of the country in general, and vulnerable children in particular. A reorganization involving the building of a strong primary care infrastructure with good linkages to other levels of care is imperative.

Social, environmental, and political characteristics of the United States, combined with the heightened physical and physiological vulnerability of young people, create the conditions for inequity in the achievement of good health in different population subgroups. The absence of a federal role in the direct provision of public health services creates the conditions for even greater inequities across states and local jurisdictions, each of which bears responsibility for provision of its own public health activities, which often run counter to local economic interests. Only an aware, ever-vigilant, and concerned populace can create the conditions under which children can thrive and develop as healthy, productive adults with a sense of life's worth and their potential to contribute to the progress of humankind.

References

Bearer C. 1995. Environmental health hazards: How children are different from adults. The Future of Children 5:11–26.

Billings J, Zeitel L, Lukomnik J, Carey TS, Blank AE, Newman L. 1993. Analysis of variation in hospital admission rates associated with area income in New York City. Health Affairs 12(1):162–73.

Blendon R, Rogers D. 1983. Cutting medical care costs. Journal of the American Medical Association 250:1880–5.

Brennan T, Leape L, Laird N. 1991. Incidence of adverse effects and negligence in hospitalized patients: Results of the Harvard Medical Practice Study I. New England Journal of Medicine 324:370-6.

Casanova C, Starfield B. 1995. Hospitalization of children and access to primary care: A cross-national comparison. International Journal of Health Services 25:283–94.

Centers for Disease Control. 1990. Mercury exposure from interior latex paint—Michigan. Morbidity and Mortality Weekly Report 39:125–6.

Gergen PJ, Turkeltaub PC. 1986. Percutaneous immediate hypersensitivity to eight allergens. U.S. 1976–80 Vital & Health Statistics, Series 11, No. 235, DHHS Pub. No. (PHS), p. 17. Washington: Public Health Services.

Homel R, Burns A. 1989. Environmental quality and the well-being of children. Social Indicators Research 21:133–58.

Kogan M, Alexander G, Teitelbaum M, Jack B, Kotelchuck M. 1995. The effect of gaps in health insurance on continuity of regular source of care among preschool-aged children in the United States. Journal of the American Medical Association 274:1429–35.

Lissau I, Sorensen T. 1992. Prospective study of the influence of social factors in childhood on risk of overweight in young adulthood. International Journal of Obesity 16:169–75.

McDowell I, Newell C. 1996. Measuring health: A guide to rating scales and questionnaires. New York: Oxford University Press.

McGauhey P, Starfield B. 1993. Child health and the social environment of white and black children. Social Science and Medicine 36(7):867–74.

National Health Policy Forum. 1996. Emerging and re-emerging infectious diseases: A major public health challenge. Issue Brief No. 686. Washington: The George Washington University.

Nelson M. 1992. Socioeconomic status and childhood mortality in North Carolina. American Journal of Public Health 82:1131–3.

Nersesian W, Petit M, Shaper R, Lemieu D, Naor E. 1985. Childhood death and poverty: A study of all childhood deaths in Maine, 1976 to 1980. Pediatrics 75:41–50.

Newacheck P, Hughes D, English A, Fox H, Perrin J, Halfon N. 1995. The effect on children of curtailing Medicaid spending. Journal of the American Medical Association 274:1468–71.

Parchman ML, Culler S. 1994. Primary care physicians and avoidable hospitalizations. Journal of Family Practice 39(2):123.

Rainwater L, Smeeding T. 1995 Fall–Winter. U.S. Doing poorly—compared to others. News and Issues, National Center for Children in Poverty: 4–5.

Starfield B. 1985. Effectiveness of medical care: Validating clinical wisdom. New York: Oxford University Press.

Starfield B. 1989a. Child health care and social factors: Poverty, class, race. Bulletin of the New York Academy of Medicine 65:299–306.

Starfield B. 1989b. Child health and public policy. In: Kopelman L, Moskop J, editors. Children and health care: Moral and social issues, pp. 7–21. Dordrecht: Kluver Academic Publishers.

Starfield B. 1991. Childhood morbidity: Comparisons, clusters, and trends. Pediatrics 88:519–26.

Starfield B. 1992. Effects of poverty on health status. Bulletin of the New York Academy of Medicine 68(1):17–24.

Starfield B. 1993. Primary care. Journal of Ambulatory Care Management 16(4):27–37.

Starfield B. 1994. Primary care: Is it essential? The Lancet 344:1129–33.

Starfield B, Shapiro S, Weiss J, Liang K, Ra K, Paige D, Wang X. 1991. Race, family income, and low birthweight. American Journal of Epidemiology 134(1):1167–74.

Starfield B, Riley A, Green B, Ensminger M, Ryan S, Kelleher K, Kim-Harris S, Johnston D, Vogel K. 1995. The adolescent CHIP: A population-based measure of health. Medical Care 33:553–6.

Stein REK, Jessop D. 1990. Functional status II(R). A measure of child health status. Medical Care 28:1041–55.

Stewart J, Ware J. 1992. Measuring functioning and well-being. Durham, NC: Duke University Press.

Weissman J, Gatsonis C, Epstein A. 1992. Rates of avoidable hospitalization by insurance status in Massachusetts and Maryland. Journal of the American Medical Association 268:2388–94.

4

Children's Access to Health Care: The Role of Social and Economic Factors

Paul W. Newacheck, Jeffrey J. Stoddard,
Dana C. Hughes, and Michelle Pearl

Introduction

Children's Access to Care

IN THE UNITED STATES, access to needed health care is not afforded equally to all children. Vast differences exist in children's ability to obtain care, and in the number and quality of services they receive (Butler et al., 1985; Guendelman and Schwalbe, 1986; Hahn, 1995; Holl et al., 1995; Kleinman et al., 1981; Kogan et al., 1995; Levey et al., 1986; Lieu et al., 1993; Newacheck and Halfon, 1988; Newacheck and Starfield, 1988; Rosenbach, 1989; St. Peter et al., 1992; Starfield, 1982; Stoddard et al., 1994; Wood et al., 1990). When access to care is denied, there are implications for people of all ages, but the impact can be especially profound for children, who undergo rapid growth and development. When these processes are interrupted by illness or injury, permanent consequences may ensue. Indeed, untreated childhood illness and injury may affect a child's lifelong health and well-being. The social costs of untreated illness include both direct costs, such as added long-term medical expenses, and indirect costs, such as lost economic productivity. Thus, ensuring that all children have access to timely and appropriate care is a critical public policy and programmatic goal.

Support for the preparation of this chapter was provided by the Maternal and Child Health Bureau, U.S. Department of Health and Human Services (Grant MCJ-113A18-03).

Despite the importance of assuring that children have access to care, wide disparities in access have been identified among children of different social and economic classes. In particular, large differences by race/ethnicity, income, and health insurance status have been documented for a variety of measures of access, utilization, and quality. Several studies have examined the role of insurance status as an independent risk factor for diminished access to and utilization of basic health care. Evidence demonstrates that compared to insured children as a group (Wood et al., 1990), uninsured children as a group have fewer annual physician visits, are more likely to go without any physician contact in a given year (Guendelman and Schwalbe, 1986; Kogan et al., 1995), and are significantly more likely than both privately and publicly insured children to receive inadequate preventive services (Holl et al., 1995) and to be inadequately immunized (Kogan et al., 1995; Mustin et al., 1994). Moreover, uninsured children are less likely than insured children to be seen by physicians when symptomatic with a variety of illnesses for which office visits are warranted (Stoddard et al., 1994).

Likewise, poor children have fewer physician contacts (Levy et al., 1986; Newacheck and Halfon, 1988; Newacheck and Starfield, 1988), are less likely to receive preventive care on a timely basis (St. Peter et al., 1992), and obtain routine care in qualitatively different settings than nonpoor children (Butler et al., 1985; Lieu et al., 1993). Similarly, children in racial and ethnic minority groups are less likely than white children to identify regular sources of care (Stoddard et al., 1994) and report qualitative differences in the sites of routine care (Cornelius, 1993). Minority children also receive fewer physician services (Guendelman and Schwalbe, 1986; Newacheck and Starfield, 1988; Stoddard et al., 1994; Rosenbach, 1989), and are less likely to receive adequate early preventive care (Mustin et al., 1994).

Children's Access to Primary Care

Children's access to primary care is of particular concern because primary care is medical care that should be available to all children. While primary care has been variously defined, the American Academy of Pediatrics defines it as "accessible and affordable, first contact, continuous and comprehensive, and coordinated to meet the health needs of the individual and the family being served" (American Academy of Pediatrics, 1993). According to the Academy, pediatric primary care also encompasses "health supervision and anticipatory guidance, monitoring physical and psychosocial growth and development; age-appropriate screening; diagnosis and treatment of acute and chronic disorders; and provision of first contact care" (American Academy of Pediatrics, 1993).

Research demonstrates that poor, minority, and uninsured children fare consistently worse than nonpoor, white, and insured children in access to primary care. For example, one study, conducted using national survey data from the late 1980s, revealed that poor, minority, and uninsured children were twice as likely as nonpoor, white, insured children to lack usual sources of care, were nearly twice as likely to wait 60 minutes or more at their sites of care, and used only about half as many physician services after adjusting for health status (Newacheck et al., 1996).

Improving children's access to health care requires a thorough under- standing of the wide range of factors that facilitate and impede that access. Studies show that access is a function of a wide range of influences, includ- ing financial and nonfinancial barriers to care (Aday et al., 1993; Currie and Gruber, 1996; Halfon et al., 1995; Kasper, 1987; Kogan et al., 1995; Monheit and Cunningham, 1992; Rosenbach, 1989; St. Peter et al., 1992). Although knowledge about these factors is growing, understanding about how they actually operate in relation to the process of receiving care is still in the for- mative stages. Moreover, even if the precise role of these determinants was clearly understood, not all of them are subject to public policy or program- matic interventions, and even fewer may have politically palatable solu- tions. Thus, the true scope of opportunities for improving children's access to health care may be far more limited than it first appears.

The purpose of this chapter is to add to our knowledge about factors af- fecting children's access to health care generally, and primary care in par- ticular, by analyzing the most recent data available on the subject, the 1993 National Health Interview Survey (NHIS). (See Appendix for full descrip- tion of the methodology of analysis.)

Definitions of At-Risk Children

For the purposes of this study, we examined access and utilization patterns for four groups of children:

- those in families with incomes below the poverty level;
- those belonging to minority ethnic or racial groups;
- those without health insurance; and
- those exhibiting none of the above characteristics (i.e., nonpoor, white, and insured children).

The first three groups are referred to as *at-risk groups* and the latter as the *reference group*. Membership in the first three groups can overlap, that is, some children are represented in more than one at-risk group. (See Appendix for full definitions of poverty, race/ethnicity, and insurance status.)

A limitation of NHIS data, and indeed a shortcoming in the access to care literature generally, relates to special populations at particularly high risk for impaired access to care. Homeless children, institutionalized children, children in foster care, children of migrant farm workers and other highly mobile populations, undocumented immigrant populations, children of non-English-speaking parents, and children of highly dysfunctional parents are typically not captured in traditional household surveys, including NHIS, and remain high-risk groups for which little information relating to access to care exists. In addition, sample size considerations in this and other studies preclude separate analysis of important racial and ethnic subgroups.

Several key elements of primary care as outlined in the American Academy of Pediatrics' definition were measured in our analysis (American Academy of Pediatrics, 1993). First contact was ascertained by way of the presence of a usual source of care. Accessibility and affordability were measured in several ways: qualitative aspects of sites of care (particularly accessibility of after-hours care), reported inability or delay in obtaining care, and aggregate and health-status-adjusted utilization (number of visits). Continuity was assessed by whether or not a regular clinician was identified. The data do not allow for detailed analyses of specific health care services (e.g., comprehensiveness of preventive care or health supervision, age-appropriate screening, diagnosis and treatment of acute and chronic disorders), nor do they provide rich information on delivery processes and interactions (e.g., coordination and family-centeredness), other than what can be ascertained from dissatisfaction measures. However, they do provide insight into salient system-level differences across a variety of measures as they are experienced by children and families from population risk groups.

Population Characteristics

In 1993 an estimated 12.6 million children under the age of 18, or 19 percent of all children under 18, lived in families with incomes below the poverty level (Table 4.1). Some 22.6 million children, or 33 percent of the total child population, were from minority racial and ethnic groups. The re-

Table 4.1
Sample Distribution and Population Estimates
United States
1993

Population characteristic	Actual sample size	Estimated population (in thousands)	
		N	SE
Children from poor families	3,319	12,639	642
Minority children	5,882	22,621	909
Uninsured children	1,873	7,418	369
Children from nonpoor, white, insured families	8,035	32,780	859
All children	16,907	67,718	1,497

Source: Microdata from the 1993 National Health Interview Survey.

maining at-risk group, uninsured children, was the smallest of the three groups, with approximately 7.4 million members, or 11 percent of all children. Membership in the three at-risk groups overlaps, and together these three population subgroups accounted for a majority of the population. In fact, the reference group of nonpoor, white, insured children accounted for only 48 percent of the U.S. civilian noninstitutionalized population of children in 1993.

Usual Source of Care

While nearly 95 percent of U.S. children reported having a usual source of health care in 1993, considerably smaller proportions of children from the at-risk groups reported having a usual source for obtaining routine care and medical advice (Table 4.2). Children without health insurance coverage were eight times more likely than children from nonpoor, white, insured families (the reference group) to report *not* having a usual source of care (24 percent vs. 3 percent). Children from poor families and minority groups were also less likely than children in the reference group to have a usual source of care, but the discrepancies were smaller: minority children were three times more likely and poor children four times more likely to be reported as not having a usual source of care than children from the reference group. Hence, while membership in any of the three at-risk groups puts

Table 4.2
Children with a Usual Source of Care and Their Site of Care
United States
1993

| Population characteristic | Percent with a usual source of care (N = 15,734) | | Percent distribution by site of care (N = 14,560) | | | | | | | |
| | | | Physician's office, private clinic, and HMO | | Hospital outpatient clinic | | Community and other health centers | | All other locations[a] | |
	%	SE	%	SE	%	SE	%	SE	%	SE
Children from poor families	88.7	0.9	66.3	1.9	4.5	0.8	22.9	1.8	6.3	1.0
Minority children	90.4	0.7	70.4	1.4	4.9	0.6	18.1	1.4	6.7	0.8
Uninsured children	76.1	1.6	75.0	1.9	3.0	0.7	17.7	1.8	4.3	0.9
Children from nonpoor, white, insured families	97.1	0.3	93.4	0.7	2.0	0.3	1.5	0.3	3.2	0.6
All children	93.7	0.3	85.1	0.7	2.8	0.3	7.7	0.5	4.4	0.5

Source: Microdata from the 1993 National Health Interview Survey.
Note: Percentages may not total 100 due to rounding.
[a]Includes emergency room.

children at a significant disadvantage, absence of insurance coverage is the most important barrier to having a medical home and reasonable access to primary care.

For those children who reported having a usual source of care, more than eight in ten identified physician's offices, private clinics, or health maintenance organizations (HMOs) as the site for that care (Table 4.2). Much smaller proportions of children were reported to use hospitals, health centers, and other locations for their care. Reference group children were identified as having physician's offices, private clinics, or HMOs as their usual site of care about 40 percent more frequently than children from poor families and about 30 percent more frequently than minority children. While children without health insurance were less likely to report having a usual source of care than children from poor families or minority children, those uninsured children who had a usual source were more likely to have a physician's office, private clinic, or HMO as the site for care.

In contrast to the results showing greater use of private physicians, clinics, and HMOs by nonpoor, white, insured children, children in the three at-risk groups were at least 10 times more likely than children in the reference group to use community and other health centers for their ambulatory care. Children from impoverished families were 15 times more likely than reference group children to use health centers for their routine care. Differences were also found between the at-risk and reference groups in use of hospital outpatient clinics and other sites of care, but these differences were less pronounced and, in some cases, statistically insignificant.

Qualitative Aspects of Care

Given the substantial differences in sites of care for children in the at-risk and reference groups, significant differences would be expected among the groups in the qualitative aspects of the care provided. Indeed, more than twofold differences were found between the at-risk and reference groups in the proportion of children for whom a regular medical provider could *not* be identified (Table 4.3). Although only about one-tenth of nonpoor, white, insured children were without a regular practitioner at their usual source of care, about one-quarter of poor, minority, or uninsured children were reported to see different practitioners when they visited their usual source of care. The differential was similar for each of the three at-risk groups. Even larger differences were apparent among the at-risk and reference groups for

Table 4.3
Access Indicators for Children's Usual Source of Care
United States
1993

Population characteristic	Percent not identifying a regular clinician (N = 14,339)		Percent without after-hours medical care (N = 12,091)		Percent not satisfied with at least one aspect of their care[a] (N = 4,559)	
	%	SE	%	SE	%	SE
Children from poor families	24.8	1.7	14.3	1.5	17.9	2.2
Minority children	23.5	1.3	13.0	1.2	15.2	1.3
Uninsured children	25.1	1.8	13.2	1.5	18.9	3.8
Children from nonpoor, white, insured families	11.2	0.7	4.8	0.4	12.8	0.9
All children	15.7	0.7	7.8	0.5	14.3	0.7

Source: Microdata from the 1993 National Health Interview Survey.
[a]Question asked only for children visiting their usual source of care within the previous three months; aspects of care include waiting time to get an appointment, waiting time to see the doctor, satisfaction with the way questions were answered and with the overall care received.

access to after-hours care, that is, services on weekends and evenings at the usual source of care. Poor, minority, and uninsured children were each almost three times as likely as nonpoor, white, insured children *not* to have access to after-hours care. Again, the differential is very similar for each at-risk group.

Finally, approximately one in seven respondents overall expressed dissatisfaction with at least one of three elements of the care their children received: waiting times for appointments or seeing the practitioner, the way questions were answered by the practitioner, or the overall care received. Once again, higher levels of dissatisfaction were reported for children in the at-risk groups compared to children in the reference group. The highest rates of dissatisfaction were for uninsured children.

Delayed or Missed Care

Overall, approximately one in every ten children was reported unable to get medical care, dental care, prescriptions, eyeglasses, or mental health care in the past year (Table 4.4). Two-thirds of these children were unable to get dental care and about one-quarter were unable to get medical care. Some children were reported to need multiple types of services but were unable to get them.

Children in the three at-risk groups were more likely than children in the reference group to be reported as unable to get needed services of all types. Uninsured children faced the greatest obstacles to gaining needed care. Fully one in every four of them was unable to gain access to needed services

Table 4.4
Missed Care Among Children
United States
1993

Population characteristic	Percent unable to get needed medical care (N = 15,756)		Percent unable to get needed dental care (N = 15,737)		Percent unable to get needed prescriptions, eyeglasses, and/or mental health care (N = 15,732)		Overall percent unable to get needed care (N = 15,634)	
	%	SE	%	SE	%	SE	%	SE
Children from poor families	3.5	0.6	8.5	0.8	4.3	0.5	12.8	1.0
Minority children	2.4	0.3	5.5	0.5	3.3	0.3	8.7	0.7
Uninsured children	7.2	1.1	17.6	1.3	7.4	0.8	24.0	1.6
Children from nonpoor, white, insured families	1.0	0.1	4.5	0.4	1.9	0.2	6.4	0.4
All children	1.9	0.2	6.2	0.3	2.9	0.2	9.0	0.4

Source: Microdata from the 1993 National Health Interview Survey.

in 1993. Uninsured children were nearly four times as likely as nonpoor, white, insured children to report going without at least one needed service. Children from poor families faced smaller, but still significant, barriers to obtaining care. Overall, poor children were about twice as likely as nonpoor, white, insured children to miss needed services. Minority children were more likely than children in the reference group to have missed needed care, excluding dental care. In general, families were much more likely to report that the cost of medical care resulted in a delay in getting needed care rather than in preventing them from getting care at all (4.1 percent vs. 0.9 percent) (Table 4.5). Once again, poor, minority, and uninsured children were each more likely than reference group children to delay or go without needed medical care due to cost concerns, and again, the largest differentials were for uninsured children, followed by poor and then minority children.

Table 4.5
Delayed Care Among Children
United States
1993

Population characteristic	Percent delaying medical care due to cost (N = 15,777)		Percent unable to get needed medical care due to cost (N = 16,883)		Percent delaying and/or unable to get medical care due to cost (N = 15,778)	
	%	SE	%	SE	%	SE
Children from poor families	5.3	0.6	2.0	0.5	6.1	0.7
Minority children	3.6	0.5	1.1	0.2	3.9	0.5
Uninsured children	14.2	1.1	5.2	1.0	15.9	1.3
Children from nonpoor, white, insured families	2.8	0.2	0.2	0.1	2.9	0.2
All children	4.1	0.2	0.9	0.1	4.4	0.2

Source: Microdata from the 1993 National Health Interview Survey.

Volume of Ambulatory Care

Another indicator of access is *realized access to care*, measured by the volume of physician care received by children adjusted for need, as indicated by bed days, perceived health status, and disability status. Overall, U.S. children were reported to have approximately 1.2 doctor contacts for each day spent ill in bed (Table 4.6). Differences in the use-disability ratio were not significant for minority and poor children when compared to their non-poor, white, insured counterparts. On the other hand, uninsured children lagged significantly behind children in the reference group on this measure, using only about 70 percent as much ambulatory care as reference group children on an adjusted basis.

Among children reported to be in excellent, very good, or good health, minority children used 71 percent and uninsured children used only 57 percent as many physician services as children in the reference group (Table 4.6). The difference for poor children was not statistically significant. Larger gradients in utilization were apparent for children reported to be in fair or poor health. Minority children used only 64 percent of the ambulatory care received by reference group children in similar health, while uninsured children used just 43 percent as much physician care as their reference group counterparts. The difference between poor children and reference group children was not statistically significant.

Similarly, minority and uninsured children with long-term limitations in their activities or disabilities used consistently fewer physician services than reference group children. The gaps in service use were greater for children with disabilities than for children without disabilities. The differences between poor children and reference group children were not statistically significant.

Taken together, these findings show that somewhat greater disparities in volume of physician services existed for children reported to be disabled or in less than optimal general health compared to those without disabilities and in superior health. These results suggest that at-risk children with health problems face added hurdles in obtaining primary care.

Analysis

What can be concluded regarding the factors that affect children's access to primary medical care? First, many U.S. children fall into one or more of the risk categories. During 1993, fully 19 percent of U.S. children lived in poverty, 11 percent were uninsured, and a third belonged to a minority

Table 4.6
Average Annual Physician Contacts
United States
1993

Population characteristic	Per 100 bed days (N = 16,722)		For children in excellent, very good, or good health (N = 16,261)		For children in fair or poor health (N = 467)		For children without limitation of activity (N = 15,741)		For children with limitation of activity (N = 1,100)	
	Mean	SE	Mean	SE	Mean	SE	Mean	SE	Mean	SE
Children from poor families	113.9	11.0	2.9	0.2	10.5	2.1	2.9	0.2	8.1	1.2
Minority children	116.6	8.1	2.5	0.1	9.6	1.6	2.5	0.1	6.8	1.0
Uninsured children	87.1	8.1	2.0	0.1	6.5	1.5	1.9	0.1	5.4	0.9
Children from nonpoor, white, insured families	126.1	4.9	3.5	0.1	15.0	1.5	3.2	0.1	10.4	1.1
All children	118.0	3.9	3.1	0.1	11.4	1.1	2.9	0.1	8.8	0.6

Source: Microdata from the 1993 National Health Interview Survey.

group. Fewer than half of U.S. children experienced none of these risk factors. Thus the scope of the risk is vast. With respect to measurable differences in access to and use of medical care, children in any of the risk groups continue to experience problems relative to children from nonpoor, white, insured families. The magnitude and dimensions of the problems experienced by poor, uninsured, and minority children appear to have changed little since 1987, the last time in-depth access data were collected on a national household sample of children (Newacheck et al., 1996). Caution must be taken when comparing the data presented in this chapter with older data, such as that from the 1987 National Medical Expenditure Survey (Newacheck et al., 1996), however. Differences between the survey instruments, sampling frames, and the wording of questions limit exact comparisons between the two.

Financial Barriers to Care

Our results suggest that absence of health insurance remains the predominant risk factor affecting children's entry into the health system, identification of a regular clinician, rate of dissatisfaction with care, likelihood of delaying or foregoing needed care, and volume of services received.

These results are particularly disturbing because the population of uninsured children will likely grow even larger in coming years due to a continuing decline in employment-related health benefits. Although Medicaid coverage of poor children has increased steadily since the mid-1980s, this growth has failed to compensate entirely for the rapid deterioration of employer-based coverage, as indicated by a 10 percent increase in the proportion of uninsured children from 1992 to 1993 (unpublished data from the 1993 Current Population Survey; Newacheck et al., 1995a). Because the downward trend in private employer-based coverage is unlikely to cease in the near future, access barriers for uninsured children will require greater attention.

Family income appears to have diminished somewhat as a barrier to care, although poverty shows the strongest effect of the three risk factors on lack of after-hours care. The gap in use of physician services between poor children and reference group children appears to have narrowed since the late 1980s (Newacheck et al., 1996), which may reflect the effect of Medicaid expansions that provided many poor children with insurance coverage (unpublished data from the 1993 Current Population Survey; Newacheck et al., 1995a). With regard to poverty's association with diminished availability of after-hours care, qualitative differences in the characteristics of the sites of routine care relied upon by poor children (in comparison with those used by nonpoor children) have been demonstrated in prior work (Levey et al., 1986; St. Peter et al., 1992). This suggests that the care available at the sites visited by poor children continues to be more restricted than that at sites used by nonpoor children, possibly forcing poor families to rely more heavily upon emergency departments for after-hours care.

Our data indicate that poverty and insurance status are both related to satisfaction with health services. Other studies of satisfaction with children's medical care across different types of ambulatory settings have shown that mothers' satisfaction with children's health care generally had far more to do with differences among practice settings (i.e., system features) than with patient characteristics (Dutton et al., 1985). The empirical study by Dutton et al. (1985) did however demonstrate that, among a lengthy set of patient characteristics, income was independently and strongly associated with most satisfaction measures.

Nonfinancial Barriers to Care

Nonfinancial barriers to care include a host of family and health system characteristics. Race and ethnicity are often considered barriers to care because they are powerful predictors of access. In this study, as in others, children in racial and ethnic minorities are less likely to have a usual source of care, more likely to miss needed care, and less likely to use services than their white counterparts. Despite the abundance of evidence of the importance of race and ethnicity, the precise role that they play in influencing access to care is not clear. Differences in access and use of care are, in part, attributable to differences in other factors that are correlated with race and ethnicity, such as income and insurance coverage. Cultural norms (e.g., attitudes and beliefs about health care) that are associated with population groups may also play a role here, as may discrimination against racial and ethnic minorities (Newacheck et al., 1996). Further study is needed, however, to fully understand the complex role of race and ethnicity in influencing access and utilization of health services.

Two recent reviews have summarized the structural, personal, and other nonfinancial barriers to care for disadvantaged children (Halfon et al., 1995; Margolis et al., 1995). These and other authors (Andersen and Aday, 1978; Weissman and Epstein, 1993) have categorized nonfinancial barriers to care using Andersen and Aday's theoretical models of access to care:

- *predisposing factors*, including sociodemographic characteristics such as age, gender, ethnicity, education, occupation, and family structure;
- *health need components*, including perceived need, health risk, and health status; and
- *enabling characteristics*, encompassing both family characteristics and system characteristics.

Family characteristics include not only financial indicators but also attitudes and beliefs, social support, identification of a regular provider and a regular source of care, residential location, transportation time to appointment, and convenience of services, whereas system characteristics encompass delivery system and organizational structural issues related to personal medical care. Relevant system characteristics include benefits and funding sources; cultural competence of providers; provider type, training, and attitudes; geographic distribution and location of sites of care; service capacity; models of care; and system and service integration, co-location, and collaboration. Many of these sorts of barriers have been notoriously difficult to measure, and as a result little empiric evidence is available describing the impact of these factors on children's access to care. Case studies and anecdotal reports have, however, documented the importance of many of these features as barriers to care (Halfon et al., 1995; Margolis et al., 1995).

Focusing on nonfinancial barriers to care, Margolis et al. (1995) have outlined several suggested approaches to improving access to care including:

1. developing home- and community-based services to address the environmental and personal factors associated with poor health outcomes among socially disadvantaged children;
2. improving the organization of practice to provide preventive services and patient education more efficiently; and
3. sharing of resources among physicians and health departments.

With respect to geographic distribution of health care providers, it has long been known that populations at highest risk for poor or no access to health care services are those in rural or inner-city areas. Whereas the shortage of child health providers in rural areas has been well documented (Budetti et al., 1982; Newacheck et al., 1996), data on provider availability in the inner cities have been far more limited and additional studies are needed. Studies of physician supply in underserved geographic areas are hampered by methodologic issues including geographic boundary determinations, as well as uncertainty regarding willingness of physicians located in underserved areas to treat Medicaid and uninsured patients (American Academy of Pediatrics, 1996; Budetti et al., 1982; Yudkowsky et al., 1990).

Community health centers serve an important role as a source of primary care for many at-risk children. Among poor children who indicated that they had a regular source of health care, nearly one-fourth identified community centers and other health centers as the source of that care. Similarly, relatively large proportions of minority children and uninsured children identified community health centers as a source of usual care, especially compared to the reference group. Because federally funded community health centers must, by law, be located in medically underserved areas and offer services on a sliding fee scale, their importance for these groups is not surprising. However, the future role of federally funded health centers in providing care to these groups of children is uncertain. In particular, the expansion of Medicaid managed care in most states could threaten the current central role of health centers for many children. To the extent that health centers are not involved in the provider networks with which state Medicaid agencies contract for managed care, health centers will no longer serve Medicaid patients and therefore would lose one of their most significant sources of revenue. Even when health centers are contained within the networks under contract, managed care can threaten their funding. Under traditional fee-for-service arrangements, state Medicaid agencies are required to reimburse federally qualified health centers at levels that reflect the cost of care (including a portion of the cost of providing uncompensated care to uninsured patients), even if the costs are higher than standard reimbursement rates. Such cost-based reimbursement policies do not apply to capitated managed care arrangements and health centers therefore are paid the negotiated rate, which is typically lower not only than the cost-based rate, but than the standard fee-for-service rate. Health centers can expect to receive significantly reduced levels of reimbursement under managed care, which could threaten their ability to provide care to uninsured patients, including children.

In many major U.S. cities medical care for medically indigent children is provided predominantly by teaching hospitals and public hospitals (Whitcomb and Miller, 1995). The financial viability of these institutions is notoriously precarious, and their future looks increasingly bleak as public support dwindles and federal, state, and local budgets tighten. In many large cities, particularly in the northeastern United States, a large volume of health services are delivered to children in hospital outpatient departments by pediatric residents, many of them international medical graduates (Whitcomb and Miller, 1995). (See chapter 7 for a full discussion.) Various influential panels have recently recommended sharp reductions in the number of international medical graduates allowed to pursue training in the United States (Council on Graduate Medical Education, 1995; Institute of Medicine, 1996; Whitcomb and Miller, 1995). Unless replacement funding is provided to subsidize service delivery to medically indigent urban residents as has been recommended (Institute of Medicine, 1996), the elimination of this health work force would almost certainly translate into sharply diminished access to care for many urban children.

Additional Considerations and Future Trends

Other private sector and public policy trends will affect the availability of health services for disadvantaged children. Enrollment of Medicaid beneficiaries into managed care plans has risen dramatically, although there is no evidence that Medicaid managed care fulfills its promise for children. Its shortcomings seem to be attributable to the design of most Medicaid managed care programs, which typically are patterned after the needs of relatively healthy, mainstream, middle-class families. Moreover, Medicaid managed care programs are virtually always designed to achieve some cost savings. How such cost savings are realized, and indeed whether such cost savings can be consistently realized, remain open questions.

The impact of managed care on children is a topic under active investigation, but this area is one in which policy changes are occurring far more rapidly than the health services research literature is evolving. Studies of Medicaid managed care programs report mixed results with respect to improved access to primary and preventive health services. While there is evidence that managed care programs have reduced children's use of emergency departments and specialty services, it remains unclear as to whether or not such changes have produced a net benefit for children. Very little is known about the effect of managed care on the quality of health care services for enrolled children.

Recommendations set forth for improving access and quality of care for children under Medicaid managed care programs (Hughes et al., 1995; Newacheck et al., 1994) include the following measures:

1. limiting expectations regarding cost savings;
2. ensuring access to comprehensive services;
3. involving providers who traditionally serve low-income families;
4. ensuring access to adequately trained providers;
5. establishing fee structures adequate to minimize the risk of under-service;
6. paying careful attention to quality measures; and
7. addressing the problem of lack of continuous eligibility and coverage.

The recent enactment of welfare reform and proposed spending reductions for Medicaid have also emerged as major public policy issues. Public opinion strongly favored changing the welfare system, and some type of reform therefore became a political necessity (Blendon et al., 1995; Geltman et al., 1996). The likely impact on children's health of reducing income support for low-income families under welfare reform as enacted by Congress and being implemented by states has been outlined elsewhere (Geltman et al., 1996). Similarly, after years of sustained double-digit increases in expenditures, spending reductions appear inevitable for the Medicaid program (Newacheck et al., 1995b).

With respect to uninsured children, whose numbers may increase substantially under Medicaid reform proposals, the health system's ability to absorb the costs associated with providing uncompensated care is threatened. Whereas in the past cost-shifting was a common and tacitly accepted practice used by many health care providers, this mechanism for financing the care of poor and uninsured children is becoming progressively less viable in a health care environment that is increasingly competitive, managed, and scrutinized by payers. Competition in the marketplace has forced all payers and providers to keep costs to a bare minimum for those with coverage, thereby allowing much less leeway for providers to inflate their charges to insured patients in order to subsidize their care of uninsured individuals.

Conclusion

Depending on one's perspective, the data presented in this chapter could be construed as evidence of persistent disparities in access to care for poor, uninsured, and minority children. Others might perceive the magnitude of these problems as quite modest. Disadvantaged children in our society do not fare as well in terms of access to health care as their nonpoor, white, insured counterparts, but there is a safety net in place that provides at-risk children with a level of care that is at least minimally acceptable.

However, it is critical to understand that the fabric of social programs that constitute that safety net is a delicate one. The Medicaid program, public hospitals and other teaching hospitals, community and migrant health centers, Indian Health Service clinics, the National Health Service Corps, volunteerism, charitable and philanthropic institutions, and uncompensated care subsidized by cost-shifting are all historically important components of the U.S. health care system that have effectively helped provide services to children at risk. In turn, each of these components of the health system for vulnerable children is itself now at risk and relies on inherently unstable funding bases. Unlike other western industrialized nations, U.S. society has not chosen to guarantee access to basic health care services for its children. Until such a guarantee becomes a matter of public policy at all levels of government, disparities in access to care are likely to persist, and indeed may increase given the turmoil in our health system.

Appendix: Research Methods

Overview of the National Health Interview Survey

The National Health Interview Survey (NHIS) is a continuing nationwide household survey that is conducted by the Bureau of the Census for the National Center for Health Statistics (Benson and Marano, 1994). The purpose of the survey is to collect information on the health status and use of health services by the U.S. civilian noninstitutionalized population. Each year the survey instrument consists of a core questionnaire on health status, utilization, and demographic characteristics, and a set of supplemental questionnaires on topics of current interest. During the final two quarters of 1993 (July 1 through December 31), two special supplemental questionnaires on access to care and health insurance coverage were included in the survey. The analysis presented in this chapter draws upon the data collected in those supplements.

Our analysis included 16,907 children under age 18 years (see Table 4.1). In the NHIS, an adult member of the household knowledgeable about the health of child family members serves as the respondent. In most cases this is the mother. The overall response rate for the survey was 94.7 percent. Item nonresponse, including missing and unknown responses, for each of the dependent variables was less than 10 percent. Cases with missing item responses were excluded from relevant estimates for the access and utilization variables.

Poverty status was assessed using the Bureau of the Census definition that takes into account family income from all sources and family size. In 1993, the poverty level for a family of three was $11,890. It should be noted that because the NHIS collects income data in bands (e.g., $1,000 to $1,999), the poverty status indicator is approximate. Children from families with unknown or unreported income (N = 1,272) were excluded from the income comparisons. Classification of race and ethnicity was based on respondent self-reports. In our analysis, all persons identifying themselves as nonwhite or of Hispanic origin were classified as minority. There were no missing data for race and ethnicity. Insurance status was assessed based on responses to questions included in the health insurance supplement about coverage status during the month prior to the interview date. Persons were classified as insured if they reported coverage that month for either CHAMPUS, Medicare, Medicaid, Indian Health Service, other public assistance programs, or private insurance. Persons reporting no coverage from any of these sources were classified as uninsured. Children with unknown or unreported insurance status (N = 1,662) were excluded from the insurance comparisons.

When a child was reported to have a usual source of care, the respondent was asked whether this place was a physician's office or private clinic; company or school clinic; community, migrant, or rural health center; county, city, or public hospital outpatient clinic; private hospital outpatient clinic; hospital emergency room; HMO or prepaid practice; psychiatric hospital or clinic; Veteran's Administration hospital or clinic; military health care facility; or "other place." To ensure adequate estimate precision for our analysis, less prevalent sites of care were collapsed into larger categories. These larger categories included physician's office, private clinic, and HMOs; hospital outpatient clinic; community and other health centers; all other sites listed above (Table 4.2).

Statistical Analysis

Estimates presented in the tables and text have been statistically weighted to reflect national population totals. The weights, provided by the data collection agency, were equal to the inverse of the sampling probability for each case, adjusted for nonresponse. The statistical significance of differences between estimates for the risk groups (poor, minority, or uninsured) and the reference group (nonpoor, white, and insured) was assessed using t-tests for differences in means and proportions. Test statistics were calculated using the unweighted number of sample cases. In addition, paired comparisons were performed using the Bonferroni correction for multiple comparisons. In all cases standard errors were derived using the Taylor series linearization method that takes into account the complex survey design used by the NHIS (Shah et al., 1992). Unless otherwise noted, statistically significant differences are discussed in the text.

References

Aday L, Lee ES, Spears B, Chung CW, Youssef A, Bloom B. 1993. Health insurance and utilization of medical care for children with special health care needs. Medical Care 31(11):1013–26.

American Academy of Pediatrics. 1993 Nov. The medical home statement addendum: Pediatric primary health care. American Academy of Pediatrics News 9(11):7.

American Academy of Pediatrics. 1996. Physician workforce ratios for child health care, 1994. Elk Grove Village, IL: American Academy of Pediatrics.

Andersen R, Aday LA. 1978. Access to medical care in the U.S.: Realized and potential. Medical Care 16(7):533–46.

Benson V and Marano MA. 1994. Current estimates from the National Health Interview Survey, 1993. Vital Health Statistics 10(190):1–9.

Blendon R, Altman D, Benson J, et al. 1995. The public and the welfare reform debate. Archives of Pediatrics and Adolescent Medicine 149: 1065–9.

Budetti PP, Kletke PR, Connelly JP. 1982. Current distribution and trends in the location pattern of pediatricians, family physicians and general practitioners between 1976 and 1979. Pediatrics 70:780–9.

Butler JA, Winter WD, Singer JD, Wenger M. 1985. Medical care use and expenditure among children and youth in the United States: Analysis of a national probability sample. Pediatrics 76:495–506.

Cornelius LJ. 1993. Barriers to medical care for white, black, and Hispanic American children. Journal of the National Medical Association 85(4):281–8.

Council on Graduate Medical Education. 1995. June. 7th Report, Washington: Department of Health and Human Services, Health Resources and Services Administration.

Currie J, Gruber J. 1996 May. Health insurance eligibility, utilization of medical care, and child health. The Quarterly Journal of Economics, pp. 431–66.

Dutton D, Gomby D, Fowles J. 1985. Satisfaction with children's medical care in six different ambulatory settings. Medical Care 23:894–912.

Geltman P, Meyers A, Greenberg J, et al. 1996. Welfare reform and children's health. Archives of Pediatrics and Adolescent Medicine 150: 384–9.

Guendelman S, Schwalbe J. 1986. Medical care utilization by Hispanic children: How does it differ from black and white peers? Medical Care 24:925–40.

Hahn BA. 1995. Children's health: Racial and ethnic differences in the use of prescription medications. Pediatrics 95(5):727–32.

Halfon N, Inkelas, M, Wood D. 1995. Nonfinancial barriers to care for children and youth. Annual Review of Public Health 16:447–72.

Holl JL, Szilagyi PG, Rodewald LE, Byrd RS, Weitzman ML. 1995. Profile of uninsured children in the United States. Archives of Pediatrics and Adolescent Medicine 149(4):398–406.

Hughes D, Newacheck P, Stoddard J, Halfon N. 1995. Medicaid managed care: Can it work for children? Pediatrics 95(4):591–4.

Institute of Medicine. 1996. The nation's physician workforce: Options for balancing supply and requirements. Washington: Institute of Medicine, National Academy of Sciences.

Kasper JD. 1987. The importance of type of usual source of care for children's physician access and expenditures. Medical Care 25(5):386–9.

Kleinman JC, Gold M, Makuc D. 1981. Use of ambulatory medical care by the poor: Another look at equity. Medical Care 19:1011–29.

Kogan MD, Alexander GR, Teitelbaum MA, Jack BW, Kotelchuck M, Pappas G. 1995. The effect of gaps in health insurance on continuity of a regular source of care among preschool-aged children in the United States. Journal of the American Medical Association 274(18):1429–35.

Levey LA, MacDowell NM, Levey S. 1986. Health care of poverty and nonpoverty children in Iowa. American Journal of Public Health 76: 1000–3.

Lieu TA, Newacheck PW, McManus MA. 1993. Race, ethnicity, and access to ambulatory care among U.S. adolescents. American Journal of Public Health 83:960–5.

Margolis P, Carey T, Lannon C, et al. 1995. The rest of the access-to-care puzzle. Archives of Pediatrics and Adolescent Medicine 149:541–5.

Monheit AC, Cunningham PJ. 1992 Winter. Children without health insurance. The Future of Children 2(2):154–70.

Mustin HD, Holt VL, Connell FA. 1994. Adequacy of well-child care and immunizations in U.S. infants born in 1988. Journal of the American Medical Association 272(14):1111–5.

Newacheck PW, Halfon N. 1988. Preventive care use by school aged children: Differences by socioeconomic status. Pediatrics 82 (pt 2):462–8.

Newacheck PW, Starfield B. 1988. Morbidity and use of ambulatory care services among poor and nonpoor children. American Journal of Public Health 78:927–33.

Newacheck P, Hughes D, Stoddard J, Halfon N. 1994. Children with chronic illness and Medicaid managed care. Pediatrics 93(3):497–500.

Newacheck P, Hughes D, Cisternas M. 1995a. Children and health insurance: An overview of recent trends. Health Affairs 14(1):244–54.

Newacheck P, Hughes D, English A, Fox H, Halfon N, Perrin J. 1995b. The effect on children of curtailing Medicaid spending. Journal of the American Medical Association 274(18):1468–71.

Newacheck PW, Hughes DC, Stoddard JJ. 1996. Children's access to primary care: Differences by race, income and insurance status. Pediatrics 97(1):26–32.

Rosenbach ML. 1989. The impact of Medicaid on physician use by low-income children. American Journal of Public Health 29:1220–6.

St. Peter RF, Newacheck PW, Halfon N. 1992. Access to care for poor and nonpoor children: Separate and unequal? Journal of the American Medical Association 267:2760–4.

Shah BV, Barnwell BG, Hunt PN, LaVange LM. 1992. SUDAAN user's manual: Professional software for survey data analysis for multi-stage sample designs, Release 6.0. Research Triangle Park, NC: Research Triangle Institute.

Starfield B. 1982. Family income, ill health and medical care of U.S. children. Journal of Public Health Policy 3:244–59.

Stoddard JJ, St. Peter RF, Newacheck PW. 1994. Health insurance status and ambulatory care for children. New England Journal of Medicine 330:1421–5.

Weissman JS, Epstein AM. 1993. The insurance gap: Does it make a difference? Annual Review of Public Health 14:244–70.

Whitcomb ME, Miller RS. 1995. Participation of international medical graduates in graduate medical education and hospital care for the poor. Journal of the American Medical Association 274(9):696–9.

Wood DL, Hayward RA, Corey CR, et al. 1990. Access to medical care for children and adolescents in the United States. Pediatrics 86:666–73.

Yudkowsky BK, Cartland JDC, Flint SS. 1990. Pediatrician participation in Medicaid-1978 to 1989. Pediatrics 85:567–77.

II

THE ORGANIZATION OF CHILDREN'S HEALTH SERVICES

In the United States, health care is provided to children through multiple, largely uncoordinated service delivery structures. The mix of public and private care that has evolved consists largely of population-based programming provided through the public sector and medical care for individuals provided through a market-driven private sector or safety net providers. Child and adolescent health services are delivered in public health departments, private physician offices, community health centers and other nonprofit community agencies, schools, and hospitals. Insurance coverage patterns for children and adolescents are uneven and mirror this mix of public and private health service delivery.

The major market-driven change in recent years has been an increased focus on cost containment and decreased expenditures by means of increasing participation in managed care. Associated with the growth in managed care is a shift from fee-for-service medicine to capitated arrangements with the prospect of large, integrated service delivery systems. The fee-for-service model was not conducive to the development of a coordinated system of health care for children. One potential benefit of managed care is that capitation may be translated into somewhat greater coordination of services, more effective prevention programs, but it is not clear that changing the insurance mechanism alone can accomplish this goal.

Perhaps the greatest obstacle to building a truly comprehensive system of health care for children stems from a lack of consensus about the proper scope of health policy interventions: Should public programs be limited to specific health problems (the categorical approach) or should they be more compre-

hensive, addressing broader factors that predispose individuals to health problems? To date, federal child health legislation has been largely categorical, with separately enacted pieces of legislation aimed at filling gaps in service availability and access to personal health services. Because funding usually comes tied to categorical objectives and individual program specifications, initiatives designed to pull together the public and private service sectors are often doomed from the beginning—even though such cooperation is vital to building a sustainable health care delivery system in this country.

5

A History of Child Health
and Pediatrics in the United States

Vince L. Hutchins

We cherish belief in the children and hope
through them for the future.
—Lillian Wald, Founder,
Henry Street Settlement

THE HISTORY OF CHILD HEALTH in America is a tale of two sectors, the private and the public, and how they interact, resolve disagreements, collaborate, sometimes work at cross purposes, and often complement each other. Public programs for children, with their focus on the health of populations, were historical latecomers to the field; the private sector has always operated from an individual patient or family base. Both sectors have worked toward the goal of optimal physical, mental, and social health for all infants, children, adolescents, and young adults. Their joint struggle with the health system and with society to attain these goals is not unlike historian Marshall C. Pease's description of the American Academy of Pediatrics as "an adventure in practical idealism" (Pease, 1952, p. 9).

This chapter reviews, with commentary, the roles of pediatricians and public health officials in the health care of children in this country and

Special thanks to Susan Marshall, librarian, and John Zwicky, archivist, at the Drs. Harry and Ruth Bakwin Library, and to Gretchen Fleming, also at the American Academy of Pediatrics, and to Joe Lockhart and Peter Hutchins—all for their manuscript location and retrieval—and to John Hutchins for his general manuscript assistance.

notes how their evolving partnership can benefit the future health of the nation's children.

Early Days

The primary provider of care for the child has always been the family, particularly the mother or, in many instances, the mother surrogate. In seventeenth century America she was assisted by other female family members, midwives, wet nurses, and wise old women in the community. Physicians and other male practitioners of the healing arts were rarely involved, providing little assistance. Herbs, purgatives, emetics, blisters, and bleeding did little to ameliorate the epidemics of communicable and infectious diseases. The most common ailments of children were worms, teething, and convulsions. Infant mortality, largely unreported officially, took a heavy toll among the colonists. Salem reported a high of 313 per 1,000 for female children in the 1600s. The average number of children born per family in colonial Andover was 8.8. As many as 10 or 20 children per colonial family was not unknown. Because of the scarcity of physicians in the seventeenth century, children were often treated by other community leaders such as preacher-physicians (including Samuel Fuller, a Mayflower passenger, and Thomas Thacher, author of the first medical publication in the colonies) or by governor-physicians (for instance, John Winthrop, Sr., governor of the Massachusetts Bay Colony, and John Winthrop, Jr., governor of Connecticut). *Acute Diseases of Infancy* (1689) by Walter Harris was the most popular pediatric treatise until it was supplanted a century later by Michael Underwood's *A Treatise on the Diseases of Children* (1784) (Cone, 1979, pp. 7–17; Pease, 1952, p. 9; Radbill, 1979).

Aside from quarantines, public health activities in the seventeenth century are little noted. The public effort for children was focused on education and family life, ranging from the 1642 requirement in Massachusetts that parents teach their children to read to the state's 1660 ruling that men proved to be the fathers of bastards be held liable for the children's support, to Virginia's 1675 provision for removing children from unsuitable homes (Bremner, 1970, pp. 3–6, 817–818).

In the early eighteenth century, the concept of child health hardly existed. Children were treated no differently than their elders. Young and old alike fought sickness by drinking exotic concoctions of herbs and other vegetable and animal matter and by alternately dieting and bleeding, purging and sweating. Smallpox, diphtheria, and yellow fever were epidemic. Smallpox caused the most terror. Inoculation (variolation) against smallpox was introduced in 1721, when at Reverend Cotton Mather's suggestion, Zabdiel Boylston inoculated his son; this was the first significant advance in American medicine (inoculation smallpox, smallpox resulting from the direct purposeful transfer of smallpox virus from a patient to a well person, was widely practiced before the advent of vaccination). However, the prevailing belief that original sin was the ultimate cause of illness often discouraged lifesaving inoculation of children. On the plus side, maternal deaths in childbirth decreased after the 1750 introduction of English obstetrical methods.

During the last half of the eighteenth century, some children in urban centers benefited from the availability and improved quality of hospital care. In 1751, the first charter for a hospital was issued to the founders of Pennsylvania Hospital. Similarly, children profited from the improved professional standards that resulted from the founding of medical schools at the College of Philadelphia (1765), King's College (1767), and Harvard University (1782). Benjamin Rush, the leading clinician of his time, wrote influential treatises on cholera infantum (1773), scarlet fever (1784), and insanity in children (1812). His pupil Charles Caldwell wrote the first monograph on pediatrics to be submitted as a dissertation for a medical degree.

Unfortunately, physicians were still in short supply. When a yellow fever epidemic hit Philadelphia in 1793, 6,000 men, women, and children ill with fever were treated by only three physicians, "who were able to do business out of their homes." Postcolonial parents depended on a plethora of almanacs as mostly unreliable sources of medical information for the diseases that plagued children (BCHS, 1979, p. 1; Bremner, 1970, pp. 282–285, 818–819; Cone, 1979, pp. 7–17).

Public efforts for children continued to focus on education and family life, rather than health, for example, by establishing public schools and public orphanages (Cone, 1979, pp. 29–45).

Early Nineteenth Century

The beginning of the nineteenth century brought the early Industrial Revolution and with it the movement of citizens from farms to the cities. Ill children were still cared for almost exclusively by family and neighbors. Physicians were rarely consulted nor did they seek out infants and children as patients. In matters relating to health, the children benefiting most from the welfare movements of the early nineteenth century were the deaf-mute, the blind, and the "feeble-minded." However, efforts on behalf of these children had more to do with the general movement of humanitarianism and the growing concern with education than with medical care. Nevertheless, during the first half of the century, hygiene and medical care of children received more attention than ever before. Benjamin Waterhouse introduced smallpox vaccination in 1800, when he vaccinated his son and six other members of his household with samples of the new vaccine from Sir William Jenner. Two years later, after President Thomas Jefferson vaccinated more than 70 members of his family with a supply of cowpox vaccine from Waterhouse, vaccination spread throughout Virginia and other parts of the United States.

The first American book on the management and feeding of infants, *The Maternal Physician*, written by an anonymous mother, was published in New York City in 1811. Scientific works on the diseases of children also appeared. Epidemics of yellow fever, smallpox, typhoid fever, and cholera appeared about 1820. Mortality from tuberculosis was increasing, and diarrhea was the chief cause of death among children. In Boston, between 1840 and 1845, 40 percent of all deaths were among children under 5 years of age. Proportionally more children and youths between 5 and 19 years of age died in the mid-nineteenth century than at the end of the eighteenth. After 1850, based on the model established in Europe 50 years earlier, the first U.S. hospitals exclusively for children were founded in Philadelphia, Boston, and New York; arguments continue today as to which was established first. In 1860, Abraham Jacobi of New York Medical College was appointed to the first special chair of diseases of children and established the first children's clinic. Esteemed today as the founder of American pediatrics, Jacobi commented on the emerging view that children's health needs are special: "Therapeutics of infancy and childhood are by no means so similar to those of the adult that the rules of the latter can simply be adopted to the former by reducing doses. The differences are many" (BCHS, 1979, p. 9).

Progress in medical treatment of children was accompanied by growing interest in public health and a new awareness of the relationship between child health and sanitary conditions. John H. Griscom's study of tenement conditions in New York City (1845), Lemuel Shattuck's survey of sanitation in Massachusetts (1850), and Stephen Smith's authorship of the New York Metropolitan Health Law (1866) helped prepare the groundwork for the public health movement of the later nineteenth century (Bremner, 1970, pp. 758–760, 821; Cone, 1979, pp. 73, 79, 84–85).

Late Nineteenth Century

The population of the nation more than tripled from 1850 to 1900, growing from slightly more than 23 million, with 42 percent of the population under 15 years of age, to almost 76 million, with 34 percent under 15 years of age. Urbanization, industrialization, and immigration were the broad social factors that reshaped American life during these years.

In the half century after the end of the Civil War, the subject of child health became defined, and pediatrics emerged as a distinct branch of medicine. Social action for the welfare of children was one source of the gradually emerging concept of child health. A second stimulus came from the more rapid pace of advances in medicine, especially in pediatrics and obstetrics, and in medical education. A third element was the development of state and local health departments, which provided the governmental framework within which pediatric knowledge and the broad concern with social action for children could be joined to form programs (Cone, 1979, pp. 99–104; Schmidt, 1973, pp. 5–10).

Social action for children's welfare sometimes arose from unusual sources. The Society for Prevention of Cruelty to Animals (SPCA), established in 1866, was the only agency in New York City to take responsibility for helping a child who had been brutally beaten by her foster parents in 1874. The story of "little Mary Ellen," widely reported in contemporary newspapers, led to the formation of The Society for the Prevention of Cruelty to Children (SPCC) in 1874.

The most significant child-oriented social and public health milestones of the late nineteenth century were:

- the establishment of milk stations, where safe milk could be purchased at or below cost or, if necessary, be given away;
- the concern with the spread of communicable disease after compulsory school attendance laws were passed;
- the movement to outlaw child labor; and,
- the opening of Settlement Houses (charitable institutions founded among congested, impoverished city populations to supply various educational, recreational, health, and other services to the community).

These events evolved during the early years of the Progressive movement. (Bremner, 1971, pp. 185–192, 811–815; Hutchins, 1994, p. 695).

Pediatrics—"pediatry" or "pedology," as the field was called in the nineteenth century—was officially designated as a specialty in 1880, when the Section on Diseases of Children was founded by Jacobi at a meeting of the American Medical Association (AMA). During these years, more than a third of all infants born in most cities died before reaching the age of 5 years. Most of these deaths were attributed to improper bottle-feeding: "(inadequate) selection and care of cow's milk, its preparation and use in infant feeding" (Holt, 1903, p. 5). Overcoming this major contributor to infant mortality became the raison d'être of pediatrics for the 60 years between 1870 and 1930.

Pediatrics, in the 1880s, was an underrecognized, underserved academic area. The AMA's Section on Diseases of Children had lapsed into inactivity by 1887, and only a half dozen children's hospitals had been established nationwide. If pediatrics was taught at all, it was under the aegis of internal medicine or obstetrics. In the 1880s, only a few academic pediatricians and barely 50 physicians identified themselves as interested and involved in the medical problems of infants and children—and none limited their practice to the care of children. In 1888, these few physicians, under the leadership of Job Lewis Smith, formed the American Pediatric Society (APS) because there was a perceived need for medical organizations independent of the AMA. (The AMA's position on a national code of medical ethics and concerns about its policies regarding academic medicine and education had caused dissatisfaction and controversy.) Jacobi, in the first APS presidential address (referred to by S. McC. Hamill as "Jacobi's first epistle to the pediatrists"), delineated the field of pediatrics as separate, saying that the "development and maturation of the whole child was key," and emphasized the responsibility of the pediatrician to preventive medicine.

Job Lewis Smith's *Treatise on the Diseases of Infancy and Childhood*, published in 1869, went through eight editions in the next 27 years. By the end of the century, there were more than two dozen children's hospitals scattered across the country, and out of 119 medical schools, 64 had special chairs of pediatrics. The *Archives of Pediatrics*, launched in 1884, was the first English-language journal dealing specifically with the medical problems of children (Cone, 1979, pp. 99–104; Pearson, 1988, pp. 2–5, 20, 41, 44).

In 1869, Massachusetts became the first state to have a permanent Board of Health and Vital Statistics, and by 1877, 14 states had established state health departments. By 1890, a few counties and larger cities had established their own public health authorities. These state and local departments advocated and secured adoption of health legislation at the state level and provided a forum for discussions of public health. Soon the possibility of extending the work of health agencies to include services for mothers and children began to develop. In 1872, the first New York City Commissioner of Health, Stephen Smith, surgeon and brother of Job Lewis Smith, established the American Public Health Association (APHA) to help increase the regulatory authority of these departments. Most members were physicians who were officials in local and state health departments. By 1898, 19 states and New York City maintained public institutions for feeble-minded children. Greater knowledge of the nature of children's mental illness had to wait for the next century, however. Minnesota, in 1897, was the first state to undertake work with crippled children; Massachusetts and New York soon followed (Alexander et al., 1996; BCHS, 1979, p. 9).

By the end of the nineteenth century, through the emerging cooperation of three groups—social reformers, pediatricians, and individuals from the public health arena—a sense of public responsibility for mothers and children was taking hold. Jacobi had said in his first APS presidential address, "Questions of Public Hygiene and Medicine are both professional and social. Thus every physician is by destiny a 'political being' in the sense in which the ancients defined the term; viz., a citizen of the commonwealth with many rights and great responsibilities." Thomas M. Rotch, the first incumbent of the chair of pediatrics established by the Harvard Medical School in 1888, echoed this in 1909: "The large body of women who are connected with the Child Labor Movement has added greatly to the accomplishment of markedly successful results. . . . We physicians, however, whose mission it really is to guide the progress of the various reforms connected with early life and see that they do not go astray, should interest ourselves in curbing exaggerated ideas and in the prevention of unwisely pressing upon our legislators unsound views on which to base new laws." These were pioneering words, words that presaged the American Academy of Pediatrics' philosophy that the primary role of pediatricians is commitment to the welfare of children (Jacobi, 1889, p. 829; Rotch, 1909).

The Progressive Period and the Children's Bureau

Hillary Rodham Clinton, looking back a century, has observed:

> (at) the beginning of industrialization, immigration, and the movement from farm to city . . . three uncertainties were unleashed: fear of rapid change fueled a sentimental fervor for simpler times, just like today. Populist politics raised valuable concerns about economic exploitation and

political corruption, but also unleashed extreme reaction that gave rise to racism and ethnocentrism and isolationism. But then look at what happened next: a progressive political consensus was achieved that addressed genuine concerns about economic and political equality . . . . Americans of all political stripes began to think differently about what politics and government could do. Progressive politics at the turn of the century . . . were able to see a vision of the future. (1996)

From 1900 to 1915, during the era known as the Progressive period, the federal government expressed greater concern for the welfare of U.S. citizens and began to take a more direct interest in public health issues and concerns. As services for mothers and children began to be recognized as a public responsibility, a reform movement, "the crusade for children," engaged in efforts to improve child health and labor conditions. Three women played important roles in this movement in the decades on either side of 1900: Jane Addams of Hull House in Chicago, Florence Kelly of the National Consumers' League, and Lillian Wald of the Henry Street Settlement in New York City, who "invented" public health nursing and home visits. All three were on the board of the National Child Labor Committee, which was organized in 1904 with three goals: nationwide investigation of child labor, campaigns for more stringent child labor legislation at the state level, and enforcement of existing child labor laws. Its work culminated in the Fair Labor Standards Act of 1938, which barred the products of industrial child labor from interstate commerce.

The case of a 12-year-old boy who was excluded from school because of an untreated skin condition led Lillian Wald to discuss with the New York City health commissioner the wastefulness of medical inspection without follow-up. Wald loaned a nurse from the Henry Street Settlement, Lina L. Rogers, to be the first full-time school nurse to provide medical inspection; she was to work in six schools for a one-month demonstration in 1902. Within just a few weeks, absenteeism was reduced by 50 percent. As a result, the board of health hired 12 more nurses to work in the schools in November 1902, and an additional 33 by the end of 1903. The utility of providing nurses and health rooms in schools had been amply demonstrated.

In 1903, Wald suggested the establishment of a federal Children's Bureau to Florence Kelly of the National Consumers' League and then to President Theodore Roosevelt. A bill supported by Roosevelt was introduced in both houses of Congress in 1906 and in each of the next six years. It met with fierce opposition both from states, which argued that the federal government was usurping their responsibility for the welfare of children, and from those who feared that it would give federal employees the right to enter and regulate the homes of private citizens. Support for the bill came from parent's organizations, labor unions, health workers, social workers, and women's organizations, as well as from the first White House Conference on the Care of Dependent Children in 1909.

Finally, on April 9, 1912, President William Howard Taft signed an Act of Congress that created the Children's Bureau with the charge "to investigate and report on all matters pertaining to the welfare of children and child life among all classes of our people." The interrelated problems of child health, dependency, delinquency, and child labor were to be considered and interpreted as they affected "children in the several States and Territories." As chief of the new Bureau, President Taft appointed Julia C. Lathrop, who became the first woman to head a federal statutory agency as a presidential appointee. Lathrop had worked closely with Jane Addams for 25 years at Hull House in the slums of Chicago. At last, the federal government had an institutional representation of its responsibility to promote the welfare of the nation's children.

States and localities also began to acknowledge their corresponding responsibility. In 1908, the Division of Child Hygiene was established in the New York City Health Department, the first of its kind in the world. For S. Josephine Baker, a New York physician who faced such gender prejudice that she could not earn enough to support herself in private practice, an appointment as a medical inspector for the New York City Health Department in 1902 was a means to supplement her meager earnings. Troubled by the city's infant deaths, which climbed to 1,500 a week in the summers, she designed a program of education on the value of breastfeeding, ventilation, and sanitation. In recognition of her achievement in lowering the infant death rate, she was named chief of the newly created Division of Child Hygiene. She increased the number of infant milk stations and the number of trained public health nurses, already under the direction of Wald at Henry Street, available to make home visits to every infant out of reach of the health stations. She also established the Little Mothers League. League members, numbering over 20,000 schoolgirls from 12 to 14 years of age, were taught infant hygiene and feeding and helped in raising infants of mothers who were forced to work. They learned parenting skills that would later be useful in their own lives. A wellspring of interest in "baby-saving" as a public responsibility was developing.

Biomedical research in pediatrics began during the first two decades of this century with the establishment of two research laboratories. Supported by the Rockefeller Institute for Medical Research, L. Emmett Holt opened the first laboratory at Babies Hospital in New York in 1910; it dealt with problems in infant feeding. John Howland, the founder of academic pediatrics and head of the pediatric department at Johns Hopkins University Medical School, established the second research laboratory in 1912. His studies on acidosis, rickets, and tetany are landmarks in the history of pediatrics. The staff he collected at Hopkins made enormous contributions to pediatrics. "Howland's influence changed the whole course of pediatrics from the proprietary to the academic approach," commented Martha May Eliot, fifth chief of the Children's Bureau.

From 1904 to 1922, the private sector increased its involvement in programs for the mentally and physically disabled. Voluntary organizations such as the Shriners, National Society for Crippled Children (now known as the Easter Seal Society), Rotary Club, and Lions Club each initiated new programs for disabled adults and children (Alexander et al., 1996; Baker, 1992; Bradbury, 1962, pp. 1–6; Cone, 1979, pp. 151–155, 163–166, 169–170, 202, 205–206, 218–219; Eliot, 1967; Lynch, 1983, pp. 46–47, 56–59).

Sheppard-Towner and the Birth of the American Academy of Pediatrics

During its first decade, the Children's Bureau conducted studies on infant and maternal mortality, promoted birth registration, and published booklets for the public on the care of infants, including *Infant Care* (1914), which became the government's all-time best seller, and *Prenatal Care* (1913). Using these studies, the Bureau, in conjunction with the emerging suffragette movement and a few socially involved physicians, began a campaign for federal legislation to provide funds for states to provide prenatal and postnatal care. Josephine Baker argued at the time: "During the nineteen months we were at war [during World War I], for every soldier who died as a result of wounds, one mother in the U.S. went down into the valley of shadow and did not return" (Cone, 1979, p. 157). A plan was proposed that maternal and child health services be established in each state, funded by federal grants-in-aid and matching state funds, a mechanism for which precedents had been set by the Department of Agriculture. Passed in 1921, the Maternity and Infancy Act, or Sheppard-Towner Act, established the national policy that the people of the United States, through their federal government, share with the states and localities the responsibility for helping to provide community services that children need for a good start in life. Forty-five states and the Territory of Hawaii accepted these grants; the holdouts were Connecticut, Illinois, and Massachusetts, where the organized medical lobby in opposition to the Act was strongest. The Sheppard-Towner Act was allowed to lapse in 1929, due primarily to opposition from influential people in the Catholic Church, the Public Health Service, and the AMA.

The first steps toward the formation of the American Academy of Pediatrics really began at a meeting of the AMA Section on Diseases of Children in St. Louis in the spring of 1922. After a day of discussion, the Section voted to approve the Sheppard-Towner Act. However, on the same day, the AMA House of Delegates condemned the Act as "an imported socialistic scheme." Incensed at the Section's action, the House of Delegates reprimanded it, but the Section refused to recant, convinced that the Act was for the welfare of mothers and children. The ensuing discontent of Section members made the formation of a new national pediatric society almost inevitable. In June 1930, 34 pediatricians met in the library of Harper Hospital in Detroit and drew up a constitution and bylaws for a new organization, the American Academy of Pediatrics (AAP or "the Academy"). Isaac A. Abt was elected president. At this first meeting, the Academy defined its purposes: "to create reciprocal and friendly relations with all professional and lay organizations that are interested in the health and protection of children [and] to foster and encourage pediatric investigation, both clinically and in the laboratory, by individuals and groups" (BCHS, 1979, p. 34). The AAP claimed a specific focus on education, public health, and social issues affecting children. Not all involved agreed, however. Some leaders thought it was ill-advised to engage in activities of sociological interest. They believed that enhanced private cooperation rather than the expansion of public agencies was what was really needed to bring about a complete program of child health services (BCHS, 1979, pp. 28–34; Beaven, 1955; Bradbury, 1962, pp. 5–13, 21–28; Bremner, 1971, pp. 1003–1025; Cone, 1979, pp. 156–157, 203–204; Emerson, 1923; Hughes, 1980, pp. 1–2, 1993; Hutchins, 1994, p. 696; Pearson, 1995; Pease, 1952, p. 9; Schlesinger, 1967; Schmidt, 1973, pp. 12–14).

Title V of the Social Security Act

With the end of the Sheppard-Towner Act and the beginning of the Great Depression, the states' abilities to continue useful child health work eroded while needs grew. Based upon data collected during the first years of the depression, the Children's Bureau prepared a plan for children's health and welfare programs that included three major proposals: aid to dependent children, welfare services for children needing special care, and maternal and child health services, including services for crippled children. The first proposal, aid to dependent children, an expansion of the states' mother's pension system, became Title IV of the Social Security Act—Aid to Dependent Children (ADC). ADC evolved into Aid to Families with Dependent Children (AFDC), recently ended by Congress in its efforts to reform welfare.

The latter two proposals in the plan were enacted in 1935 as Title V of the Social Security Act, and within nine months, all 48 states, Alaska, Hawaii, and the District of Columbia were cooperating. Extensive programs for maternity care and the care of infants and children were created, including, for the first time, a full range of federally funded medical care for handicapped children. For the next 60 years, Title V was the foundation upon which notable advances in child health were made under the leadership of the Children's Bureau and its successors.

In its early days during the depression, the AAP focused on education, standards, publications, and government relations. Within its first year, the AAP launched a medical education program, which included scientific sessions at its annual meetings, and contributed to the general welfare of children through the work of its voluntary committees. One of the first acts of the AAP's Executive Board was to initiate action that culminated in 1933 with the formation of the American Board of Pediatrics, in collaboration with the APS and the AMA Section on Diseases of Children. The creation of a national board to certify competency of pediatricians did much to improve pediatric education. Certification became a mandatory requirement for membership in the AAP after 1937. The *Journal of Pediatrics*, published by C.V. Mosby Co. under contract to the AAP, first appeared in 1932. It was succeeded by the AAP-owned and published journal *Pediatrics* in 1948.

During its first 20 years, the AAP had its ups and downs with its efforts to affect federal health legislation. While the AAP never swerved from its ideal to improve the health of the nation's children, there was a continuing fear that the government, through influence and the control of large sums of health care money, would gradually intrude on private medical practice. It was the Emergency Maternal and Infant Care program of the Children's Bureau that broke the pattern of friendly relations on health legislation, and caused one of the greatest conflicts of opinion the AAP has ever known (BCHS, 1979, pp. 42–45; Bremner, 1974; Hill, 1948; Hughes, 1980, pp. 3–8; Hutchins, 1994, p. 697; Schmidt, 1973, pp. 18–21).

Emergency Maternal and Infant Care Program
In the early 1940s, the pregnant wives of servicemen often found themselves far from their hometowns and familiar medical resources; as nonresidents, most were ineligible for medical services in the states in which they were living, and military hospitals were unable to accommodate them. When this situation reached a crisis stage for the families of servicemen at Fort Lewis in Washington State, the base's commanding officer appealed to the state health officer, who turned to the Children's Bureau for permission to rebudget federal maternal and child health funds for the care of these women. Martha May Eliot, then the associate chief of the Children's Bureau and, for most pediatricians, the living symbol of the Bureau, took the opportunity to develop a program to respond to this national emergency. Congress initiated the Emergency Maternal and Infant Care (EMIC) program as an emergency wartime measure in 1943 for the wives of servicemen in the four lowest pay grades, who accounted for three-fourths of the armed forces. It immediately became the largest public medical care program the country had ever known; state health departments quickly proved their ability to administer such programs. At its peak, EMIC covered one of every seven U.S. births, exerting its influence upon virtually every community in the country. By the end of the program in 1949, 1.5 million mothers and their infants had received necessary health supervision and medical care through EMIC. EMIC was also the first federally funded national health program to be formally evaluated (Sinai and Anderson, 1948).

Although individual obstetricians, pediatricians, and hospitals cooperated with EMIC, organized medicine suspected that EMIC was an opening wedge for "socialized medicine" and a postwar national health care program in the United States. The AAP struggled with EMIC, some members dutifully supporting it because of the war crisis, but others considering it an intrusion of state medicine that might well be extended in peace time. Where the Children's Bureau saw the implementation of quality care, some providers saw onerous administrative rules dictating conditions of medical practice in which they had no consultative role. These concerns, combined with the lack of a means test (meaning anyone of any income qualified), the belief that federally determined financial formulas led to inadequate compensation for providers, and the view that the Bureau exerted too much control over local and state programs, convinced the AAP Executive Board that it could not approve "measures established by a government bureau . . . (to) arbitrarily control medical practice" (Alexander et al., 1996; BCHS, 1979, pp. 46–47; Bradbury, 1962, pp. 65–68; Bremner, 1974; Hughes, 1980, pp. 8–11; Hutchins, 1994, p. 697; Schmidt, 1973, p. 22).

The First National Study of Child Health Services
When Senator Claude Pepper introduced the Maternal and Child Welfare Bill in 1945, which was strongly backed by the Children's Bureau, the simmering disagreement between the AAP and the Bureau moved toward confrontation. There were accusations that the Pepper bill was really just the EMIC disguised and that the Children's Bureau had deliberately deceived the AAP. Wegman (1988) notes: "Although Dr. Eliot insisted that it was not 'written by the Children's Bureau,' neither Dr. Joseph Wall, who was then President of the AAP, nor some of his colleagues in the Academy's leadership accepted this . . . (leading) to a discussion by the Executive Board of the AAP in June 1944 as to whether the Academy should 'withdraw their support from the Children's Bureau.'" Many on both sides of the disagreement were concerned that such a break would be detrimental to both organizations' shared goal of better child health. Eliot contacted Henry Helmholz, past-president of both AAP and APS and chair of the Bureau's Medical Advisory Committee, who offered to get the APS to propose to the AAP a joint study, with the Bureau, of the nation's health services for children in order to forestall a schism. "Let them set themselves to work on getting the facts," Helmholz said (Wegman, 1988, p. 87).

With APS playing the role of mediator, a survey of all child health services in the United States got underway. The AAP, the Children's Bureau, and the Public Health Service all contributed funds—as did the National Foundation for Infantile Paralysis and other private sources—totaling $1.04 million over the three years of the study. Helmholz was appointed chair of the new AAP Committee for the Study of Child Health Services. The core staff eventually grew to nearly 100 individuals. State health departments and the state chapters of the AAP were also intimately involved with the study. Although individual pediatricians had worked closely with the Bureau on advisory committees over the years, this was the first joint project between the AAP and the Bureau; it prefigured future collaborations.

The survey produced many significant findings, as well as a few controversies. Theories were substantiated about the inadequacy of child health care, but new information was discovered as well: the large proportion of hospital admissions that were children; the frequently inadequate educational background of those treating children; and five-fold child mortality rates in areas with poor medical facilities. Katherine Bain conducted the first nationwide survey of infant feeding practices in American hospital nurseries, reporting that only 38 percent of the mothers left the hospital nursing their infants. The resulting study publication, *Child Health Services and Pediatric Education* (RCSCHS, 1949), which assembled the facts and presented considered opinions on postwar planning for children, pointed out the inadequacies of the nation's child health care and strengthened the case for better pediatric education. Both the AAP and the Bureau rallied around the report and worked to implement its recommendations. The 1949 study had a significant impact on child health care services and pediatric education in the United States. In reviewing the history of this period in 1952, Pease wrote:

> There is no gain-saying the fact that the Children's Bureau and the American Academy of Pediatrics are mutually necessary to each other. No matter what the nature of their quarrels, they are ordained by fate to seek for a mutually agreeable working relationship.

(See also Bain, 1948, 1996; Beaven, 1954, unpublished; Bremner, 1974, pp. 1269–1288; Hill, 1948; Hutchins, 1994, p. 697; Pease, 1952, pp. 153–210; Wegman, 1988.)

Great Society Days
The 1960s brought legislation for the mentally retarded, projects of comprehensive maternity and infant care (MIC), comprehensive health services projects for children and youth (C&Y) in low-income areas, regional intensive infant care projects, family planning services projects, and projects to improve the dental health of children. The last five initiatives, administered by the Children's Bureau, were responsive to the growing needs in congested slums of large urban areas.

In 1965, the enactment of Public Law 89-97 provided for the Medicare (Title XVIII) and Medicaid (Title XIX) amendments to the Social Security Act. Since its enactment, Medicaid has become the major source of health insurance for poor and near-poor children. Medicaid, like Title V, is a federal-state program. State agencies have authority to structure the program within overall federal requirements and guidelines. Eligibility of children for Medicaid was originally linked to eligibility for AFDC. When Medicaid was passed, it was seen simply as an extension of the role of the federal government in providing medical care benefits within the context of welfare programs. Eventually Medicaid eligibility was broadened to include two-parent families and citizens who were not on welfare but met income standards at certain levels above poverty. These changes have led to a dramatic increase in Medicaid coverage for children. The percentage of all children through 21 years of age covered by Medicaid increased from 16.9 percent in 1990 to 20.1 percent in 1992 (Fleming, 1995). Medicaid provides physicians, hospitals, and other health care providers with direct reimbursements for their services to recipients. The distinction between public and private services was blurred.

Another key program for children is Head Start, which for more than 30 years has delivered a comprehensive child development program to preschool children from low-income families. Administered by the Head Start Bureau of the Department of Health and Human Services, Head Start programs are funded through grants to local public agencies, private nonprofit organizations, and public school systems. All Head Start programs must offer four major service components: education, social services, parent involvement, and health care. The health component provides comprehensive medical, dental, nutrition, and mental health services, including a broad array of preventive, diagnostic, treatment, and rehabilitative services for enrolled children. Head Start health services have a long history of arranging for training and technical assistance through public and private health professional entities, including the AAP and individual pediatricians (Wallace et al., 1996).

For many years the Public Health Service had maneuvered to get control of the Bureau's health programs. In 1968, Secretary Wilbur Cohen of the Department of Health, Education and Welfare (DHEW) created a major new component of the Public Health Service, the Health Services and Mental Health Administration. Assistant Secretary of Health and Scientific Affairs Philip R. Lee said it was established "to associate all agencies responsible for the provision of health care to individuals." The 1968 reorganization was used as the rationale for an August 1969 administrative order that radically changed the organization, structure, and program authority of the Children's Bureau. The Bureau, which could only be abolished by an Act of Congress, was transferred to the Office of Child Development to carry out the provisions of the Act of 1912. Child Welfare Services and the Juvenile Delinquency Service were retained in the Social and Rehabilitation Service. The Maternal and Child Health and Crippled Children's programs (Title V of the Social Security Act) were transferred together to DHEW's Public Health Service, and, after a series of organizational changes over the years, became the Maternal and Child Health (MCH) Bureau. Family planning projects administered by the Children's Bureau were transferred to the National Center for Family Planning Services, established in 1970. These name and organizational changes occurring after the breakup of the Children's Bureau in 1969 will not be referred to and, for simplicity, MCH will be used in the text for events that occur after 1969 (Hutchins, 1994).

Successors to the First National Study of Child Health Services
Almost two decades after the 1949 publication of *Child Health Services and Pediatric Education*, it was generally acknowledged that although U.S. children in general were healthier because of advances in medical knowledge, many were still not receiving optimal care. The rapid increase in the pediatric population, new migration patterns of U.S. families, the proliferation of child health programs, the continually changing status of child health legislation, and variations in the distribution of the increasing number of pediatricians throughout the nation made it necessary to evaluate regularly the delivery of child health services. In 1967, in response to the need for standards recognized as early as the 1949 report, the AAP published *Standards of Child Health Care*, presenting guidelines for the optimal care of children and a review of the changing scope of pediatrics.

In 1968, the AAP's Executive Board approved a new two-year study, directed by Carl C. Fischer and funded, in part, by the Children's Bureau. The resulting study, *Lengthening Shadows: A Report of the Council on Pediatric Practice of the American Academy of Pediatrics on the Delivery of Health Care to Children* (1971), stated:

> Within the last decade there has appeared a new set of child health problems, some related to, if not caused by, the social upheaval that started in the early '60s (increased use and abuse of drugs, adolescent pregnancies, increase in venereal disease and child abuse), and some related to current socioeconomic problems (near epidemic proportions of lead poisoning in the cities, exposure to environmental pollution of our food, water and air, and increased incidence of severe accidents).

The report concluded that the factors behind the inequalities of health services were complex and that their correction would require major changes in the current health care delivery system (AAP, 1971; Bremner, 1974, pp. 1313–1317; Hughes, 1980, pp. 42–43).

In 1976, the Task Force on Pediatric Education, composed of representatives from the AAP and nine other medical organizations concerned with pediatric education, began two years of study "to examine in detail all issues pertaining to pediatric education from the undergraduate through the postgraduate years." The task force was charged with "consider[ing] the health needs of American children and how the educational process may better meet these needs." Federal funding for this project came from the National Institute of Child Health and Human Development (NICHD) of the National Institutes of Health (NIH). The task force's report, *The Future of Pediatric Education*, identified the core issues confronting pediatric education. It found the educational content of many residency programs inadequate in certain subjects, including the biosocial and developmental aspects of pediatrics and adolescent medicine, the health needs of adolescents, clinical pharmacology, and care for children with chronic handicapping conditions. The task force also found that graduates of pediatric residencies were inadequately prepared in several aspects of community pediatrics (AAP, undated; Hughes, 1980, pp. 59–60).

As this chapter is being written in 1997, a Task Force on Pediatric Education II is underway (counting the 1949 study, it is actually the third national study on pediatric professional education by the AAP) with funding from the MCH Bureau and others. The three-year initiative will address questions of the future supply and appropriate training of pediatricians and the provision of pediatric care into the next century.

Recent AAP/Federal Partnerships

Other authors in this volume recount the recent history of child health and pediatrics (see chapters 6 and 7); therefore, the remainder of this chapter focuses on certain successful collaborations for child health between the public and private sectors, particularly the AAP and the federal government. In 1985, at the time of the 50th anniversary of Title V, it was written: "Each (current and emerging) issue involves interagency coordination and collaboration. This interagency partnership gives some sense of order to the issues. In MCH each issue, in a sense, is everybody's business and thus the various 'bodies' need to be involved in the resolution" (HRSA, 1985).

Research and the Creation of NICHD
In the early days of the Children's Bureau, a child research entity had been proposed but nothing developed legislatively. However, the Bureau conducted research studies under its own general authority. In its first decades, individual studies proposed by the Bureau were reviewed and approved or disapproved by Congress through the budget process.

Despite continuing resistance in some quarters to the need for pediatric research, Robert Cooke, chair of pediatrics at Johns Hopkins University Medical Center, led the way in creating a National Institute for Child Health, overcoming opposition from the NIH administration, the National Institute of Mental Health (because of some turf problems regarding mental retardation), and the Children's Bureau. The opposition of the Children's Bureau was overcome by the development of a memorandum of understanding that allocated research on the delivery of services to the Bureau, basic research to the new NICHD, and psychosocial research to the welfare component of the DHEW; an ex officio member from the Children's Bureau was to serve on the NICHD council (Cooke, 1993, p. 868).

Soon after the NICHD was established by President John F. Kennedy in October 1962, a series of planning sessions was arranged for professionals from a variety of fields to discuss developing programs appropriate for the new institute. Children's Bureau staff, with their experience in child research and government operations, were particularly helpful in getting NICHD organized (Bain, 1996; Cooke, 1993).

NICHD has continued with its broad mandate without a focus on a specific disease. It has fostered research in developmental biology, perinatal medicine, population studies of mothers and children, biological aspects of mental retardation, and the interface between biological and behavioral issues as they relate to mothers and children. NICHD has maintained close contacts with the field of pediatrics: its leaders and advisors are pediatricians, and the majority of its grants are awarded to pediatric academic institutions.

In 1986, the Pediatric Research in Office Settings (PROS) network was established by MCH to provide research opportunities for AAP fellows engaged in office-based practice (or similar primary care settings). MCH has provided core funding for the network since 1987; other governmental and foundation sources fund individual studies. The PROS network, made up of 378 practices and 1,177 practitioners in 56 smaller "networks" organized at the chapter (state) level, is committed to generating new knowledge about the basic pediatric issues of prevention and medical effectiveness—knowledge that can have a significant impact on the health of children (Wasserman, 1995–96).

Efforts to Encourage Diversity in Pediatrics

The health of children of minority groups received scant attention until the twentieth century. Citing "surprising gaps in the literature" about minority children, Katherine Bain noted in 1940 "that communities fail[ing] to provide public health facilities for Negro citizens is one of the major causes of difference in racial health records" (Bain, 1941). She added that "hospital facilities for Negroes are inferior, and in some communities nonexistent. Clinics are fewer and are less well equipped and less well-manned." She reported a high infant mortality rate for Mexican-Americans and found statistics of American Indian children unreliable. She called tuberculosis "the great killer of all three groups." Bain prophesied that "until a positive attitude is taken toward all health problems of minority groups in this country and until all groups are provided with equal opportunities for practicing the 'art of life,' the health of these minority groups will remain below the national average."

The first black pediatrician to become a member of the AAP was Roland B. Scott, an eminent pediatric researcher and early worker in the field of sickle cell anemia at Howard University Medical School. He became a member of the AAP in 1945, after having been denied membership in the AAP (as well as in the District of Columbia Medical Society) in the early 1940s.

As late as the 50th anniversary AAP annual meeting in Detroit in 1980, there were no women among the cap and gown procession of 200 current and past officers and officials from the national and state AAP organizations. The percentage of women AAP members was increasing, yet few were in leadership positions, reflecting the situation in organized medicine in general. Although the AAP had conducted one leadership course for women in pediatrics in 1980 and several women's gatherings during its annual meetings, it was apparent that a further stimulus was needed. It was provided that autumn with MCH funds to the AAP to support a Task Force on Opportunities for Women in Pediatrics. After reviewing the historical role of women in health care and pediatrics, as well as the current status of women in medical school, pediatric residencies, academia, and practice, the task force presented its report in October 1982. Among its findings, it reported that women were less likely than men to enter pediatric subspecialties. To point out the opportunities for women in pediatrics, the report cited adolescent medicine and public health as subspecialties that presented special challenges and new frontiers for women pediatricians. The report also described the barriers faced by women of ethnic minorities. The Executive Board immediately implemented the task force's first recommendation, by establishing a Provisional Committee on Opportunities for Women in Pediatrics, which was charged with implementing the task force's seven other recommendations.

These two defining events not only increased diversity in the AAP membership but encouraged diversity in its leadership positions. In 1989, Birt Harvey became the first African-American to head the AAP. He was succeeded by Antoinette P. Eaton, the first woman president (Bain, 1941, 1996; BCHS, 1979, pp. 62–63; Task Force, 1982).

Standards and Guidelines for Pediatric Practice
Other important public-private initiatives have focused on the development of standards for pediatric practice. They include:

- A 1981 AAP conference supported by MCH and the Ford Foundation to explore the ethical and legal ramifications of consent, confidentiality, and health record privacy for adolescents, which resulted in the development and publication of 12 broad guiding principles (AAP, 1982).
- Expansion of MCH's agreement with Head Start. In addition to support for dental services, MCH began in the 1980s to provide professional expertise, technical assistance, and training for Head Start's medical, mental health, and nutrition services.
- Joint development and promulgation of standards by MCH and the Administration on Children, Youth and Families. Together the two organizations funded meetings of state licensing and regulatory staff

with health staff to discuss current child care practices and provided partial support for the development of *Health in Day Care: A Manual for Health Professionals* (1987) by the AAP's Committee on Early Childhood, Adoption, and Dependent Care.

- A study of nine states with state-of-the-art day care programs with a strong health emphasis, which culminated in the publication of *Health of Children in Day Care: Public Health Profiles*, supported by MCH.

- A 1987 joint AAP/APHA project examining all current state licensing requirements, resulting in the report *Caring for Our Children: National Health and Safety Performance Standards—Guidelines for Out-of-Home Child Care Programs.* This MCH-funded work serves as a set of reference standards about health and safety in out-of-home child care settings to guide regulatory agencies, child care providers, accreditation and credentialing agencies, trainers, and health and safety consultants, and as a consumer information tool for parents (APHA/AAP, 1992; CCB/MCHB, 1996; Hutchins, 1995).

- The Healthy Tomorrows Partnership for Children Program, begun in 1989 and jointly sponsored by AAP and MCH, which brings together local communities and local pediatric leadership to form a unique coalition that includes the federal and state governments, professional organizations, foundations, corporate leaders, and families for collaborative problem solving (NCEMCH, 1995).

MCH and AAP also share a history of working together to assist children with special needs and their families, which is exemplified by their cooperation following passage of P.L. 99-457 (the Education for All Handicapped Children Act Amendments of 1986), especially Part H, which provides for services for children with disabilities from birth to 3 years. These efforts have included

- A joint MCH/AAP Surgeon General's Conference in 1986, at which Surgeon General C. Everett Koop released the Surgeon General's Report on Children with Special Health Care Needs, outlining a national agenda to promote family-centered, community-based, coordinated care, with examples of coordination among the public sector, the private sector, and parents. This conference was followed in 1987 by a second Surgeon General's conference, which highlighted innovative community-based systems.

- Two working conferences, in 1988 and 1989, jointly sponsored by MCH and AAP, on "The Participating Pediatrician and Family-Centered, Community-Based Health Care for Children with Chronic Illness and Disabling Conditions," which culminated in an issue paper.
- A national conference in 1988 on Part H of P.L. 99-457 for pediatricians in private practice.
- A 1991 conference to alert pediatricians to recent legislative changes in MCH programs and to support a national effort to enhance the development of coordinated systems of health and medical care through teams of private pediatricians, public MCH officials, and parents.

These jointly sponsored initiatives for children and families with special health care needs informed both the public and private sectors and worked through state leadership to promote community partnerships. The process underscored former AAP president Robert Haggerty's maxim: "We do have a role in pushing the boundaries of health beyond traditional medical care" (AAP, 1991; Bureau of Maternal and Child Health, Resource Development and the American Academy of Pediatrics, 1989; Gittler, 1988; Haggerty, 1992; Hutchins, 1992; Magrab, 1988; Shonkoff and Meisels, 1990; U.S. Department of Health and Human Services, 1987).

Conclusion

Once considered little more than chattel, children began to be recognized as individuals in the latter half of the nineteenth century—although mostly as sources of family income until this century. Children's issues, tied to the women's and social reform movements, came to the forefront during the early days of this century. Though not as swift or as thorough as most child advocates desire, progress in children's health has been steady through the twentieth century, despite occasional setbacks. In the same graduation speech quoted above, Hillary Rodham Clinton (1996) reflected on the opportunities of a new century:

> Just as every other generation met its challenges, we will do the same. I know that if we do that and enter into this new century and millennium with that American spirit of confidence and optimism, that a hundred years from now, someone will be standing on this campus talking about the challenges that we confront then as well. And they will look back and say, "Once again, in a time of great change and turmoil, Americans who value what we inherited made the right choices for themselves and their future."

Collaboration between the private and public sectors, represented by partnership of the AAP and MCH described in this chapter, has increased by leaps and bounds since the first official alliance between the two institutions for the 1945-1948 Child Health Services Study. Their 50-year history of working together demonstrates that both the public and the private sectors can reaffirm the statement contained in the preamble to the AAP constitution (AAP, 1996; Clinton, 1996):

> Together with those who share this purpose, [we pledge our] efforts and expertise to a fundamental goal—that all children and youth have the opportunity to grow up safe and strong, with faith in the future and in themselves.

References

Alexander GR, Oglesby AC, Hutchins VL. 1996. History and philosophy of maternal and child health. Unpublished internal training materials.

[AAP] American Academy of Pediatrics. 1971. Lengthening shadows: A report of the council on pediatric practice of the American Academy of Pediatrics on the delivery of health care to children, 1970. Evanston, IL: American Academy of Pediatrics.

[AAP] American Academy of Pediatrics. 1982. American Academy of Pediatrics conference on consent and confidentiality in adolescent care. Evanston, IL.

[AAP] American Academy of Pediatrics. 1991. Proceedings from a national conference on supporting children and families through integrated services. Elk Grove Village, IL: American Academy of Pediatrics.

[AAP] American Academy of Pediatrics. 1996. Fellowship directory. Elk Grove Village, IL: American Academy of Pediatrics.

[AAP] American Academy of Pediatrics. Undated. The future of pediatric education: A report by the Task Force on Pediatric Education. Evanston, IL: American Academy of Pediatrics.

[APHA/AAP] American Public Health Association, American Academy of Pediatrics. 1992. Caring for our children: National health and safety performance standards: Guidelines for out-of-home care programs. Washington, DC: APHA/AAP.

Bain K. 1941. Racial aspects of maternal and child health. The Child V:273–7. In: Bremner RH, editor. 1974. Children and youth in America: A documentary history, Vol. III: 1933–1973, pp. 1207–10. Cambridge, MA: Harvard University Press.

Bain K. 1948. The incidence of breast feeding in hospitals in the United States. Pediatrics 2:313.

Bain K. 1996. Personal communication.

Baker SJ. 1992. Fighting for life. In: Conway JK. Written by herself: Autobiographies of American women: An anthology, pp. 143–170. New York: Vintage Books.

[BCHS] Bureau of Community Health Services. 1979. Child health in America. Rockville, MD: Department of Health, Education and Welfare.

Beaven PW. 1954. The weapon of truth: The influence of the study of child health services conducted in 1946–1948. Pediatrics 14(1):64–76.

Beaven PW. 1955. For the welfare of children, pp. v–xvi. Springfield, IL: Charles C Thomas.

Beaven PW. Unpublished. Background and activities of the American Academy of Pediatrics: 1951–1956, pp. 48–50, 116–26.

Bradbury DE. 1962. Five decades of action for children. Washington: US DHEW, Children's Bureau. Pub # 358-revised 1962.

Bremner RH, editor. 1970. Children and youth in America: A documentary history, Vol. I: 1600–1865. Cambridge, MA: Harvard University Press.

Bremner RH, editor. 1971. Children and youth in America: A documentary history, Vol. II: 1886–1932. Cambridge, MA: Harvard University Press.

Bremner RH. editor. 1974. Children and youth in America: A documentary history, Vol III: 1933–1973, pp. 1207–10. Cambridge, MA: Harvard University Press.

Bureau of Maternal and Child Health, Resource Development and the American Academy of Pediatrics. 1989. Establishing a medical home for children served by Part H of Public Law 99-457: An issue paper. Washington: Georgetown University Child Development Center.

[CCB/MCHB] Child Care Bureau, Maternal and Child Health Bureau. 1996. Healthy child care America, pp. iv–ix. Washington: CCB/MCHB.

Clinton HR. 1996 May 23. Unpublished commencement address. University of Maryland at College Park.

Cone, Jr. TE, editor. 1979. History of American pediatrics. Boston: Little, Brown and Company.

Cooke RE. 1993. The origin of the National Institute of Child Health and Human Development. Pediatrics 92(6):868–71.

Eliot MM. 1967. The United States Children's Bureau, the John Howland Award Address. American Journal of Diseases of Children 114:565.

Emerson H. 1923. The part of the general public in bringing about a complete program of child health services. Transactions, American Child Health Association 1923:63–70. Quoted in: Schmidt WM. 1973. The development of health services for mothers and children in the United States, p. 13 in: Wallace HM, Gold EM, Lis EF, editors. Maternal and child health practices: Problems, resources and methods of delivery. Springfield, IL: Charles C Thomas.

Fleming G. 1995. The health insurance status of children: 1990 to 1992. Elk Grove Village, IL: American Academy of Pediatrics.

Gittler J. 1988. Community-based service systems for children with special health care needs and their families. Iowa City, IA: National MCH Resource Center.

Haggerty RJ. 1992. Physician envisions child health in next century. American Academy of Pediatrics News 8:19.

Hill LF. 1948. The American Academy of Pediatrics—its growth and development. Pediatrics 1(1):1–7.

Holt LE. 1903. The care and feeding of children. 3d ed. New York: Appleton Press.

[HRSA] Health Resources and Services Administration. 1985. A look to the future. In: Health Resources and Services Administration (HRSA) Chronicle, special issue: Maternal and child health anniversary. Rockville, MD: HRSA.

Hughes JG. 1980. American Academy of Pediatrics: The first 50 years. Chicago: American Academy of Pediatrics.

Hughes JG. 1993. Conception and creation of the American Academy of Pediatrics. Pediatrics 92(3):469–70.

Hutchins VL. 1992. Federal policy for early childhood: Evaluation of services for children with disabilities. In: Gallagher JJ, Fullagar PK, editors. The coordination of health and other services for infants and toddlers with disabilities: The conundrum of parallel service systems. Chapel Hill, NC: The Carolina Policy Studies Program, Frank Porter Graham Child Development Center, The University of North Carolina.

Hutchins VL. 1994. Maternal and Child Health Bureau: Roots. Pediatrics 94(5):695–7.

Hutchins VL. 1995. Reflections on the past, vision for the future. Presentation at the National Child Care Health Forum; 1995 May 10–11; Washington, DC.

Jacobi A. 1889. The relations of pediatrics to general medicine. Transactions of the American Pediatric Society, 1:17. In: Bremner RH, editor. 1971. Children and youth in America: A documentary history, Vol. II: 1886–1932. Cambridge, MA: Harvard University Press.

Lynch A. 1983. Redesigning school health services. New York: Human Sciences Press.

Magrab P, editor, 1988. The practicing pediatrician and family-centered, community-based health care for children with chronic illness and disabling conditions. Washington: Georgetown University Child Development Center.

[NCEMCH] National Center for Education in Maternal and Child Health. 1995. Healthy Tomorrows partnership for children: Abstracts of active projects FY 1996. Arlington, VA: NCEMCH.

Pearson HA, with assistance of Brown AK. 1988. The centennial history of the American Pediatric Society, 1888–1988. American Pediatric Society.

Pearson HA. 1995. The American Pediatric Society. Pediatrics 95(1):149

Pease MC. 1952. A history of the American Academy of Pediatrics: A forum where discussion should be free, intelligent and continuous, June, 1930–June, 1951. Chicago: American Academy of Pediatrics.

Radbill SX. 1979. Preface. In: Cone, Jr TE, editor. History of American pediatrics, pp. viii–ix. Boston: Little, Brown and Company.

[RCSCHS] Report of the Committee for the Study of Child Health Services, The American Academy of Pediatrics with the cooperation of the United States Public Health Service and the Children's Bureau. 1949. Child health services and pediatric education, pp. vi–xv, 251–5. The Commonwealth Fund. New York: Oxford University Press.

Rotch TM. 1909. The position and work of the American Pediatric Society toward public question. Transactions of the American Pediatric Society 21:8–10. In: Bremner RH, editor. 1971. Children and youth in America: A documentary history, Vol. II: 1886–1932, p. 821. Cambridge, MA: Harvard University Press.

Schlesinger, ER. 1967. The Sheppard–Towner era: A prototype case study in federal–state relationships. American Journal of Public Health 57(6): 1034–40.

Schmidt WM. 1973. The development of health services for mothers and children in the United States. In: Wallace HM, Gold EM, Lis EF, editors.

Maternal and child health practices: Problems, resources and methods of delivery. Springfield, IL: Charles C Thomas.

Shonkoff JP, Meisels SJ. 1990. Early childhood intervention: The evolution of a concept. In: Meisels SJ, Shonkoff JP, editors. Handbook of early childhood intervention. New York: Cambridge University Press.

Sinai N, Anderson OW. 1948. EMIC (emergency maternity and infant care): A study of administrative experience. Bureau of Public Health Economics, Research Series No. 3. Ann Arbor, MI: School of Public Health, University of Michigan.

Task Force. 1982. Report of the task force on opportunities for women in pediatrics. Evanston, IL: American Academy of Pediatrics.

U.S. Department of Health and Human Services, Public Health Service. 1987. Children with special health care needs, campaign '87. Iowa City, IA: National MCH Resource Center.

Wallace HM, Biehl RF, MacQueen JC, Blackman JA. 1996. Mosby's resource guide to children with disabilities and chronic illness. St. Louis: Mosby-Year Book.

Wasserman RC. 1995–96 Winter. The Network News; 8:2. Elk Grove Village, IL: American Academy of Pediatrics.

Wegman ME. 1988. The American Pediatric Society, The American Academy of Pediatrics and the Children's Bureau: 1944–1945. In: Pearson HA, with assistance of Brown AK. The centennial history of the American Pediatric Society, 1888–1988, pp. 86–9. American Pediatric Society.

6

Health Services for Children and Adolescents: A "Non-System" of Care*

Holly Grason and Madlyn Morreale

HEALTH SERVICES FOR CHILDREN in the United States are characterized by fragmentation, not organization. The "non-system" of health care comprises a mix of public and private care, largely divided along the lines of population-based programming under the aegis of the public sector and medical care for individuals provided within the market-driven private sector.

While the pervasive forces within U.S. culture emphasize individualism, market economics, and local and state sovereignty—and therefore private sector medical care—such care is only one component of the system needed to address the health needs of children and adolescents. Socioeconomic, environmental, psychosocial, and developmental aspects of child and adolescent health require a multidisciplinary and multisector approach, with a number of interventions—such as efforts to reduce alcohol consumption or exposure to lead—implemented both at the individual treatment level and on a population basis. Neither public nor private sector efforts alone have been sufficient to address the broad spectrum of child and adolescent health care needs, and policymakers face significant challenges in developing a coordinated and integrated system of care for this population.

In this chapter, we argue that children and adolescents have unique health service needs that require a comprehensive and coordinated array of medical care, linked with community-based services. We then chart the

*Madlyn Morreale's work on this chapter was partially funded by the Prevention Centers Program, National Center for Chronic Disease Prevention and Health Promotion, Centers for Disease Control and Prevention.

evolution of the public sector response to child health needs and explore, in brief, how and why we have the system we do. We demonstrate that while the United States has elements of the full spectrum of services needed to address the specific health needs of children and adolescents, these components are not organized as a cohesive system. We further characterize the fragmentation of health care delivery for children and youth as they relate to three significant factors. We next discuss "wraparound" approaches to linking service components for children and youth in this country, and note models of systems seen in other industrialized countries as well as in services for the elderly in the United States. In conclusion, we discuss the implications of current trends in the organization of health services—such as evolving managed care strategies in the private sector and the move to consolidation in the public sector—for efforts to improve the manner in which children and adolescents are served.

Unique Characteristics of Child and Adolescent Health

As described in chapter 1, children and adolescents have health service needs distinct from adults', requiring different types of prevention, diagnosis, and treatment strategies. Jameson and Wehr (1993) have argued for a special standard of medical necessity for children with respect to clinical services, based on children's developmental vulnerability in the context of rapid growth and development, their dependency on adults and social institutions for both financial and nonfinancial support in accessing health care, and the differential epidemiology of disease whereby health problems in children and adolescents differ in prevalence and scope from illnesses in adults. Similar arguments can be made for special standards for health care system structures and functions for children and adolescents. Such standards would recognize the extent to which development influences the medical needs of children and the special opportunities to avoid or reduce the potential impact of disease or disability through early, aggressive, and ongoing prevention.

These standards would also recognize the importance of flexibility. Although an adult's health profile may stabilize for many years, children's medical needs are constantly and often rapidly evolving as children grow and develop. Health and development are intertwined in complex ways that have potential long-term impact. For example, even moderate injuries resulting from the use of child passenger restraints can cause irreversible developmental and cognitive impairments with long-term costs and consequences. Lead poisoning, particularly as it is linked to mouthing behavior in young children, can cause irreversible developmental and cognitive impairments.

The dependency of children and adolescents, which makes them a uniquely vulnerable population, also has implications for the structure of health systems. For young children, preventive initiatives need to be implemented indirectly through parents, child care providers, protective environmental legislation, and the social institutions on which children depend. As children move into adolescence, the extent of their dependence lessens, but it does not disappear entirely for some years. Special skills are required of clinicians who serve children and adolescents in establishing partnerships with others in order to implement interventions.

The unique characteristics of adolescence as a discrete life stage provide an apt example of how biological and social as well as environmental contexts interact in complex ways to pose threats to health that require linked medical and community-based care. For adolescents, the biological changes introduced by puberty are joined with newly emerging risk-taking behaviors that may result in a variety of preventable morbidities and mortalities, including injuries due to violence and motor vehicle accidents; the consequences of unprotected sexual behavior; and the deleterious impact of alcohol, tobacco, and other drug abuse. The risk factors for these issues are strongly associated with complex environmental and social influences that are unlikely to be resolved in visits to medical clinicians. Igra and Millstein's (1993) analysis of 1990 data from the National Ambulatory Medical Care Survey found that screening for behaviorally related health conditions occurs in less than half of physician office visits by adolescents. However, increasing the delivery of these services during office visits alone may be insufficient. Adolescents' increasing reliance on peer norms and the relative importance of the environmental and social context compared to the biological context mean that interventions may be most effective if fashioned for community settings.

Thus, a health services system predicated on adult health care needs— relatively few and unchanging health problems generally treatable in a traditional clinical setting—is insufficient for meeting the health needs of children and adolescents. Drawing on these concepts of development, dependency, and differential epidemiology, effective health systems for children and adolescents demand:

- medical care that is responsive to developmental factors and emphasizes prevention;
- practitioners with special knowledge of pediatrics and adolescent health, including medical specialties;
- special strategies for intervention that include interactions with caregivers—parents, child care providers, and school staff—as well as peers during adolescence; and
- an array of interventions that extend beyond office- or clinic-based medical care, and include other health, social, and educational strategies.

A balanced focus on population-based prevention and community-based interventions as well as coordination of health services delivery along a number of continuums is needed. Inherent in this view is a partnership between the pediatric practitioners who provide health supervision and medical care to individual children and adolescents, and the public entities that guide, develop, and organize the planning and delivery of complementary population-based health services such as screening, disease control, environmental interventions, nutrition programming, and health education. A brief look at the evolution of the current system, however, demonstrates that such principles have not consistently guided the development of the U.S. health care system for children and youth.

Brief History of the Development of Public Health Programs for Children and Adolescents

The evolution of the current system has been influenced by economics and politics as much as by the assessed health needs of children and adolescents. The child health problems that evoked national concern in the late nineteenth and early twentieth centuries were related primarily to hygiene and infectious diseases. Because many of these problems were concentrated in densely populated urban areas, the health of mothers and children became the concerns of the then newly organized city public health agencies (Lesser, 1985). A linkage between health services and social welfare concerns coalesced in the creation of the Children's Bureau in 1912 (see chapter 5 for full account). Charged with a broad mandate to investigate and report on critical children's health and welfare concerns, including infant mortality, orphanages, juvenile courts, child labor issues, and child health and injuries, the Bureau adopted a population approach to child health concerns.

In 1921 the Maternity and Infancy Act, or Sheppard-Towner Act, was passed to provide resources for state health agencies to establish and improve health services for women and children. When this legislation expired in 1929, a service infrastructure had been developed in most states, providing a foundation for the national Maternal and Child Health (MCH) program established in 1935 through Title V of the Social Security Act. Under Title V, states received formula grant funds to establish units to develop and oversee clinical preventive health services for the broad population of mothers and children, and treatment services for "crippled children." Case finding and a comprehensive multidisciplinary approach to service delivery were emphasized. In addition to service provision, the Act stimulated the development of a system of high-quality services with a mandate to "extend and improve services," and a requirement that state plans be developed.

This governmental response to child health recognized: the need for 1) prevention services organized on a population basis, 2) state planning and gap-filling responses to the maldistribution of pediatric providers, especially in rural areas, and 3) a public response to health problems requiring highly specialized services not adequately addressed by organized medicine, such as specialized care for "crippling conditions" resulting primarily from poliomyelitis. For many years, the federal-state Title V MCH partnership was the predominant means by which public, and to some extent private, health services for women and children were organized. The scope and nature of health services in both sectors changed little between the late 1930s and the early 1960s.

Some 30 years following the creation of Title V, the "Great Society" agenda of the Kennedy and Johnson administrations spurred the development of health, social welfare, education, and economic opportunity programs for children and families. Between 1963 and 1965, a variety of programs were launched, including the Maternal and Infant Care projects, Comprehensive Children and Youth projects, and the Office of Economic Opportunity Neighborhood Health Centers. In 1965, Medicaid (Title XIX of the Social Security Act) and its Early and Periodic Screening, Diagnosis and Treatment (EPSDT) program were enacted. As a result of these federal initiatives, public funding streams and program authority for services began to bypass state government, and the threads of the state-based infrastructure for planning, organizing, and monitoring the system began to unravel.

In the 1960s, the growth of categorical funding for special programs was fueled by a number of complex and interacting forces, including the civil rights movement and consequent distrust of states' abilities to address important social problems. In addition, significant advances in medical technology provided new venues for treatment for highly vulnerable, small subsets of the child population (for example, children with cardiac conditions and low-birthweight infants).

Small but vocal constituencies—of both providers and consumers of health care—began to advocate and ultimately compete for resources to support their preferred new programs. Moreover, as the national economy began to weaken relative to the boom of the post-war years, incremental or sequential public health programming approaches developed as the most viable means by which to secure congressional approval of public funding requests. Over the next 15 years, additional expansions in categorical services for special populations and problems, such as for family planning, dental care, child development (through the Head Start program), and nutrition (through the Special Supplemental Food Program for Women, Infants and Children, or WIC), continued, and little or no attention was paid to the relationships among programs. Similar trends in child welfare and education program development occurred during this period.

In the 1970s and early 1980s, the Nixon and Reagan administrations sought significant change in governance through a "New Federalism," which attempted to return authority to states. Though not as far reaching as originally proposed (Combs-Orme and Guyer, 1992), the resulting block grant approach initially produced significant reductions in resources for public services and all but eliminated federal agency responsibilities for program administration. While some child health program consolidation occurred with the creation of the MCH Services Block Grant, the federal role in organizing the health services system for women and children was diminished by virtue of lack of authority, funding, capacity, and, at times and places, credibility.

In short order, however, the consolidation goals of the Nixon and Reagan administrations were eroded as Congress responded to the concerns of national advocacy groups about the lack of accountability of block grant programs by legislating earmarks and set-asides for categorical activities. Concurrently, fiscal constraints and conservative political trends demanded that reforms be implemented incrementally rather than comprehensively. These factors led to the reemergence of a categorical approach to health services funding and programming. Medicaid expansions and enhancements, although significant, were implemented through multiple annual changes for discrete subpopulations and services. More recently, the emergence of new morbidities, such as AIDS, youth violence, and other risk-related morbidities, contributed to the development of new categorical initiatives including the Ryan White Comprehensive AIDS Resource Emergency (CARE) Act, pediatric AIDS programs, Children of Substance Abusers Act, Program for Pregnant Substance Abusing Women and Their Infants, and fetal alcohol syndrome programs administered by the Centers for Disease Control and Prevention. In addition, new categorical programs were established for lead poisoning prevention and immunization services, which were believed to have been neglected by states when incorporated into block grants in 1981. The early 1990s also brought significant expansions of school health centers as a source of health care for children and adolescents.

The Current Context of Child and Adolescent Health Services

And so today, health and related care for children is provided through multiple and uncoordinated service delivery structures, which evolved from several decades of separately enacted pieces of legislation aimed at filling gaps in service availability and in access to personal health services through a variety of financing mechanisms and through the provision of services such as outreach or transportation. In addition, legislation has created public health programs to add services not otherwise provided within the context of private-office pediatric care.

Mix of Public and Private Sector Personal Health Care Delivery

Child and adolescent health services are delivered in public health departments, private physician offices, community health centers, and other nonprofit community agencies, schools, and hospitals (Table 6.1), with no centralized source of information, intake, or coordination at the service delivery level. Particularly problematic over the years has been the geographic maldistribution of practicing pediatricians, with far too few in rural and inner-city areas (Perloff, 1992; Schroeder, 1992). The government response to resulting access problems has been the establishment of personal health services in local health departments, community/migrant health centers, and more recently, school facilities. Notwithstanding the broad array of potential providers, more than 12 percent of all children reported having no source of routine care in 1988 (National Center for Health Statistics, 1988).

Further complicating this picture, children's involvement with the health services system is rarely limited to only one source of care. Most children and

Table 6.1
Source of Routine Health Care for Children and Adolescents
United States
1988

Age	No source of routine health care	Physician office/private clinic[a]	Community, neighborhood, or other family health center[b]	Hospital outpatient clinic	Other source[c]
0–17	12.1%	73.4%	5.4%	4.1%	5.1%
0–11	10.2	74.3	5.2	4.2	5.5
12–17	16.2	71.5	3.5	3.8	4.6

Source: National Center for Health Statistics (1988).
[a]Includes HMO/prepaid group practices.
[b]Includes migrant, and rural health centers, which each is reported as a source of routine care for less than 1 percent of children and adolescents.
[c]Includes company, school, or other clinics; walk-in emergency care centers; home; or other place. Less than 1 percent of children and adolescents (in each age group) reported using each of these sources.

adolescents obtain care in the private pediatric sector, and interact infrequently with publicly funded health services. Their contact with public health services may be limited to seeing a school health nurse for hearing or vision screening, or for acute care because of a school playground injury. Another group of children, however, receives care from the private sector, but because of a particular condition or problem, has more extensive interactions with the public system. For example, children with chronic health impairments may receive medical attention in specialty clinics administered by state programs for children with special health care needs (Title V/MCH) or in school settings. There is also a group of children who are quite intensely involved with the public sector. These children and youth often live in low-income households in disadvantaged urban or rural areas where private care is scarce and unaffordable. These children and youth therefore rely heavily on the public sector for needed care and are among the most intensive users of services. Nevertheless, children who routinely use a broad array of both public and private services represent a minority of the population.

Mix of Public and Private Insurance Strategies
Insurance coverage patterns for children and adolescents mirror the mix of private and public health service delivery. Most children are covered through dependent care coverage of their parents' employer-based health

plans (Employee Benefits Research Institute, 1996; U.S. General Accounting Office, 1996a). Trends in health care coverage over the last decade, however, show a decline in employer-based coverage for children and adolescents (Newacheck et al., 1995a; Rosenbaum, 1992; U.S. General Accounting Office, 1995b, 1996a). Children whose parents are unemployed, as well as those whose parents' employers do not include coverage for dependents in their benefits packages, must rely on public coverage. Neither employment nor low income guarantees insurance coverage, however. As a case in point, approximately two-thirds of uninsured adolescents live in families with incomes above the poverty level (National Research Council, 1993).

Further, underinsurance (limitations in benefits) has long been a problem for children covered under traditional employer-based indemnity insurance plans. Gaps in employer-subsidized benefits persist, both for preventive care, including well-child visits and immunizations, and for specialized care, such as mental health and substance abuse treatment for adolescents and medical and habilitative specialty care for children with chronic health impairments (Elster et al., 1993; Hughes et al., 1995; McManus and Hertz, 1995; Short and Banthin, 1995; U.S. Congress, Office of Technology Assessment, 1991). Thus, even when children are insured through their parents' employer-based coverage, they may need publicly financed coverage and/or services.

Medicaid and its EPSDT component represent the single most important source of financing and programmatic guidance for public child health programs. (EPSDT requires states to periodically screen Medicaid-eligible children under 22 years for illnesses, abnormalities, or treatable conditions, and to refer them for definitive treatment.) Originally, Medicaid and EPSDT served only very low-income women and children. Expansions of the Medicaid program in the 1980s, however, weakened the link between welfare and Medicaid, first with legislation allowing for optional extension of coverage to pregnant women and infants who were not receiving Aid to Families with Dependent Children (AFDC), and ultimately with a mandate in the Omnibus Budget Reconciliation Act of 1989 (OBRA '89), to extend coverage to pregnant women and infants to 133 percent of the federal poverty level, and to young children in families with incomes under 100 percent of the federal poverty level. OBRA '89 also provided important expansions to the EPSDT program, requiring states to provide any federally reimbursable service that is "medically necessary" to diagnose or treat a problem that is identified in the screening, regardless of whether that service is included in the state's Medicaid plan. Eligibility for children over age

6 was subsequently phased in, one year at a time, so that (assuming no changes in federal policy) all poor adolescents under age 19 will be covered in the year 2001 (Omnibus Budget Reconciliation Act of 1990).

These Medicaid expansions, coupled with state public and private child health insurance programs in some states, have mediated the extent of uninsurance (Newacheck et al., 1995a; U.S. General Accounting Office, 1996a, 1996b). By 1994, more than 16 million children and adolescents were covered under Medicaid, or about 23.2 percent of the population under 18 years of age (Employee Benefits Research Institute, 1996). Eligibility for Medicaid, however, remains complex, with a myriad of age, income, and medical criteria for enrollment.

Uncoordinated Public Sector Programming

For those children and adolescents who rely on public programs to meet their health needs, families must sort through many small and often inconsistent rules and procedures to find their way to the frequently overlapping public programs and services that might assist them. All too often, inconsistent and rigid eligibility requirements confound or preclude access to care. Efforts of policymaking bodies, public program administrators, and the public to address children's needs are similarly thwarted by the sheer numbers of programs, as well as by the complete absence or the complexity of linkages among them.

Federally legislated child health programs implemented today represent a mix of income-based entitlement programs (e.g., Medicaid and EPSDT), quasi-entitlement programs (e.g., WIC), categorical population or disease-specific programs (e.g., immunization, pediatric AIDS, lead poisoning, health care for the homeless, and family planning programs), age-specific entitlement programs (e.g., early intervention services for infants and toddlers with disabilities), as well as "gap filling" formula grant funded programs (e.g., Title V prenatal and child health services, and categorical grants to localities for community and migrant health centers. Health services also are embedded in entitlement and categorical programs for education (e.g., special education and school health services) and social services (e.g., Head Start, family preservation programs). This array is even more complex when one looks beyond to income maintenance, employment, housing, and justice programs. By and large, this body of federal authorizing legislation and its implementing regulations are not coordinated (National Commission on Children, 1991; Reingold and Frank, 1993; U.S. General Accounting Office, 1995a).

More recent legislative initiatives to improve services to children, such as those found in the Child and Adolescent Service System Program and the Individuals with Disabilities Education Act early intervention program for infants and toddlers, attempt to redress some of these problems through a "systems" focus, incorporating requirements for interagency coordination of policy development, planning, service provision, and financing. However, states and localities are now grappling with the overlap among complex systems as well as the overlap among complex programs.

Service System Snapshots

Although linking individual (private sector) and population-based (public sector) care makes sense in terms of meeting child and adolescent needs, it is clear that the current system has evolved in response to a host of other influences and rationales that have undermined the goal of developing a coherent and organized system of care for children and adolescents. As described below, the services available to children and families depend on a variety of factors such as age, area of residence, and definition of need (health or developmental risk and/or impairments, financial status, etc.), and fail to meet the needs of many families in many ways.

Understanding the scope and complexity of service programs, eligibility criteria, and the pathways to access can be a formidable challenge. While a child's needs may remain constant, changes in family status or age may lock a child out of needed services; conversely, a child may remain ineligible for needed services despite changing or intensifying needs. Paradoxically, the complex array of services may result in a child being technically eligible for many similar programs but unable to get help because limited program funding has resulted in long waiting lists, or because programs are completely absent in many localities (U.S. General Accounting Office, 1995a). To illustrate these points, three scenarios are outlined below.

The Story of Kelli: How Changes in Income Status Impact Service and Program Eligibility

> *Kelli is four years old. She lives with her mother, who has never worked outside the home. Kelli's parents divorced two years ago. Kelli's father has been living apart from the family since her birth without providing child support or other financial assistance. Kelli and her mother recently lost their eligibility for dependent coverage through her father's employer-sponsored health insurance. Kelli has not seen a medical provider in the past year. Her mother*

Table 6.2
How Income Status Impacts Service/Program Eligibility: The Case of Kelli

	Program or service	Program/service orientation or function	Comments
Kelli while her mother has no earned income	Private physician care	Medical services.	Such care is likely to be paid for by Medical Assistance (see below). Local physicians, however, may limit the number of Medical Assistance patients they see.
	Temporary Assistance to Needy Families (TANF)	Income support, with work requirement that provides assistance with child care expenses.	Each state sets eligibility criteria. TANF benefits are unlikely to raise a family's income to more than 50 percent of the federal poverty level
	Medical Assistance	Payment for medical care for very low income individuals/families, and those with disabilities.	As long as Kelli and her mother meet 1996 eligibility criteria for welfare, Kelli will be eligible for comprehensive preventive, primary, and specialty care through EPSDT.
	Head Start	Center-based developmental services to low-income children under age 6: primarily serves 3- and 4-year-olds. Health and screening and referral, immunizations, and nutrition are also provided.	Kelli is likely eligible to attend a Head Start center as long as one operates nearby and does not have a long waiting list for enrollment.

Kelli after her mother obtains a minimum-wage job	WIC	Nutritional supplements (food packages or vouchers) to pregnant and postpartum women, infants, and children through age 4 who are at risk of inadequate nutrition.	Kelli is unlikely to be eligible unless she has lead poisoning, anemia, or another health condition that puts her at high nutritional risk.
	Health care services	Local health departments, community health centers, and/or hospital clinics may be available to provide preventive and primary care for Medicaid beneficiaries and persons without insurance.	Kelli's mother will lose eligibility for Medical Assistance within a year of starting her new job. She is unlikely, however, to obtain private health insurance through her minimum-wage job.
	Head Start	Same as above.	A significant increase in her mother's income may make Kelli ineligible for program services.
	Child Care Block Grant	Infrastructure development to improve availability and quality of child care; some assistance for payment.	Kelli's mother is probably eligible for help in finding and paying for child care. This care will need to be coordinated with Head Start services in terms of hours and transportation.
	Earned Income Tax Credit (EITC)	"Refundable" tax credit to subsidize earnings of low-income families.	Kelli's mother may receive between $1,000 and $2,000 additional income through this program.

has relied on assistance from her church and public programs for groceries and income support. As a condition for receiving welfare payments, Kelli's mother must participate in job training courses. She has had trouble finding child care services that she can afford while attending these courses.

The health and social support services available to Kelli and her mother will vary depending on Kelli's mother's income and employment status (Table 6.2). Within a year of Kelli's mother receiving a minimum wage position, she and Kelli will lose health coverage as a result of employment. If Kelli is able to participate in Head Start, some health services may be available to her through that program. However, unless Kelli and her mother live near a community health center, or unless a private pediatrician will provide care without compensation, Kelli's health care may be available only at the local emergency room.

The Story of Naomi: How Age Impacts Service Eligibility

Naomi was born with spina bifida, a neurological condition characterized by incomplete closure of the spinal cord, with consequent paralysis of her lower extremities, and neurogenic bladder and bowel. Naomi was shunted soon after birth in an attempt to prevent hydrocephalus and related mental retardation. Over her lifespan, Naomi will need surgery to close the spinal column and for shunting. She will also need bracing and other physical and occupational therapy interventions related to her paralysis, skin care, urologic monitoring, bowel training, monitoring for scoliosis, and special attention to the potential for weight problems and learning disabilities.

Naomi's parents both work, although her mother works only part-time so that she can devote the extra hours and energy needed for Naomi's daily care. Her family has health insurance through her father's employer, although the coverage package is limited as the company he works for is small, with a limited profit margin to allocate to the employees' health benefit package.

The services that Naomi needs and that she and her family are able to access will differ markedly depending on her age (Table 6.3). The availability of services depends largely on the extent to which Naomi's medical condition impacts her cognitive development and her ability to function independently (age-appropriately) at various ages. It is also determined by her family income, program rules in her state of residency, and the variable application of parental resources to the determination of eligibility for public programs.

Table 6.3
How Age Impacts Service Eligibility: The Story of Naomi

	Program or service	Program orientation/function	Comments
Naomi at 2 years	Private physician care	Medical services.	Most routine services are covered by insurance, but specialty care may not be. Immunizations are not covered under parents' health plan.
	Title V MCH Block Grant Program for Children with Special Health Care Needs (CSHCN)	Care/service coordination for the child/adolescent; financing for medical care not covered by insurance; administration/funding for multidisciplinary specialty services (clinics).	Because this is a block grant, not an entitlement program, federal/state funds are capped. Naomi's eligibility depends on how medical and financial eligibility is defined in her state of residence.
	Part H, Individuals with Disabilities Education Act	Developmental/early intervention and special education services (center or home-based); services planning and coordination.	Free appropriate public education is provided if Naomi meets state's criteria for developmental delay, risk, or disability. Only available to age 3.
	Child Care Block Grant	Infrastructure development to improve availability and quality of child care; some assistance with payment.	Naomi's family may receive assistance until she is 13 years old, depending on state rules implementing federal requirements related to children with disabilities.

Table 6.3
How Age Impacts Service Eligibility (*cont.*)

	Program or service	Program orientation/function	Comments
Naomi at 19 years	Private physician care	Medical services.	Naomi may lose coverage under her parents' policy unless she is in school.
	Title V MCH Block Grant Program for CSHCN	Same as above.	Naomi may receive services as above, but only those Medicaid does not cover. She may be ineligible, depending on age cut-offs in her state of residence.
	Supplemental Security Income (SSI)	Income support for low-income disabled adults.	Naomi may be financially eligible because family income ceilings no longer apply after age 18. Her eligibility also will depend on the severity of her condition and her potential employability.
	Medical Assistance	Payment for medical care for very low-income individuals, and those with disabilities.	Naomi is now categorically eligible by virtue of SSI eligibility. Comprehensive EPSDT no longer applies.
	Food stamps	Coupons redeemable for retail food purchases.	Naomi is now eligible by virtue of SSI eligibility.

The Story of Peter: How Living Situation Affects Receipt of Services

Peter is 16 years old and has a history of alcohol and substance abuse and mental health problems associated with the ongoing physical and emotional abuse he experiences at home. His parents live in a small, rural town and their employer-sponsored health insurance does not cover mental health or substance abuse services for dependents. Peter does not know this, however, because he is reluctant to seek assistance. He is unaware of any publicly supported service in his community. Peter's school performance has been satisfactory until this year, but now he is considering dropping out of school and running away from home.

The health-related services available to Peter depend on whether he remains at home or runs away, as well as on where he and his family live, his parents' income, whether he becomes a ward of the state, the availability of publicly financed categorical programs or privately funded care, and Peter's knowledge of these resources (Table 6.4).

These brief stories illustrate a number of important limitations of the current system of health and social support services for children and adolescents. In each story, change in only one variable (age, residence, or income level) resulted in dramatic changes in access to services, even when the need for these services changed very little. In reality, the lives of children, youth, and families are even more dynamic, and multiple variables are likely to change over the course of a child's life, making efforts to coordinate continuous access to services difficult for both families and providers. Moreover, the scope of these and most children's needs extends far beyond what health care providers alone can provide, regardless of the adequacy of insurance coverage.

Efforts to Link Private and Public Sector Care

Notwithstanding this bleak picture, some partnerships have succeeded in enhancing and extending private office medical care. Enhancements to Medicaid and other programs enacted in the mid-1980s and early 1990s provided important new venues for public-private partnerships. For example, when Medicaid extended financial access to private sector obstetrical and pediatric care, limitations in the capacity of the market-driven private sector to meet the needs of the Medicaid-eligible population became increasingly evident and documented (Hill, 1992; Lewis-Idema, 1988; Perloff, 1992). These limitations included the lack of sufficient providers to absorb additional Medicaid beneficiaries into private practices, low reimbursement

Table 6.4
How Residence or Living Situation Impacts Service Eligibility: The Story of Peter

	Program or service	Program/service orientation or function	Comments
Peter living at home	Physician care	Medical services.	Peter may get care for acute medical problems from his family doctor, with payment made through his parents' insurance.
	Medical Assistance	Payment for medical care for very low-income individuals/families and those with disabilities.	Peter is not eligible because of family income. In most cases, an adolescent must become a ward of the state (through the child welfare or juvenile justice system) before he/she becomes eligible for Medical Assistance.[a]
	Substance Abuse Prevention and Treatment Block Grant	Prevention, treatment, and rehabilitation activities related to alcohol and other drugs, including inpatient and outpatient alcohol and drug detoxification and counseling.	The availability of services depends on the locality and the priorities of state planners. Peter is unlikely to know whether these services are available in his community unless he actively seeks assistance.
	Child Welfare Services	Services for abused, neglected, homeless, and troubled youth under age 21 and their families, including preventive interventions to keep children in their homes, family reunification, and alternative placements.	These services are administered by states and counties and have no income requirements. Peter's ability to access these services depends on his knowledge of their availability and his willingness to report the abuse he experiences at home and on the level of services in each area.

	Program	Services	Availability
	Child and Adolescent (Mental Health) Service System Program	Services for children and youth aged 0–22 years who are at risk for mental health and emotional or behavioral disorders.	The availability of services depends on the locality and the priorities of state planners. Peter is unlikely to know whether these services are available in his community unless he actively seeks assistance.
Peter living on the streets	Runaway and Homeless Youth Program, Basic Centers	Short-term emergency shelter, counseling, family reunification, direct outreach, and linkages with community agencies that provide other support services.	Peter's access to basic centers depends on his knowledge of their existence and whether one exists in the community to which he has run away. The total number of basic centers in 1995 was 366.
	Transitional Living Program for Runaway and Homeless Youth	Mental and physical health care, housing assistance, job placement services, and educational and career training for youth aged 16-21 years who cannot be reunited with their families.	Peter's access to transitional living services depends on his knowledge of their existence and whether one exists in the community to which he has run away. The total number of programs in 1995 was about 75.
	Health care services	Local health departments, community health centers, homeless centers, or organizations receiving other public or private funds.	Unless Peter becomes Medicaid-eligible, his care will likely be provided without payment. Providers are reimbursed for services to non-paying patients through categorical grants, private donations, and other unstable sources.

*The process of becoming a ward of the state varies by state. Typically, there must be either voluntary placement by the parents or substantiated abuse or neglect that results in court-ordered placement in the child welfare system. Once a child or adolescent is in the child welfare system, most states will provide Medical Assistance, regardless of the family's income.

rates, and inconsistent duration of client eligibility, which created uncertainty about payment for services provided. In addition, pediatric clinicians practicing in communities became aware of limitations in their ability to provide the full array of interventions and support needed by low-income populations. To compensate for these gaps in the private sector, the public sector offered enhancements to standard medical care through wraparound services such as outreach, follow-up for care recommendations provided during office visits, case management, additional nutritional and social work counseling services, home visiting, and health education (Association of Maternal and Child Health Programs, 1991; Balla, 1995; Bell and Simkin, 1993; Buescher et al., 1991, 1993; Hill, 1992; Hill and Bennett, 1990; Hill and Breyel, 1989, 1991; U.S. General Accounting Office, 1990).

While promising, these new public-private partnerships evolved haphazardly, often relying on the availability of unstable funding sources, and with no systematic organizational focus nationally. Our collective failure as a society to enact universal national health care legislation diminished the hopes of many child health advocates that a remedy would emerge in this century. The growth of managed care and integrated service networks within the health industry, however challenging in the intensity and magnitude of the changes they bring, may provide new opportunities to promote systemwide approaches that make sense for families and that adequately meet the full spectrum of child and adolescent health needs.

Integrated Models

While the United States may have begun to fashion an organized system approach earlier in this century with the creation of the Children's Bureau as a locus for national planning and oversight and the development of the state-federal MCH partnership program in Title V, this review illustrates the need to address the well-intentioned but haphazard manner in which health services for children and adolescents evolved over the course of this century.

Comparative studies of health systems in other industrialized countries that have organized primary care systems that link private medical and public population-based services reveal the potential for improved health outcomes for the population ("Child Health," 1990; Starfield, 1991; U.S. General Accounting Office, 1993; Williams and Miller, 1991). France, Belgium, Japan, and the Scandinavian countries all have fashioned approaches to maternal and child health services that universally assure women, children, and their families have access to preventive and curative personal and population-based health services. Public sector roles in these countries include disseminating information about health and development, outreach, providing community-based preventive services such as health screening and home visiting, and tracking and follow-up to help secure adequate health care and to promote parental participation in assuring that children receive appropriate care. Private sector physicians provide medical care for acute and chronic conditions. This is accomplished with a governmental locus of accountability on the national, regional, and/or community levels. To date, however, other countries' health systems models have not been seriously considered by most U.S. policymakers, by leaders in the private sector insurance industry or in the medical professions, or by the general public.

Models exist in this country as well. Analysis of the design of services for the elderly in the United States reveals apt policy and program design lessons for child and family health services. The Older Americans Act (OAA) establishes a high-level, visible national locus for information, policy development and coordination, advocacy, research, demonstration projects, and professional training. The OAA also provides the legislative structure for a uniform consolidated program of comprehensive, community-based planning, and preventive and social services that complement the medical care financing and income support provided to the elder population through Medicare and Social Security entitlements (Grason and Guyer, 1995b).

Organizing Care for Children and Adolescents in Ways That Make Sense—Building the Foundation for the Twenty-first Century
This review shows a history of public sector concern and private sector interest in addressing child and adolescent health needs. The private sector insurance and medical care provider responses that have evolved can address many, but not all, of the primary health needs of the majority of children and adolescents. However, in the absence of universal health care coverage, the public health safety net of publicly funded clinics and programs is needed to provide care for the most vulnerable, including those who are uninsured or underinsured. Ongoing attention to health system planning to assure capacity where the market does not develop (particularly in rural and inner-city areas) also is clearly indicated.

Population-based health services and activities—fundamental to addressing health education and promotion, environmental interventions, and

linkages among health, education, and social service professions and programs—also must be incorporated into a systems approach to improving the
health of all children and adolescents. Enhanced wraparound health services
and outreach to address underutilization of appropriate preventive and primary health care will continue to be important, particularly for the most vulnerable segments of the population—members of young families in poverty,
children and youth with chronic and disabling medical and physical conditions, and those who are culturally and/or socially isolated.

Much has been written about the need to provide coordinated and comprehensive care for children and adolescents, both at the policy level and
from the perspective of individual service providers. Increasingly, a systems
approach has been advocated for communities, where integrated networks
of providers serve children and families by linking across sites and with
non-health service providers, and by blending public and private sources of
funding (Hayes et al., 1995; Kahn and Kamerman, 1992; Kitzner and Page,
1996; Newacheck et al., 1995b; Office of Inspector General, 1991). Moreover, at this juncture an increasing proportion of populations who are publicly insured are receiving health services through private sector managed
care entities and integrated service networks. As the private sector medical
profession and the health insurance industry become more organized and
embrace greater accountability for enrolled populations, opportunities exist
to consider new ways to blend private sector medical care with population
health. Further, political support to consolidate public programming, although raising concerns about the potential erosion of financial resources
and entitlement services, provides opportunities to move forward in a
number of ways.

First and fundamental to assuring the health and well-being of children
and adolescents is adequate funding. Health insurance coverage equal in
scope to that provided for the elderly population should be universally
available to children and adolescents. In addition, support for population-
based public health and related community-based services must be better
balanced with support for clinical medical care. Access to public programming for prevention and support services, so critical to health during this
early stage of the lifespan, should not be dependent on where a child or
teenager resides.

Second, responsibilities for preventive services must be sorted rationally
among clinical medicine and public health. Questions related to the extent
of preventive and supportive care—such as nutrition services, counseling,

and case management—that can reasonably be provided in clinical versus public health settings need to be answered, and consensus established systemwide.

Third, delineation of roles and responsibilities for health promotion and supportive services—such as wraparound and enabling services including outreach, transportation, and translation services—among public health and organized medical care is needed. Geographic regions and communities must determine how responsibility for the health of populations will be shared, and how public and private health entities will work together to assess and address population-based prevention issues, particularly educational and environmental interventions. Greater linking of individual private sector clinicians, physician group practices, and hospitals under administrative umbrellas of managed care organizations should facilitate these processes in that there will be fewer but larger and more well-defined private sector providers to assume responsibility in negotiations.

Fourth, rational realignment of the public programs that serve children and adolescents is needed to promote access to the full spectrum of services needed by individual families. Such reorganization needs to occur both at the community level, through community-based planning and service and program restructuring, as well as through legislative changes at the national and state levels. The general trend in the political arena to consolidate public programming through block grants can provide the basis for such restructuring—but only if planned with a comprehensive, long-term view and implemented incrementally to allow for systematic monitoring of impact and feedback guiding future steps. We cannot afford for important supports for children and youth to be lost through hasty reconstruction. As elements of such efforts, structural changes at the local level need to assure centralized information and entry into public programs, as well as systems that allow information to move among multiple providers (public programs and private sector medical providers and managed care organizations) serving a single child or teenager while guarding sensitive and confidential information.

Finally, of critical importance in these evolving systems changes is advocacy for children and adolescents, who as a population are physically, socially, economically, and legally dependent on adults. Societal responsibility for the health and well-being of children and adolescents must be implemented at both the clinical care and governmental levels. Special standards of care for children and youth must be established for managed care entities and integrated service networks: system structures predicated on adult needs alone cannot appropriately address the health needs of our youngest citizens. Further, assuming that managed care strategies will be widely implemented with a focus on controlling expenditures, tools of government—legislation, regulation, contracting specifications, and external review and auditing of private sector services—should be used to assure that MCH-specific criteria are met and that the focus on cost savings does not harm children and adolescents (Grason and Guyer, 1995a).

This work will not be easy, but few challenges of significant importance to our country are. Implementing this vision will require a societal commitment to children not observed to date, but not, we believe, impossible if our country truly seeks a strong and secure future.

References

Association of Maternal and Child Health Programs. 1991. Making a difference: A report on Title V maternal and child health services programs' role in reducing infant mortality. Washington: Association of Maternal and Child Health Programs.

Balla P. 1995. CHIP—a community model for a comprehensive health care system. In: Grason H, Guyer B, editors. Assessing and developing primary care for children: Reforms in health systems. Arlington, VA: National Center for Maternal and Child Health.

Bell KN, Simkin LS. 1993. Caring prescriptions: Comprehensive health care strategies for young children in poverty. New York: National Center for Children in Poverty.

Buescher PA, Roth MS, Williams D, Goforth CM. 1991. An evaluation of the impact of maternity care coordination on Medicaid birth outcomes in North Carolina. American Journal of Public Health 81(12):1625–9.

Buescher PA, Larson LC, Nelson MD, Lenihan AJ. 1993. Prenatal WIC participation can reduce low birth weight and newborn medical costs: A cost-benefit analysis of WIC participation in North Carolina. Journal of the American Dietetic Association 93(2):163–6.

Child health in 1990: The U.S. compared to Canada, England and Wales, France, The Netherlands, and Norway. Pediatrics 86(suppl):1025–127.

Combs-Orme T, Guyer B. 1992. America's health care system: The Reagan legacy. Journal of Sociology and Social Welfare 19:63–89.

Elster A, Panzarine S, Holt K, editors. 1993. American Medical Association state-of-the-art conference on adolescent health promotion: Proceedings. Arlington, VA: National Center for Education in Maternal and Child Health.

Employee Benefits Research Institute. 1996. Sources of health insurance and characteristics of the uninsured: Analysis of the March 1995 current population survey. Issue Brief No. 170. Washington: EBRI.

Grason H, Guyer B. 1995a. MCH policy research brief: Quality, quality assessment, and quality assurance considerations for maternal and child health populations and practitioners. Baltimore: The Child and Adolescent Health Policy Center, The Johns Hopkins University.

Grason H, Guyer B. 1995b. Rethinking the organization of children's programs: Lessons from the elderly. Milbank Quarterly 73(4):565–97.

Hayes CD, Lipoff E, Danegger AE. 1995. Compendium of comprehensive, community-based initiatives: A look at costs, benefits, and financing strategies. Washington: The Finance Project.

Hill I. 1992. The role of Medicaid and other government programs in providing medical care for children and pregnant women. The Future of Children 2(2):134–53.

Hill I, Bennet T. 1990. Enhancing the scope of prenatal services: Strategies for improving state perinatal programs. Washington: National Governors' Association.

Hill I, Breyel J. 1989. Coordinating prenatal care: Strategies for improving state perinatal programs. Washington: National Governors' Association.

Hill I, Breyel J. 1991. Caring for kids: Strategies for improving state child health programs. Washington: National Governors' Association.

Hughes RG, Davis TL, Reynolds RC. 1995. Assuring children's health as the basis for health care reform. Health Affairs 14(2):158–67.

Igra V, Millstein SG. 1993. Current status and approaches to improving preventive services for adolescents. Journal of the American Medical Association 269(11):1408–12.

Jameson EJ, Wehr E. 1993 Fall. Drafting national health care reform legislation to protect the health interests of children. Stanford Law and Policy Review: 152–76.

Kahn AJ, Kamerman SB. 1992. Integrating services integration: An overview of initiatives, issues, and possibilities. New York: National Center for Children in Poverty.

Kitzner J, Page S. 1996. Map and track: Initiatives for young children and families. New York. National Center for Children in Poverty.

Lesser AJ. 1985. The origin and development of maternal and child health programs in the United States. American Journal of Public Health 75: 590–8.

Lewis-Idema D. 1988. Increasing provider participation: Strategies for improving state perinatal programs. Washington: National Governors' Association.

McManus MA, Hertz K. 1995. Private health insurance coverage of preventive benefits for children. In: Solloway MR, Budetti PP, editors. Child health supervision: Analytical studies in financing, delivery, and cost-effectiveness of preventive and health promotion services for infants, children, and adolescents. Arlington, VA: National Center for Education in Maternal and Child Health.

National Center for Health Statistics. 1988. National health interview survey child health supplement, 1988. Washington: U.S. Government Printing Office.

National Commission on Children. 1991. Beyond rhetoric: A new American agenda for children and families, summary final report of the National Commission on Children. Washington: National Commission on Children.

National Research Council. 1993. Losing generations: Adolescents in high risk settings. Washington: National Academy Press.

Newacheck PW, Hughes DC, Cisternas M. 1995a. Children and health insurance: An overview of recent trends. Health Affairs 14:244–54.

Newacheck PW, Hughes DC, Brindis C, Halfon N. 1995b. Decategorizing health services: Interim findings from the Robert Wood Johnson Foundation's child health initiative. Health Affairs 14(3):232–42.

Office of Inspector General, Department of Health and Human Services. 1991. Services integration: A twenty-year retrospective. OEI-01-91-00580. Washington: Department of Health and Human Services.

Omnibus Budget Reconciliation Act of 1989. Public Law No. 101-239, Section 6403.

Omnibus Budget Reconciliation Act of 1990. Public Law No. 101-508, Section 4601.

Perloff J. 1992. Health care resources for children and pregnant women. The Future of Children 2(2):78–94.

Reingold JR, Frank BR. 1993. Targeting youth: The sourcebook for federal policies and programs. Washington: Institute for Educational Leadership.

Rosenbaum S. 1992. Rationing without justice: Children and the American health system. University of Pennsylvania Law Review 140:1859–80.

Schroeder SA. 1992. Physician supply and the U.S. medical marketplace. Health Affairs 11(1):235–43.

Short PF, Banthin JS. 1995. New estimates of underinsured younger than 65 years. Journal of the American Medical Association 274(16):1302–6.

Starfield B. 1991. Primary health care: A cross national comparison. Journal of the American Medical Association 266(16):2268–71.

U.S. Congress, Office of Technology Assessment. 1991. Adolescent health, Vol. III: Cross-cutting issues in delivery of health related services. OTA-H-467. Washington: U.S. Government Printing Office.

U.S. General Accounting Office. 1990. Home visiting: A promising early intervention strategy for at-risk families. GAO/HRD-90-83. Washington: GAO.

U.S. General Accounting Office. 1993. Preventive health care for children: Experience from selected foreign countries. GAO/HRD-93-62. Washington: GAO.

U.S. General Accounting Office. 1995a. Early childhood programs, multiple programs and overlapping target groups. GAO/HEHS-95-4FS. Washington: GAO.

U.S. General Accounting Office. 1995b. Health insurance for children: Many remain uninsured despite Medicaid expansion. GAO/HEHS-95-175. Washington: GAO.

U.S. General Accounting Office. 1996a. Health insurance for children: Private insurance coverage continues to deteriorate. GAO/HEHS-96-129. Washington: GAO.

U.S. General Accounting Office. 1996b. Health insurance for children: State and private programs create new strategies to insure children. GAO/HEHS-96-35. Washington: GAO.

Williams BC, Miller CA. 1991. Preventive health care for young children: Findings from a 10-country study and directions for United States policy. Arlington, VA: National Center for Clinical Infant Programs.

7

The Role of the Individual Child
Health Care Practitioner

Michael Weitzman

MARKED CHANGES in child health services are occurring in the context of fundamental changes in the health care system for individuals of all ages. All health care arenas are affected, including hospitals, hospital ambulatory services, community health centers, private practices, and home care services. Medical and nonmedical services for children and families are being changed as part of the alteration of far more extensive and expensive services and resources for individuals of all ages. As the rate and extent of these changes increase, they will influence the content, quality, organization, delivery, and financing of health services for all children—those who are healthy and those with chronic health problems, those who are affluent and those who are poor—in virtually all communities of the United States. Amidst these changes, there is the danger of inadvertently compromising child and family services, particularly if pediatricians and other child health service providers are not involved in designing the changes and monitoring their effects on child health and functioning (Lewin, 1995; Nazarian, 1995).

The major marketplace-driven change is the increased focus on cost containment and decreased expenditures by means of increasing participation in managed care (Table 7.1). Associated with the growth in managed care is a shift from fee-for-service medicine to capitated arrangements and the development of large integrated service delivery systems. These systems are designed to meet the vast majority of medical service needs of those of all ages, with more unique or specialized needs, if covered, being provided by out-of-plan providers with whom the primary organization has contractual arrangements. For children and youth who have either private health in-

Table 7.1
Major Marketplace-Driven Changes in Children's Health Services

- Increase in number of children enrolled in managed care programs.
- Increased reliance on capitated payment and associated decrease in fee-for-service practice.
- Increased penetration of health maintenance organizations (HMOs), physician organizations (POs), physician-hospital organizations (PHOs), and large multispecialty systems, and associated decrease in small group practices.
- Increased insurance coverage for preventive health services for children.
- Increased utilization review.
- Increased pressure to reduce costs by decreasing children's hospitalizations, emergency room visits, laboratory tests, and utilization of drugs and therapies of questionable utility.
- Increased use of midlevel practitioners.

surance or Medicaid coverage, the likely result is less freedom in the choice of primary care provider, fewer referrals to subspecialists, and possibly decreased access to many services, such as social services, mental health services, early intervention programs, substance abuse programs, and home visiting services. These and other services often emanate from the public health and education sectors of local human service systems, which also are undergoing rapid changes in funding. Many local human service systems are planning and implementing changes in these nonmedical community-based services without paying adequate attention to the need for the integration of child and family services, thereby potentially exacerbating the fragmentation of child and family health services (Weitzman et al., 1994). These changes will almost certainly affect uninsured children's access to medical care, although in ways that are not yet clear.

Other significant forces also are reshaping health services for children. They include social and demographic changes; changes in government policy and support of child and family-related human services, health insurance, and entitlements; and scientific and technologic advances in areas relating to the prevention, identification, and treatment of children's and families' physical and mental health problems.

Despite the radical and still undefined nature of the changes anticipated, the basic mission of child health services in the United States will remain unchanged. As stated by Robert J. Haggerty, "The core of pediatrics . . . will continue to be providing technically competent, empathic care for children in families and communities. The continuing goal of pediatrics must be to help all children achieve their optimal function physically, mentally and socially" (Haggerty, 1995).

Who Will Provide Children's Individual Health Care Services?

Longstanding disparities persist in children's health and in their access to and utilization of health care services. Very significant differences in the percentage of children who have a regular source of primary care and who are up-to-date in having their well-child care needs met are linked to region, family income, insurance status, source of care, and child health status (Holl et al., 1995; NCHS, 1993); variations in provider, site of care, and number of ambulatory care visits are similarly linked.

In 1987, pediatricians provided approximately 50 percent of all office-based visits for children and youth aged 0-19 years in the United States (Table 7.2). This proportion has increased steadily for all age groups, from 39 percent in 1976-1977 to 50 percent in 1987 (Martinez and Ryan, 1989; Stone, 1995). Pediatricians provided 72 percent of all office-based visits for U.S. children 0-2 years of age, but only 24 percent of all office-based visits for those aged 10-19 years. There are marked geographic variations in the availability of pediatricians, with significant shortages in many rural and indigent urban areas. Family practitioners, internists, and pediatric nurse practitioners provide primary care services to the majority of children who do not receive such care from pediatricians.

In recent years, more U.S. medical school graduates have been choosing pediatric careers. The percentage of U.S. medical school graduates who

Table 7.2

Percentage of Ambulatory Child Health Service Visits Provided by Pediatricians[a]
United States
1976–1987

Age (years)	1976–1977	1983–1984	1985–1986	1987
0–2	65.0%	67.5%	68.6%	71.8%
3–9	47.4	52.4	52.8	55.4
10–19	15.6	21.3	20.9	24.4
All age groups	38.8	45.5	46.3	49.8

Source: From Stone (1995), adapted from Martinez and Ryan (1989).
[a]Defined as number of office-based patient visits to pediatricians divided by the total number of all same-age patient visits to a physician. Excludes children who do not receive ambulatory health services.

"matched" to pediatric residency positions increased from 10 percent of U.S. medical school seniors in 1992 to 12 percent in 1996 (AAP, 1996). (Matching is the process in which medical school seniors and residency programs rank and select one another.) In 1996, 1,593 seniors from U.S. medical schools matched to pediatric training programs, up from 1,315 in 1991. Approximately 98 percent of the 2,097 first-year pediatric residency positions available were filled through the National Resident Matching Program in 1996, the highest rate ever for pediatrics, compared with 82 percent in 1992. As the size of the U.S. child population has not changed significantly in the past several decades and is not anticipated to increase in the near future, these increases suggest that an increasing proportion of children will have access to pediatricians trained in U.S. medical schools, at least in the immediate future.

At the same time, proposed changes in the number of international medical graduates entering the U.S. physician workforce have implications for children's health services. Twenty-nine percent of all pediatricians are international medical graduates, compared with 22 percent of all physicians, and the number of international medical graduates entering pediatrics has been increasing rapidly. Both the *Third Report of the Pew Health Professions Commission* (1995) and the Institute of Medicine's report *The Nation's Physician Workforce: Options for Balancing Supply and Requirements* (Lohr et al., 1996) call for the total number of first-year residency slots to be reduced to match more closely the current number of graduates of U.S. medical schools. The reports suggest additional mechanisms to diminish the number of international medical graduates who train in the United States and stay to practice after training. International medical graduates, however, disproportionately enter pediatrics, and thus serve as an important part of the pediatric workforce. Moreover, a disproportionate number trains in residency programs that provide ambulatory and inpatient services for the urban poor and uninsured; many remain in these underserved communities as a vital source of pediatric care. The proposed decrease in international medical graduates allowed into U.S. training programs may further reduce access to health care for these children (see discussion below of children living in poverty and near poverty).

As of 1991, 66 percent of pediatricians were generalists, 15 percent were board-certified subspecialists, 11 percent were trained in a subspecialty but were not board-certified, and 7 percent were trained in a subspecialty for which there is no formal board certification. Nineteen percent of the general pediatricians spent some time doing subspecialty-related clinical activities, and 13 percent of those with subspecialty training practiced general pediatrics exclusively (Brotherton, 1994). The major professional activity of 90 percent of all pediatricians in 1991 was patient care in office- and hospital-based settings (AMA, 1993).

It is likely that the increasing penetration of managed care into marketplaces nationwide will result in growing pressure to increase the number of pediatricians practicing primary care pediatrics. As a result, the percentages of pediatricians practicing general pediatrics and pediatric subspecialties may change. It is likely that fewer pediatric trainees will enter subspecialties; primary care pediatricians will be asked to assume more responsibility for problems currently referred to subspecialists; and some pediatric subspecialists will increase their involvement in primary care activities. Each of these potential changes has implications for the quality of care for children, graduate pediatric education, and the future workforce for pediatric research. In some situations, efforts to contain costs may lead managed care programs to rely on non-pediatricians to provide primary care services to children and on non-pediatric subspecialists to meet the needs of enrolled children with subspecialty-related needs. No empirical data are available to monitor the effects of these changes on the quality of care children receive, children's health status, or the quality of pediatric education and continuing medical education. Such studies are greatly needed.

There are approximately 6,000 pediatric nurse practitioners active in the United States (Eaton, 1991), the majority of whom are involved in the delivery of primary care services. More than 60 percent of the members of the National Association of Pediatric Nurse Associates and Practitioners (NAPNAP) work in urban areas with populations of more than 100,000, increasing access for many poor, underserved families (Dunn, 1993). Many managed care plans were originally reluctant to use mid-level professionals such as pediatric nurse providers or child health associates (pediatric physician assistants) to provide pediatric primary care services because of a concern that these practitioners would be perceived as providing inferior care (Stone, 1995). However, it is likely that there will be an increasing reliance on these mid-level providers in the future, as it has been shown that they can meet the majority of children's primary care needs, as currently conceived (Brown and Grimes, 1993, p. 11; DeAngelis, 1994; Sox, 1979; U.S. Congress, 1986, p. 6).

Content of Children's Individual Health Care Services
Currently, the American Academy of Pediatrics (AAP) recommends that children and youth receive, at a minimum, the following number of well-child visits:

one prenatal visit;

seven visits before 1 year of age (in hospital after birth, within first week of life, and at 1, 2, 4, 6, and 9 months of age);

visits at 12, 15, and 18 months;

yearly visits between 2 and 6 years of age;

visits at 8 and 10 years of age; and

yearly visits between 11 and 21 years (AAP, 1995b).

These visits serve as the core of children's primary care services and provide an opportunity for health promotion and disease prevention activities, including:

anticipatory guidance for behavioral, developmental, and social issues (e.g., injury prevention, smoking prevention, diet, exercise, and the prevention of sexually transmitted diseases and teenage pregnancy);

screening for occult biological or psychosocial problems, such as lead poisoning, anemia, tuberculosis, malnutrition (both under- and overnutrition), developmental delays, and vision and hearing problems;

provision of immunizations; and

counseling regarding behavioral and emotional problems.

It is during these visits that the basis for a longstanding relationship and therapeutic linkage between family and primary care provider is established. These visits also provide an opportunity to establish linkages between families and social services, nutrition support programs, or mental health services, and to provide follow-up for chronic health conditions.

In 1990, children enrolled in prepaid group practices, which frequently pay for preventive health services, had four to five preventive health care vis-

Table 7.3
Ambulatory Child Health Visits to All Physicians
United States
1990

Age (years)	Average visits per year	Recommended visits per year
0–5	4.19	13
6–10	1.56	3
11–14	1.82	4
15–21	2.03	7

Source: From AAP (1996).

its per year, compared to only three visits per year for children in fee-for-service arrangements (Smoller, 1992; Valdez et al., 1989), which typically do not cover the cost of preventive services (see Table 7.3 for average visits to all physicians). Uninsured children made fewer visits than those who were insured (Holl et al., 1995), and chronically ill children visited the physician at least twice as often as the overall child population (Ing and Tewey, 1994). To the extent that prepaid health insurance plans attempt to control costs by supporting preventive services, it is likely that children's utilization of preventive services will increase as growing proportions are covered by such plans. On the other hand, it is possible that some insurers or managed care plans may question the content or frequency of currently recommended well-child visits, and may try to eliminate some well-child visits and activities.

The incentives to educate parents and children to promote health are likely to increase. Immunizations, counseling regarding injury prevention (Bass et al., 1993), and smoking prevention and cessation programs (Epps and Manley, 1990) have clearly demonstrated utility. Although there is likely to be pressure on primary care providers to increase the volume of patients seen, there is also consensus that time spent in anticipatory guidance should be increased, according to new clinical guidelines for children (Green, 1994) and adolescents (Elster and Kuznets, 1989) developed by expert committees. Although many pediatric counseling interventions lack a strong empirical base because few randomized clinical trials have been carried out to evaluate their effectiveness, the absence of empirical evidence should not be construed as evidence of absence of efficacy (Perrin et al., 1992; Starfield, 1985), and there is substantial professional and parental consensus about their importance.

The issue of how much can be accomplished in a 15-minute pediatric visit cannot be ignored. Pediatricians are being asked increasingly to provide anticipatory guidance and therapeutic interventions for a very large number of behavioral problems, school difficulties, risk-taking behaviors, and environmental threats to children's well-being. In addition, there are issues related to responsibility and level of expertise for infrequently encountered problems, such as relatively rare medical problems, many of which currently are cared for by pediatric subspecialists, as well as for frequently encountered mental health and school-related difficulties for which many pediatricians are poorly trained. While these issues raise questions about how best to alter the training of pediatricians-to-be and how to make continuing medical education of pediatric practitioners more relevant, they also raise questions about whether individual encounters between children and families and primary care pediatricians are the best way to meet the primary care needs of many children and families. Potential approaches that already have been tried or suggested include:

1. expanded roles for pediatric nurse practitioners as children's primary care providers;
2. increased reliance on home visiting services for primary care;
3. development and utilization of community-based alternatives to office-based primary care services for groups of children and adolescents who underutilize office, community health center, or hospital-based primary care clinics;
4. use of family resource centers for health education and anticipatory guidance of parents and families;
5. expanded reliance on written and audiovisual materials to provide needed information; and
6. group well-child care.

It is likely that still other approaches will be conceived and implemented in the foreseeable future.

As noted, the mission of pediatrics will remain the same. However, the content of children's individual health services will undergo changes driven by the continuation of existing trends, medical and technological advances, and the pressure of managed care. All of these changes will occur in the context of a drive by insurers, businesses, and governments to contain costs, and new financial pressures on medical schools and pediatric training programs.

Medical and Technological Advances

The incidence of infectious diseases is likely to decrease as new vaccines are developed for such conditions as rotavirus diarrhea and respiratory syncytial virus. Continued advances in the ability to manage conditions in outpatient settings will mean that less time will be spent in the care of hospitalized children (Menna, 1990), although pediatricians and other primary care providers will continue to play a critical role in the identification of children requiring hospitalization, and transferring patients into and out of the hospital (Nazarian, 1995). Continuing developments in genetics will lead to increasing prenatal diagnosis of health conditions and identification during childhood of asymptomatic individuals who are at increased risk for developing certain conditions later in life.

Telecommunications is likely to affect rural practice, and all practices will be influenced by increasing computerization of records, appointments, prescriptions, billing, and educational materials.

Changes in Society and Family Structure

Continuing immigration will require an understanding of ethnic and cultural diversity, while changes in family structure will require familiarity in handling issues of single parents, divorce, blended families, and gay and lesbian couples.

The Impact of Cost-Containment Efforts

The growth of capitation will lead to increasing pressure to reduce referrals to subspecialists, with pediatricians increasingly being asked to serve as gatekeepers, monitoring and limiting emergency room use, subspecialist referrals, and hospitalizations. There will also be pressure to reduce in-office care. There is likely to be increased telephone management of care and communitywide systems of after-hours telephone coverage (Poole et al., 1993), after-hours care sites, and home care alternatives to prolonged hospitalizations.

A great deal of attention is currently being paid to decreasing emergency room use, not only because reliance on the emergency room for care fragments care, but because of the belief that significant savings can be achieved by decreasing emergency department use. However, recent data suggest that deflecting patients with nonurgent problems from the emergency department to physicians' offices will have only a very modest effect on health care costs because the marginal cost of seeing these patients in the emergency department is actually quite low (Steinbrook, 1996; Williams, 1996). Moreover, many emergency department patients, especially those who are uninsured or on Medicaid and living in urban settings, have no alternative source of care. Restricting emergency department use could threaten the safety of these children and families.

There is also pressure to decrease hospital length of stay for many conditions. Much attention recently has been paid to early discharge of newborns, with concerns raised about cases of bilirubin encephalopathy and severe dehydration in newborns discharged after short hospital stays; potential negative effects on rates and duration of breast-feeding; and possible delays in diagnosis of serious infections, cardiac anomalies, and metabolic conditions (AAP, 1995a; Braverman et al., 1995; Britton et al., 1994; Lee et al., 1995).

Congress has enacted legislation mandating coverage for minimum length of stay of 48 hours. Clearly, as the length of stay for newborns decreases, the importance of outpatient follow-up increases. The traditional follow-up visit at two weeks is inadequate in cases of early discharge, and the AAP, as part of routine preventive care, recommends a follow-up visit two to four days after discharge for any newborn who goes home before 48 hours of age (AAP, 1995b). There are difficulties, however, in implementing this service. Some insurers currently do not cover an office visit in the immediate newborn period, and some parents have trouble with transportation at this time. Home visits by nurses have therefore been widely endorsed, especially in the lay press (Thilo and Townsend, 1996), and many insurers who mandate 24-hour discharge include a home nurse visit in the reimbursement package. There are problems with these home visits, however, including a lack of standardization in the training and experience of the personnel performing these duties and a lack of consistency in the evaluation of the infant. As insurers attempt to decrease the number and length of hospitalizations for conditions such as osteomyelitis, meningitis, and asthma, similar problems are certain to surface, and reliance on home care and primary care is sure to increase. These changes may have profound implications for the quality of care children receive, and it is essential that clinicians with expertise in child health service needs have a voice in shaping these changes and in monitoring their effects.

Special Populations

Children in Poverty and Near-Poverty

There are significant differences in the source of primary care services by a number of socioeconomic and demographic characteristics for children overall in the United States (Table 7.4) and for the more than 10 million children and youth who live in the 44 urban centers with populations of more than 1 million (Table 7.5).

Thirty-five percent of poor and 27 percent of near-poor children in the largest U.S. cities rely on hospital-based clinics and community health centers for care. Significant reductions in spending on public hospitals and clinics are likely, and those associated with academic medical centers will be especially vulnerable. Children using these sources of care are five times as likely as children who use private physicians to have one of the following characteristics known to be independently associated with increased rates of physical, mental health, educational, and social problems: maternal age at child's birth less than 17 years, one-parent household, maternal education less than high school, or living in poverty. These children also are twice as likely to have behavioral problems, 2.5 times as likely to have repeated a grade, and 1.7 times as likely to have been suspended or expelled from school (Weitzman et al., 1996).

Medicaid managed care programs may choose to include hospital-based clinics or community health centers in their panels of primary care providers. What will happen to the quality of primary care services for poor and near-poor children, both for those who continue to use hospital clinics and health centers and those who use private sources of care, as increasing percentages are enrolled in public (i.e., Medicaid) and private managed care programs? On the one hand, such programs are likely to result in altered benefit packages, and to enable many who currently use public sources of care to access the private sector. On the other hand, the failure of rapidly growing public and private managed care plans to cover screening, counseling, referrals to related child health professionals, case management, care coordination, and social work, mental health, and health education services could have extremely detrimental effects on very large numbers of socially and economically disadvantaged children and families. If substantial numbers of children move from health centers and hospital clinics to private-sector physicians, assuming that these providers are available, quality of care may decline, both for those who leave and for those who stay behind.

Table 7.4

Insurance and Health Status, and Source of Routine Health Care by Poverty Status among Children in Big Cities[a]
United States
1988

	Total population	Percent poverty level		
		≤ 100%	101–150%	> 150%
Sample Number	2,961	617	307	2,037
Weighted Number	10,175,213	2,363,539	1,053,534	6,758,140
Total big city child population	100.0%	23.2%	10.4%	66.4%
Insurance				
Private	59.1	13.6*	49.0*,**	76.7
Medicaid	25.2	69.7*	22.7*,**	9.8
None	15.8	16.7	28.3*,**	13.5
Health status				
Fair/poor health status	3.5	6.7*	3.8**	2.3
Chronic health conditions	26.1	25.5	23.8	26.7
Severity				
Mild	17.0	7.4	16.0	18.1
Moderate	7.6	9.6	5.3**	7.3
Severe	1.5	1.5	2.5	1.3
Utilization of primary care services				
Has routine source of care	86.7	85.3	83.3	87.8
Source for routine care				
Private sources[b]	62.7	41.0*	51.1*,**	72.1
Community health center	7.9	13.7*	15.8*	4.7
Hospital clinic	10.1	21.3*	11.3*,**	6.0
Other	6.0	9.3*	5.1	5.0

Source: From Weitzman et al. (1996). Child Health Supplement to the 1988 National Health Interview Survey.

[a]Big cities are the 44 Metropolitan Statistical Areas in the United States with 1 million or more people.

[b]Private sources of care are private physicians and health maintenance organizations/prepaid groups.

*p-value <.05 for comparisons with children living > 150% of poverty.

**p-value <.05 for comparisons of children living ≤100% of poverty with 101–150% of poverty.

Table 7.5
Sources of Children's Routine Health Care
United States

	Private sources[a]	Community health center	Hospital clinic	Other[b]
Total U.S. child population	73.3%	4.7%	4.1%	5.9%
Large MSAs[c]				
Urban	62.7	7.9	10.1	6.0
Suburban	79.1	2.7	2.7	3.9
Smaller metropolitan				
and rural areas	73.9	4.6	3.1	6.7
Insured	76.6	4.0	3.7	5.2
Uninsured	52.1	8.7	7.0	10.5
Poor				
<150% Poverty	55.0	10.4	8.0	10.1
>150% Poverty	80.1	2.6	2.7	4.4
Black	54.8	12.0	9.7	9.9
White	78.3	3.1	2.4	4.8
Other	60.4	5.3	10.0	9.3
0–4 Years	72.7	5.9	5.0	8.2
5–9 Years	76.6	4.8	3.6	5.0
10–18 Years	71.7	3.7	3.9	5.0

Sources: Data from Holl et al. (1995) and Weitzman et al. (1996).
[a]Private sources of care are private physicians and health maintenance organizations.
[b]Other refers to home, company/school clinic, migrant, other clinic, hospital emergency department, walk-in/emergency care center, rural health center, other place.
[c]Large MSAs are metropolitan statistical areas with 1 million or more people.

This situation may be complicated by changes in pediatric training programs; to the extent that ambulatory care training moves out of the hospital to community-based sites, hospital primary care capacity may be threatened.

Approximately 10 million (14 percent) of children and youths in the United States are uninsured. These children are less likely to have a regular source of routine or sick care, make fewer physician visits, and are less likely to be up-to-date with well-child care than those with Medicaid or private insurance coverage (Holl et al., 1995). It is not at all clear how market-driven reform will influence the care these children receive, and current policy priorities do not include serious public or private strategies to assure universal health insurance coverage of children and families. Any changes that endanger hospital-based clinics or community health centers, upon which poor, near-poor, and uninsured children disproportionately rely for their primary care needs, may result in significant negative effects on the quality of care they receive and their health status.

Children with Special Health Care Needs

Also of concern are the implications of these health care delivery changes for children with special health care needs. There is likely to be an increased reliance on the primary care provider as the coordinator of care and gatekeeper for more specialized services for the 10 to 30 percent of U.S. children with chronic health impairments. Also likely is a decrease in referrals to pediatric subspecialists and child health professionals in related fields, such as physical therapy, occupational therapy, social services, and mental health. At the same time, there will be many developments that facilitate the provision of services at home or in the community, rather than in hospitals.

There has been a near doubling in the number of children with chronic health conditions that limit their daily functional activities in recent decades (Newacheck et al., 1984, 1986a). This growth is due to the increased survival rate of low-birthweight infants and others with a wide range of chronic medical and surgical conditions such as cystic fibrosis, sickle cell anemia, and congenital heart defects. While improvements in the understanding of the genetic, environmental, and nutritional basis and prenatal diagnosis of many chronic health conditions ultimately will translate into a reduction in many of these conditions, improved therapeutic modalities and technologies will result in prolonged survival of those with chronic conditions. The health care of many children with these conditions is extremely expensive, and the quality of care they receive may be greatly influenced by the changes underway.

Most chronic conditions among children in the United States are mild and have little impact on their daily functioning or utilization of health services. Approximately 10 percent of children with chronic conditions, however, an estimated 2 million children, have severe conditions that result in extensive use of health services. An estimated 2 percent of the children with severe health conditions account for approximately 25 percent of all child health expenditures (Butler et al., 1985). It is estimated that about 70 percent of all childhood hospital admissions are for chronic health conditions (Homer et al., 1982). Data from the National Health Interview Survey indicate that 3.8 percent of children with chronic health conditions account for 9 percent of outpatient visits and 30 percent of inpatient days (Newacheck et al., 1986b). It has been reported that among a sample of children with chronic conditions, 10 percent of the sample were responsible for 60 percent of total expenditures (Newacheck and McManus, 1988). One recent study of a large managed care organization found that at least one group of children documented to have extensive use of inpatient and ambulatory services under fee-for-service medicine—ex-premature infants discharged from special care nurseries—continued to have high rates of utilization for hospital and outpatient services (Cavalier et al., 1996). How such children and their families, as well as children with other chronic health conditions and their families, will fare under managed care arrangements will depend on many factors, including:

1. The effectiveness of advocacy efforts on behalf of such children and their families;
2. The financial rates negotiated by managed care groups, physicians' individual practice arrangements, pediatric subspecialists, and academic departments of pediatrics with third-party payors for the care of children with relatively rare, but complicated and costly, medical problems;
3. Whether children with such medical problems are exempted, or "carved out," of managed care capitation arrangements and continue to receive care on a fee-for-service basis, or are in fact capitated, and, if so, at what rate;
4. Whether primary care providers or pediatric subspecialists are designated as case coordinators for such children;
5. The comprehensiveness of the benefit packages for these children, in terms of health-related ancillary services such as occupational, physical, and speech therapy; community health nursing services; and early intervention, social, and mental health services; and
6. The quality of research relating various new service and financing arrangements to health outcomes of children with special health care needs and their families.

There are myriad areas for concern for these children and their families. These include the potential for restricted access to needed medical and non-medical services, such as limited numbers of visits to subspecialists or hospitalizations per time period; the possibility that restrictions would be placed on needed ancillary services or medications, or on referrals to nonpediatric rather than pediatric subspecialists. There also is the danger that during the period in which communities shift from usual fee-for-service to managed care coverage, relationships between children and families and their health care providers may be disrupted. These relationships often are central to the quality of care provided and the quality of life of children and families.

Opportunities

The changes that are occurring in health care have the potential both to improve and to hinder the care children receive. Listed below are some of the opportunities for improved care.

1. The need for integrated service delivery systems to have a requisite number of "covered lives" may lead to a much improved community orientation. There will be an explicit mandate to consider the well-being of large numbers of children and families and the best ways to meet their needs, which may result in improved health services planning. It is essential that pediatricians have a voice in decisions being made by insurers and architects of integrated service delivery systems, managed care programs, and physician organizations, so that child health services are considered at all levels of change.

2. The nature of the financing of many managed care programs holds great potential for an increased pediatric voice in decision making. Many integrated service systems are contracting with large employers to offer comprehensive services for their employees. Many of the individuals enrolling in these programs are adults of child-bearing age, or parents, and the quality of pediatric services available to their children is extremely important to them. Thus, pediatricians may have a greater say in the development of such systems than would otherwise have been the case.

3. The large size of many integrated service delivery systems may result in economies of scale that lead to cost savings (such as the bulk purchase of immunizations or other essentials) and the consolidation of services so that duplication and fragmentation of services are diminished.

4. Large service systems and the focus on cost savings may provide the opportunity and impetus to monitor the quality of care delivered, to establish patterns of use, and to identify providers who are outside the mean of average practice. Such efforts may also facilitate the development of outcomes research and the study of the effectiveness of various preventive and therapeutic interventions.

5. Large service systems may facilitate the regionalization of many pediatric services. The size and community-wide orientation of many of these systems may also result in new services, such as community-wide after-hours telephone triage systems and related after-hours services for non-emergencies outside of emergency room settings. This may improve the care provided and the quality of life of pediatric providers.

6. The focus on primary care, cost containment, and gatekeeping may result in increased coordination of care and a greater role for the general pediatrician in the care of children with chronic health impairments. This will result in improved care if needed services that primary care providers cannot provide themselves are available to such children and families and if pediatricians and other primary care providers are educated for these new roles; provided appropriate continuing education so that their skills remain current; and adequately reimbursed for such efforts, rather than penalized for the increased time spent and resources utilized in the care of such children.

7. Integrated service systems may provide the requisite number of primary care providers to facilitate enhanced community-based education of medical students and pediatric house officers. To the extent that systems are truly integrated, "town-gown" issues may be diminished, leading to better communication and true faculty roles for community practitioners.

Dangers
The health care changes that are occurring also threaten the quality of health care for children.

1. If pediatricians are not involved at the highest levels in the design of integrated service delivery systems or in the design and implementation of utilization review programs, child health services may suffer. It is especially difficult to measure child health status or the quality of care children receive

(see chapter 2), and methodologies for evaluating adult care are inappropriate for assessing children's health services.

2. The focus on cost containment may erode support for many of the most vital child health services. Primary care providers seeing increasing numbers of children may have less opportunity to provide anticipatory guidance, behavioral assessment and interventions, and counseling regarding health promotion and disease prevention. Some insurers or integrated service delivery systems may limit availability or coverage of mental health or social services, referrals for subspecialty evaluation or care, or ancillary services such as occupational or physical therapy, thus diminishing the quality of care received by children challenged by social adversity or chronic physical health impairments.

3. Delays in diagnosis or treatment, which may result from policies adopted to contain costs, may impair the health of children with both acute and chronic conditions.

4. The creation of integrated health service delivery systems and Medicaid managed care plans may have a negative effect on the quality of care for children and families who rely on hospital-based clinics or community health centers, whether they transfer to private physicians or continue to rely on these sources of care. These market-driven changes are designed primarily to cut costs and serve those who already are insured, and there is little or no data about their effects on those living in or near poverty. The fragile safety net system of health services for children and families may be greatly damaged by these changes.

5. Should too many primary care pediatricians be trained, there may be a shortage of pediatric subspecialists, which would have potentially negative implications for pediatric care, education, and research. This problem may be exacerbated by downsizing of many medical centers and the anticipated closing of many community hospitals.

6. If those primary care pediatricians who are asked to assume a greater role in the care and coordination of care of children with chronic health conditions and with behavioral or emotional problems do not receive adequate training, continuing medical education, and specialized back-up, the quality of care received by these children could be significantly compromised.

7. The development of competing integrated health service delivery systems in particular regions could significantly disrupt doctor-patient and doctor-doctor relationships. If employers sign up with a system that does not include families' previous physicians, families may have to change the sources of their care, in many cases disrupting long-standing relationships. Similarly, in many communities, referral patterns and professional support networks may be disrupted. For example, it is possible that prenatal and obstetrical services will not be aligned with emerging and exclusive service delivery systems in exactly the way that pediatric services are. In such cases, there may be significant constraints on pediatric providers visiting and examining newborns while in hospital.

8. Pressure to see an increasing volume of patients may limit the involvement of community-based primary care providers in medical students' and pediatric trainees' clinical training (Weitzman et al., 1996). It may also serve as a disincentive for pediatrician involvement in community activities, such as the AAP's Community Access to Child Health (CATCH) Program.

9. Decreased income, administrative overload, paperwork, and increased meetings may leave significant portions of the pediatric workforce disenchanted and demoralized.

10. Increased use of adult subspecialists, rather than pediatric subspecialists, could negatively affect children's health care and health.

Implications
Important as it is, the need to constrain medical spending must not be allowed to distort the proper role of prevention (Russell, 1993), or result in less effective care of the very large numbers of U.S. children at risk by virtue of social adversity or chronic health impairments. Managed care arrangements may result in care that is more coordinated and integrated, and that deals with the prevalent and frequently devastating problems of low-income and special needs children. Anything that results in care that is less comprehensive, accessible, or culturally sensitive, however, or that penalizes primary care providers for helping children and families access health-related preventive and supportive services, will have extremely detrimental effects.

How can we assure that managed care arrangements provide comprehensive service packages and sufficient reimbursement for the time health care providers spend identifying the common behavioral and educational problems of children, and in communicating and collaborating with related human service providers? How can we make the private sector better able to accommodate a potential influx of currently excluded low-income children with their prevalent constellation of associated social, mental health, and educational difficulties? How can we protect and enhance the capacity of the already fragile and inadequately supported network of hospital clinics and community health centers? These questions raise still other questions about how best to reform medical education so that sufficient numbers of appropriately trained primary care providers can be recruited for underserved urban and rural areas. What strategies are to be considered for recruiting and retaining professionals in these areas, and how is it possible to enhance the general pediatrician's care of children with special health care needs? To answer these questions, it is necessary to recognize the unique and often multiple needs of a very large percentage of our children; the central role that primary care services play or could play in the early identification of children who are at risk for, or already evidencing, functional impairment and in linking them to appropriate community-based services; and the importance of forcefully and effectively articulating the needs of children and families in the midst of health services changes affecting the entire U.S. population.

References

AAP Committee on Fetus and Newborn. 1995a. Hospital stay for healthy term newborns. Pediatrics 96:788.

AAP Committee on Practice and Ambulatory Medicine. 1995b. Recommendations for preventive pediatric health care. Pediatrics 96(2):insert.

AAP Committee on Careers and Opportunities. 1996. Committee report: Population to pediatrician ratio estimates: A subject review. Pediatrics 97:597–600.

AAP Division of Pediatric Practice. 1996. Pediatric residency fill rate approaches 100 percent. Pediatric News 12:7.

[AMA] American Medical Association, Department of Physician Data Services, Division of Survey and Data Resources. 1993. Physician characteristics and distribution in the United States. Chicago, IL: American Medical Association.

Bass JL, Christofell DD, Widome M, Boyle W, Scheidt P, et al. 1993. Childhood injury prevention counseling in primary care settings: A critical review of the literature. Pediatrics 92:544–50.

Braveman P, Egerter S, Peral M, et al. 1995. Early discharge of newborns and mothers: A critical review of the literature. Pediatrics 96:716.

Britton JR, Britton HL, Beebe SA. 1994. Early discharge of the term newborn: A continued dilemma. Pediatrics 94:291.

Brotherton SE. 1994. Pediatric subspecialty training, certification, and practice: Who's doing what. Pediatrics 94:83–9.

Brown SA, Grimes DE. 1993. Nurse practitioners and certified nurse-midwives: A meta-analysis of studies on nurses in primary care roles. Washington: American Nursing Association.

Butler JA, Budetti P, McManus MA, et al. 1985. Health care expenditures for children with chronic illnesses. In: Hobbs N, Perrin JM, editors. Issues in the care of children with chronic illnesses. San Francisco: Jossey-Bass.

Cavalier S, Escobar GJ, Fernbach SA, Quebsberry CP, Chellino M. 1996. Postdischarge utilization of medical services by high-risk infants: Experiences in a large managed care organization. Pediatrics 97:693–9.

DeAngelis CD. 1994. Nurse practitioner redux. Journal of the American Medical Association. 271:868–71.

Dunn AM. 1993. 1992 NAPNAP membership survey, part II. Practice characteristics of pediatric nurse practitioners indicate greater autonomy for PNPs. Journal of Pediatric Health Care 7:296–302.

Eaton AP. 1991 Feb. 12. Testimony on behalf of the American Academy of Pediatrics. Presented before the Subcommittee on Manpower of the Council on Graduate Medical Education. Elk Grove Village, IL.

Elster AB, Kuznets NJ. 1989. Guidelines for adolesent preventive services. Baltimore, MD: Williams & Wilkins.

Epps RP, Manley MW. 1990. A physician's guide to preventing tobacco use during childhood and adolescence. Rockville, MD: National Cancer Institute.

Green M, editor, 1994. Bright futures: Guidelines for health supervision of infants, children, and adolescents. Arlington, VA: National Center for Education in Maternal and Child Health.

Haggerty RJ. 1995. Child Health 2000: New pediatrics in the changing environment of children's needs in the 21st century. Pediatrics 96:804–11.

Holl JL, Szilagyi PG, Rodewald LE, Byrd RS, Weitzman M. 1995. Profile of uninsured children in the United States. Archives of Pediatric and Adolescent Medicine 149:398–406.

Homer CJ, Perrin JM, Bloom SR, Evans A. 1992. Hospital use by children with chronic illness. Abstracts: 28. Washington: Ambulatory Pediatric Association.

Ing CD, Tewey BP. 1994. Summary of data on children and youth with disabilities. U.S. Dept. of Education Publ. HN 93027001. Washington: National Institute on Disability and Rehabilitation Research.

Lee K-S, Perlman M, Ballantyne M, et al. 1995. Association between duration of neonatal hospital stay and readmission rate. Journal of Pediatrics 127:758.

Lewin LS. 1995. Adapting your pediatric practice to the changing health care system. Pediatrics 96:799–803.

Lohr KN, Vangelow NA, Detmer DE. 1996. The nation's physician workforce: Options for balancing supply and requirements. Washington: Institute of Medicine, National Academy Press.

Martinez GA, Ryan AS. 1989. The pediatric marketplace. American Journal of Diseases of Children 143:924–8.

Menna VJ. 1990. Inpatient care: The general pediatrician's future. Pediatric Review 12:165–6.

Nazarian LF. 1995. A look at the private practice of the future. Pediatrics 96:811–2.

[NCHS] National Center for Health Statistics. 1993. Health, United States, 1992 and Healthy People 2000 Review. U.S. Dept. of Health and Human Services Publ. PHS 93-1232. Hyattsville, MD: Public Health Service.

Newacheck P, McManus P. 1988. Financing health care for disabled children. Pediatrics 81:385–94.

Newacheck P, Budetti P, McManus P. 1984. Trends in childhood disability. American Journal of Public Health 74:232–6.

Newacheck P, Budetti P, Halfon N. 1986a. Trends in activity limiting chronic conditions among children. American Journal of Public Health 76:178–84.

Newacheck P, Halfon N, Budetti P. 1986b. Prevalence of activity limiting chronic conditions among children based on household interviews. Journal of Chronic Disease 39:63–9.

Perrin J, Guyer B, Lawrence JM. 1992 Winter. Health care services for children and adolescents. The Future of Children 2:58–77.

Pew Health Professions Commission. 1995. Critical challenges: Revitalizing the health profession for the twenty-first century: The third report. San Francisco, CA: The Pew Health Professions Commission.

Poole SR, Schmitt BD, Carruth T, Peterson-Smith A, Slusarski M. 1993. After-hours telephone coverage: The application of an area-wide telephone triage and advice system for pediatric practices. Pediatrics 92:670–9.

Russell LB. 1993. The role of prevention in health reform. New England Journal of Medicine 329:352–4.

Smoller M. 1992. Telephone calls and appointment requests: Predictability in an unpredictable world. HMO Practitioner 6:25–9.

Sox HC. 1979. Quality of patient care by nurse practitioners and physician's assistants: A ten-year perspective. Annals of Internal Medicine 91: 459–68.

Starfield B. 1985. The effectiveness of medical care: Validating clinical wisdom. Baltimore, MD: The Johns Hopkins University Press.

Steinbrook R. 1996. The role of the emergency department. New England Journal of Medicine 334:657.

Stone EL. 1995. Nurse practitioners and physician assistants: Do they have a role in your practice? Pediatrics 96:844–50.

Thilo EH, Townsend SF. 1996. Early newborn discharge: Have we gone too far? Contemporary Pediatrics 13:29.

U.S. Congress, Office of Technology Assessment. 1986. Nurse practitioners, physician assistants and certified nurse-midwives: Policy analysis. Washington: U.S. Government Printing Office.

Valdez RB, Ware Jr JE, Manning WG, et al. 1989. Prepaid group practice effects on the utilization of medical services and health outcomes for children: Results from a controlled trial. Pediatrics 6:25–9.

Weitzman M, Doniger AS, Partner SF. 1994. Seeking pathways to a coordinated system of health and human services for high-risk urban children and families: The Rochester, New York Experience. Bulletin of the New York Academy of Medicine 71:267–80.

Weitzman M, Byrd RS, Auinger P. 1996. Children in big cities in the United States: Health and related needs and services. Ambulatory Child Health 1:347–66.

Weitzman M, Garfunkel L, Connaughton S. 1996. The funding of pediatric education in community settings. Pediatrics 88:1284–5.

Williams RM. 1996. The costs of visits to emergency departments. New England Journal of Medicine 334:642 (and accompanying editorial).

8

Tensions in Delivering Care to Children

Judith Palfrey

IN CHILD HEALTH, tensions in care delivery have generated what many call a "non-system." Parents speak of a maze. Practitioners are frustrated by the ever-increasing number of competing demands and requirements. Trainees, struggling to learn about a system of health and developmental services, slowly realize that there is no single system but rather a vast array of loosely configured arrangements, each with its unique peculiarities and boundaries. Families, child-serving professionals, and policymakers find themselves mired in complex controversies about how to proceed in promoting child health and development. Tensions in care delivery make progress difficult.

While tension can stultify, tension can also be healthy. When there are two ideas or two sides to a question, the proponents of each point of view must hone their arguments, examine their contentions, and assure that they are offering the very best solution. The pull may become even greater as the two sides take increasingly stark positions. Alternatively, there may be a realization of the power of a combined approach that encompasses components of the tension itself and acknowledges that it is the very disagreement that is the strength.

Tensions are everywhere in the health care environment. They are philosophical, interdisciplinary, political, and fiscal. To work constructively toward an improved health care system for children, it is valuable to acknowledge these tensions as a real part of the dynamic. This chapter out-

Adapted from Palfrey, JS. *Community Child Health: An Action Plan for Today.* Westport, CT: Praeger Press, 1994, with permission of the publisher.

lines a series of tensions that child health planners must confront: Are health issues best defined in medical terms or in social terms? Should services be categorical or comprehensive? Should programming be targeted or universal? Are child-oriented or family-oriented responses most valuable? Do prescriptive or responsive attitudes work best? Should oversight be driven by professionals or by payers? Is the best approach a pragmatic one or one that says "never say die"?

Medicalization vs. Socialization of Health Issues

The recognition of the psychological and social underpinnings of many current child health problems raises questions about whether some health concerns are best defined in medical or social terms. Are gunshot wounds medical or social problems? What is the responsibility of the emergency room doctor who sews up a laceration from a gang fight? Once a cockroach antigen is identified as the cause of severe asthma in a child, who should deal with the family's landlord? When a child goes home on a ventilator, what are the family's needs? Who should respond and how?

Increasingly, child health professionals are aware of the delicate interplay among physical, mental, and environmental factors. As a result, physicians are beginning to make forays into schools, day-care centers, and community programs and to renew their interest in home visiting and home-based care. Physicians are being called on to practice what Morris Green terms "contextual pediatrics." They are being challenged to look beyond the child into the family and community, for both risk factors and resources. For instance, the new national guidelines for health care promotion, *Bright Futures*, codify a new type of practice that stretches the traditional boundaries of the pediatric office (Green, 1995). The *Bright Futures* guidelines encourage physicians and nurses to step directly and explicitly into the social world of the child.

The benefits of the contextual approach are a more direct attack on the root causes of many current child health problems. If a child is failing to thrive, for instance, it is critical for the doctor to ask questions about maternal depression, illness, drug use, and family financial status—all awkward questions, but any one of them may hold the answer to the child's malnutrition. Such probes may have far more payoff than a week's hospitalization or the most specialized series of biomedical examinations.

How can doctors expand their practice to address social problems without being seen as imposing the so-called "medical model" in potentially unwanted ways or places? This is the tension. The typical take-charge attitude of physicians does not fit every situation. In fact, such an attitude can be counterproductive when the biggest need is the strengthening of a family's self-esteem or a community's autonomy. Physicians are unfortunately not always well informed about the actual strengths and resources of the community. Medicalization may lead to an unwanted emphasis on illness and on deficits.

Another concern is often expressed by social workers and other professionals who see social issues as their particular purview. Doctors are expensive providers of care. If the physician's time is spent dealing with social problems, limited resources for "social care" may be used up rapidly. In addition, if doctors and nurses really do probe all possible concerns with each family, the little efficiency that there is now in offices, emergency rooms, and hospitals may be sacrificed.

The debate about whether some child health problems are fundamentally medical or social forces an acknowledgment of the complex and entwined nature of child health concerns. In fact, the question is not so much whether the problems are medical or social as it is what combination of approaches will best get at the biologic, social, and psychological threats to the health and safety of children. Effective health care systems need to rely on team approaches where all team members recognize the interplay between biology, environment, and social factors.

Categorical vs. Comprehensive Services

One of the most vexing questions in child health is how much any intervention should try to achieve. Should it attack a specific problem (e.g., childhood malnutrition) or should it be more broadly conceived to encompass the factors that predispose to the problem (e.g., family and community stresses)? Should a program address a specific category of problem or should it be comprehensive? Wouldn't it be most practical to define boundaries, carefully specify client eligibility, and limit expectations? On the other hand, wouldn't it be great if a program could be flexible enough to meet all of a family's needs?

Those who have studied these questions carefully find persuasive arguments against the categorical approach. The majority of innovative ideas in community services planning for children and families are based on moving to a more comprehensive approach. In her influential book *Within Our Reach*, Lee Schorr says, "Part of this gap between knowledge and action springs from traditions which segregate bodies of information by professional, academic, political and bureaucratic boundaries. Complex, intertwined problems are sliced into manageable but trivial parts. Efforts to reduce juvenile delinquency operate in isolation from programs to prevent early childbearing or school failure. . . . Evaluators assess the impact of narrowly defined services and miss the powerful effects of a broad combination of interventions" (Schorr and Schorr, 1988, p. 6).

With the telling phrase "manageable but trivial parts," Schorr describes the limitations of the categorical approach. Programs are mounted in one sector, by one agency, with a clearly targeted, measurable outcome, for example, reducing teenage pregnancy rates, educating young people about HIV disease, or preventing childhood malnutrition. Often funding comes from a governmental agency with rigid guidelines designating both method and appointed end. The problem may be manageable in the sense that it is defined and identified, but the intervention design misses significant opportunities because of insufficient attention to the complex intertwining of related concerns. For instance, the Special Supplemental Food Program for Women, Infants and Children (WIC) provides food for poor mothers and infants, but does little to address the issues of teen pregnancy, inadequate job training, lack of child support, or other factors that accompany and perpetuate the problem of childhood malnutrition. Similarly, although a high percentage of young people in the juvenile justice system have learning disabilities, the special education services available to them are totally inadequate (Thompson, 1991).

Categorical approaches suffer from a serious theoretical flaw. Because of the focus on a specific endpoint, the program's personnel and evaluators may not appreciate the impact of the intervention on important correlated outcomes. A particular intervention, even a highly specific one, may have multiple benefits. For instance, although studies of physical therapy intervention for young children have consistently failed to show the intended child outcomes, they have demonstrated positive effects on family functioning and adaptation to the needs of the child with a disability (Shonkoff and Hauser-Cram, 1987). The outcome studies of the Head Start program have shown that its effects go far beyond the planned impact on early school performance. Not only have the programs led to long-term gains in the children, but almost more importantly, they have had enormous impact on the children's parents, with many seeking further education (White and

Buka, 1987). If the program scope is too narrowly envisioned, major opportunities are passed by.

Not only are there theoretical flaws in the categorical approach, in practice, parents and providers find it extraordinarily confusing. Parents have to fill out numerous forms to qualify for similar-sounding services. Child health providers feel they need to be experts in civics and law in order to make a referral to another service sector. Parents and community service providers consistently plea for user-friendly systems and a single intake form and process that would simultaneously qualify a family for health care, welfare, WIC, and school benefits.

If the categorical approach is so limited and flawed, why are so many programs mounted in this way (USSG, 1992)? Are there any benefits?

The best explanation for the existence of the categorical approach is that domestic planning in the United States tends to occur incrementally through a legislative process that is itself categorical. The U.S. House of Representatives and Senate committee structure is categorically organized, and, therefore, initiatives designed to pull together two service sectors are often doomed from the very beginning (Blum and Blank, 1991). Because funding comes tied tightly to categorical objectives, it is often in the best interest of service providers to follow program specifications rather than experiment with cooperative arrangements that might be criticized for failing to accomplish the requirements of the federal funding agency.

Moreover, there are some definite benefits of the categorical approach that lead to its perpetuation. By far the major benefits are the ability to specify problems precisely, to describe clear-cut interventions, to mount programs and monitor them over time, and to evaluate the impact of the particular approach. If a program is defined as an HIV prevention effort, then the evaluation can measure participants' knowledge of AIDS and count the number of condoms distributed. The defined outcomes are unequivocal and the effect of the intervention is proximate enough that the outcome can be attributed with a relative degree of accuracy to the program intervention rather than to some other cause.

There is another highly pragmatic benefit of categorical planning. Families can use all the help they can get. One would not want to turn off contributions from the Department of Housing and Urban Development, the Department of Agriculture, or other sectors simply because they represented separate categories of planning. Julius Richmond, the U.S. Surgeon

General from 1976 to 1980, says that the existence of more than 100 separate categorical federal programs during his tenure was one of the reasons that he did not push for a central overarching authority such as the old Children's Bureau. In his judgment, consolidation would have cut back on, not expanded, the services available to children and families (Richmond, 1992).

Perhaps the biggest benefit of having multiple, unconnected categorical programs is that it protects against a top-down, authoritarian approach and allows innovation in many sectors. What if we got the unifying structure wrong and were stuck with it? Categorical programming means pluralism; pluralism defends against stagnation and the long-term establishment of large vested interests. By ensuring a competitive approach to program delivery, categorical programming promotes a concern for quality and accountability, which could potentially be lost with too heavily specified and petrified administrative structures.

How will this controversy play out in the next few years? With the likely advent of state block grants for health and social programs, states and localities may have greater flexibility in designing comprehensive approaches. Already there is movement toward better articulated programming in many cities. Moreover, several of the nation's largest foundations (most prominently the Pew Charitable Trusts, Carnegie Foundation, The Robert Wood Johnson Foundation, and Annie E. Casey Foundation) are sponsoring comprehensive planning projects. The reports of a number of prominent panels have urged increased comprehensiveness in program planning (e.g., National Commission on Children, 1991). Many professional groups are calling for improved collaboration in service delivery. The Association of Teachers of Education has established a national commission to explore collaborative models of service delivery and to consider the training needs for professionals entering the child-serving fields.

The proposed changes cannot occur overnight nor should the tension between specific and general goals ever be completely eliminated. It is critical for the programs to articulate goals and areas of expertise, and to monitor and determine outcomes. The challenge in program development is to weave the specific interventions of categorical programs into more generally conceived and coordinated community service networks so that families and children can have access to those preventive and management services that are effective at fostering child health and combating the threats to children's development.

Targeted vs. Universal Programming

Given limited resources, many people argue that services should be targeted to children with the greatest needs. Society has placed some children at an unfair disadvantage and therefore, the argument goes, child-serving programs should aim to level the playing field. The premise behind the highly successful Head Start program is exactly this. Even the program's name conjures up the image of a racing handicap in the early competition of primary school life.

As logical as this argument is, there is serious controversy about the benefits of delivering targeted rather than universal services. Concerns have been raised about the potential for stigmatization, the effects of separation from the mainstream, and lack of clarity about who should receive targeted services.

Targeting can be stigmatizing and may perpetuate the very patterns the interventions are trying to break. If programs are designed for one group of families because they are "poor," "minority," "disadvantaged," or "disabled," the recipients are forced to accept a label as a condition of receiving benefits (Hobbs, 1975). Systems for particular at-risk groups can take on the quality of a vested interest, existing as long as the state of need lasts. This can be seen in the institutionalization of programs for homeless families.

When groups of children are targeted for services, the project activities are often held in separate locations with special staff and facilities. Many benefits are available, but the children are separated from the mainstream. If the services are not targeted but are universally available, there is greater opportunity for children of different cultures, socioeconomic groups, and ability levels to interact with each other in the presence of teachers and parents who can promote attitudes of respect and tolerance among children of different backgrounds.

Perhaps the most serious concern about the targeted approach is that entrance criteria may exclude children and adolescents who could derive equal benefit. For instance, if health education about eating disorders is targeted only to youngsters with overt anorexia and bulimia, the young people who are in the early stages of these problems and are flirting with unhealthy nutritional patterns will be missed. Classroom modifications for children with learning disabilities have been shown to have positive spillover effects for the rest of the class that are not experienced when the children with learning disabilities are taught separately (Ciborowski, 1992; Slavin et al., 1990).

Another important argument for universal programming is that the larger and more mainstream the constituency, the more likely the long-term support for the program. Having a large and vocal stakeholder group has been the salvation of programs like Social Security and Medicare.

Those who argue against universal services base their concerns predominantly on economic issues. Why should money be spent on children who are not at risk? Shouldn't every penny go to the children who need it most? Moreover, when services are universally available, advantaged families tend to be more adept at accessing them than less advantaged families, which defeats the fundamental aim of equalizing opportunities.

Child-Oriented vs. Family-Oriented Services

Child health clinics, schools, and day-care centers are designed in large measure to deliver services to a single patient or child at a time. The services are oriented toward making changes for, or in, the child, and indeed the outcomes of child health, education, and day care should be *child* outcomes. Child care professionals should be child experts. But there is a close link between child health and developmental outcomes and community and family factors, and it may well be asked whether services should be expanded to include whole families.

Child health care providers sometimes find themselves treating the wrong patient. Why should a youngster be treated for hyperactivity when the problem is really maternal depression and the mother's inability to cope with the normal rambunctiousness of childhood? Why should an adolescent be seen in psychotherapy when the problem is really her father's alcoholism and his determination not to face it? Why should a child be treated for school phobia when racial slurs are hurled at him every time he gets on the school bus? Why should a child be admitted to the hospital with repeated bouts of asthma exacerbated by the mother's smoking? or the family cat? or the ineffective air filter in the apartment or house? Clinical experiences like these argue for an expanded focus on children in the context of family life.

Perhaps the area where a family orientation is most needed is in maternal and child health, where there are problems relating to poor coordination of obstetric, perinatal, and pediatric programs. Because each discipline has its own area of expertise, over the past 10 to 20 years, there has been a tendency for practitioners to concentrate on the technical aspects of particular disciplines. There has been relatively little cross-talk among obstetricians, neonatologists, and general pediatricians.

Financing services over the course of pregnancy is so dependent on the categorical streams that a woman may need to turn to six or seven different sources of funding during one childbearing experience. Marie McCormick has delineated an all too common scenario:

> . . . a woman with no dependent children would generally not be eligible for Medicaid until she becomes pregnant, and is thus dependent on Title X–funded family planning services. When she becomes pregnant (and desires to continue the pregnancy), she would be referred to Title V–supported public health clinics (should there be openings) and apply for Medicaid. With a Medicaid card, she could then transfer her care to a private or hospital-based obstetrician. The latter may be required should her pregnancy develop complications, although such referrals are limited by inadequate reimbursement levels and malpractice concerns. Prenatal care at a public health clinic or with Medicaid does not automatically confer WIC services, which require a separate application. Should the child be born with problems, health care may be covered by Medicaid and provided by some combination of hospital based and public health clinic providers. Seriously handicapping childhood conditions may require resources not covered by Medicaid, and be dependent on a variety of public and private payers, such as SSI, Crippled Children's programs, Easter Seals, and March of Dimes, each with different eligibility criteria. WIC certification is also separate for the child and for the mother. Meanwhile, the mother has been referred from her post-partum check back to family planning and/or general medical services (if, in fact, she has a usual source of care). (McCormick, 1989, unpublished manuscript)

Much of the problem in excess infant mortality can be attributed to the lack of a family focus; there are clear benefits to maintaining such a focus.

In health promotion, it is critical to bridge the gaps among clinic, school, and family. For example, obesity prevention cannot succeed if there are not significant adaptations at home and at school. If parents are stocking the kitchen with high-fat, high-calorie foods, it will be difficult for health providers to institute any program of weight reduction. Also, children will be much more likely to participate in fitness activities if the family supports such activities.

If there is so much to be gained by a family focus, where is the resistance? The two major barriers are training and financing. Traditional training of child health and educational professionals centers on the child. Lip service is given to the child's family contacts, and child health providers certainly deal with families to deliver services, but child health providers really do not consider themselves trained or licensed to step beyond certain contractual bonds with families. At Children's Hospital in Boston, a group of practicing pediatricians meets every month with child developmentalists and a child psychiatrist to discuss difficult cases as part of a nationwide Maternal and Child Health Bureau–sponsored Collaborative Office Rounds process. Over and over, the group discovers that the cases that are most troubling are the ones where the family is the patient, not the child. They feel constrained by current practice modes from opening the Pandora's Box of Parental Problems. However, if new pediatric approaches like those outlined in *Bright Futures* are going to succeed, child health providers must confront those problems and develop partnerships and referral networks with colleagues who care for adults and who can provide the needed counseling and support services.

Beyond inadequate training, the major barrier to providing expanded services is the lack of payment mechanisms for contextual family-oriented services, particularly those of a preventive nature. The fee-for-service model is not a conducive payment mechanism, and there are too few family health resources in place to cover such coordinated programming. Moreover, in a period of constrained resources, child-oriented health providers are anxious to preserve the basic services such as immunizations and well-child care. They are reluctant to experiment with delivery systems that may increase their workload with no increase in compensation. One potential benefit of managed care is that the emphasis on prevention may translate into the recognition that the best way to avoid expensive childhood morbidity is through responding early to family concerns and strengthening communities to address the needs of young parents.

Prescriptive vs. Responsive Attitudes

Patient, client, or consumer? Parent or colleague? Community organizer, community agitator, or team member? How should the various roles be defined, and who is the real expert?

Who really knows what children and families need and what will work for them? Should families be given preprogrammed, neatly packaged services, or should there be a dialogue between recipients and providers? Is the distinction between recipient and provider itself artificial?

The debate about whether it is best to set agendas to work for families and children or to derive agendas from families and communities troubles those who are committed to comprehensive, community-based, family-centered care. Professionals tend to be definitive, prescriptive, and task-oriented. Families and communities may be far more in touch with realities and needs, but they speak a language that is not easily translated into tasks, goals, and objectives. Parents know, and very much want, what is best for their children, but they can't always work through the arcane systems that restrict services as frequently as they deliver them.

In individual encounters, time constraints often force a prescriptive approach to health care delivery. Unfortunately, though the one-size-fits-all system is efficient, both parents and professionals are frequently dissatisfied because although they have addressed the same issues, they have not connected. The physician may feel that he or she has delivered a clear message outlining the importance of prophylactic medicine the child should take and follow-up appointments that are critical, but family members may come away feeling that no one has responded to their questions about their child's disease and their fears about the future.

In the larger context, there are currently few, if any, formal opportunities for groups of parents and young people to make their needs known to the managers of health care programs. The increasingly competitive health care environment is raising the stakes for a more family-centered and responsive approach. Parent advisory groups and consumer surveys offer two mechanisms for obtaining such formal input. The challenge is to pay more than lip service to such input and to give a partnership role to parents and adolescent patients.

Professional-Driven vs. Payer-Driven Systems

The shuffling and reshuffling of the U.S. health care system has created considerable tension about control. From moment to moment, it is not obvious who is in the driver's seat. Are health professionals driving or are payers steering by remote control? Do consumers have a say in the route that is chosen? Who is directing the traffic?

Child health care professionals want significant input in the health care policy decisions because they desire to maintain high-quality care. They also wish to ensure the proper training of child health providers. Payers also want to direct the process. They want to purchase appropriate, high-quality services *and* they want to keep costs in line. Said simply, professionals and consumers share the desire for high-quality services, but come from very different orientations with respect to cost.

Despite consensus on the importance of quality, it is a concept that eludes definition. The lack of a common conceptual frame exacerbates the tension between professionals and consumers. On the one hand, professionals maintain quality through professional guidelines and credentials. On the other, consumers demand information about outcomes and are often unimpressed by the professional calls for standards and monitoring. For example, organizations such as the American Academy of Pediatrics and the American Board of Pediatrics argue that children will receive the highest quality of care from pediatrically trained physicians. Consumers often look at these credentials less closely and accept care from adult-trained subspecialists as adequate for all patients.

While consumers may miss the nuances related to child-specific training, payers do not miss the distinctions between highly experienced physicians and those in training. With the shift toward a payer-driven health system, there has been an increasing insistence on patient access to care from senior physicians rather than trainees. The effect of this shift is to uncouple training and service, leaving unanswered questions of how the education of the future health care work force is to be financed. Professionals care deeply about this issue. Consumers, at least for now, appear relatively unconcerned about the potential consequences.

The training concern reflects fundamental differences in orientation among consumers, payers, and professionals. Consumers, who are most concerned with what is happening here and now, don't want to be taken care of by trainees. What they don't completely appreciate is that the trainee of the present is the experienced attending physician of the future. At the same time, professionals have turned a deaf ear to patients' pleas for better "customer service." No one wants to be "practiced upon." This tension requires a great deal of honest talk and planning and the recognition of the desirability of fundamental changes in the way that everyone—professionals and payers alike—thinks about training.

Beyond the issue of training, there are also differences in the degree of appreciation for the underlying ingredients required to attain and sustain high-quality health care. Health professionals value basic biologic research as the gateway to the ultimate protection of the public's health. Payers are often skeptical that what happens in the lab has any immediate returns. This tension is felt each year as Congress makes its decisions about the core support for the National Institutes of Health. In the public discussions of the utility of the basic biologic effort, health professionals emphasize the importance of basic research, while consumers demand more immediate and direct returns from the scientific enterprise.

In addition, health professionals and payers differ fundamentally on their orientation to patient services. Health professionals are responsible to one patient at a time. The doctor is trained to provide the fullest service to each patient, to cure or manage his or her condition. Payers are responsible for the health of large groups of people. A driving force for them is cost containment, but they are also concerned about the equitable distribution of care. What makes this tension increasingly real in the U.S. health care system is the growing availability of services for a growing variety of circumstances. There were less tension and fewer ethical concerns when there was not extra corporeal membrane oxygenation, when there were no intensive care unit beds, when colony-stimulating factors were not available, and when bone marrow transplants worked only for identical twins. The availability of these and other technologies makes it increasingly difficult to deny high-cost services to a given patient. Once precedents are set, payers and providers find themselves far apart regarding the offering of a given therapy.

Pragmatism vs. Never-Say-Die Approaches

This most difficult conflict underlies all the others: Who should decide the extent of an intervention? Who should decide when intervention is efficacious and when it is not? The controversy in Oregon over explicit rationing of health care brought these issues to national attention in the early 1990s, with a resolution that emphasized a verbal commitment to civil rights. The question was, however, whose civil rights were upheld: those of all citizens or those of citizens with enough savvy to wind their way through the health care system with its implicit rationing barriers.

In child health, providers face this issue daily: Should a youngster who is struggling because of his parent's alcoholism be counseled to get on with his own life, or should there be intensive outreach to cure the parent and resolve all family conflicts? At what point should Social Services cut the family ties of a child who has been abused? How much physical therapy, occupational therapy, and language intervention should be given to a child in a persistent vegetative state? The question very simply is, are there lost causes? Certainly in traditional medicine it has been the most complex cases—the cancers, the most severe immunodeficiencies, and the complex metabolic disorders—that have been pursued. But these intensive interventions occur within the context of disciplined, protocol-based approaches and clear-cut evaluation strategies. A strong political will would be needed to approach social and community issues in this way.

Recognizing that these tensions exist helps explain many of the boundary lines that become drawn in health care. Program directors often find it easier to limit services than to take on new problems and new partners. Once a mode of operations is established, it often becomes a fixed structure with its own rules, language, and customs. Nonetheless, the complex needs of children and families will not be met until more serious attention is given to the implementation of new policies and systems that acknowledge these tensions, and also strive to address the basic problems underlying them.

Summary and Implications

By definition, a health care system is the amalgamation of multiple components, points of view, needs, and resources. Place such a health care system in the United States, where authority shifts depending on who is exerting the most force, and tension results: the pull of interest groups, the pull of equally vital demands and needs, the pull of competing philosophies of care, the pull of disciplinary approaches.

For practitioners, these tensions have important implications. No longer is it possible for a physician or nurse practitioner to study medicine in a vacuum. Trainees must be provided with a full understanding of the framework of the world in which they will practice.

Once in practice, child health professionals will continue to confront the tensions. For a small few, the tensions will be overwhelming. For most, they will be an annoyance. And for some they will present a genuine challenge. These last will work to use the inherent strength that tension brings to improve health care delivery for children. They will find ways for physicians to collaborate with other child-helping professionals so that not only are the root social causes of childhood morbidities identified, they are addressed. They will experiment with service delivery systems until they find the ones that provide their own patients with the most comprehensive and up-to-date services, and they will work with payer groups to ensure the highest-quality care. We must hope that there are enough of these child health care leaders to ensure that the tensions are not destructive, but rather, that they enrich and strengthen.

References

Blum BB, Blank S. 1991. Children's services in an era of budget deficits. American Journal of Diseases of Children 145:575–8.

Ciborowski J. 1992. Textbooks and the students who can't read them: A guide to teaching content. Cambridge, MA: Brookline Books.

Green M. 1995. Bright Futures: Guidelines for health supervision of infants, children and adolescents. Arlington, VA: National Center for Education in Maternal and Child Health.

Hobbs N. 1975. The futures of children: Recommendations of the project on classification of exceptional children. San Francisco: Jossey-Bass.

National Commission on Children. 1991. Beyond rhetoric. Washington: U.S. Government Printing Office.

Richmond J. 1992 Winter. Personal communication with this former U.S. Surgeon General and Assistant Secretary for Health.

Schorr LB, Schorr D. 1988. Within our reach: Breaking the cycle of disadvantage. New York: Anchor Press/Doubleday.

Shonkoff J, Hauser-Cram P. 1987. Early intervention for disabled infants and their families—quantitative analysis. Pediatrics 80:650–8.

Slavin RE, Karweit L, Madden NA. 1990. Effective programs for students at risk. Boston: Allyn & Bacon.

Thompson LS. 1991. The forgotten child in health care. In: Children in the juvenile justice system. Washington: National Center for Education in Maternal and Child Health.

[USSG] U.S. Surgeon General's Conference on Health of Children: Ready to Learn. 1992 Feb. Washington.

White SH, Buka SL. 1987. Early education: Programs, traditions and policies. Review of Research in Education 13:43.

III

MANAGED CARE AND
CHILD HEALTH SERVICES

One of the most potent forces reshaping the health care landscape is managed care. More than 16.7 million children in the United States were enrolled in some form of managed care or health maintenance organization in 1994, and that number is growing rapidly, particularly as states seek to make managed care enrollment mandatory for their entire Medicaid populations.

Despite the fervent embrace of managed care, very little is known about its impact on children as a group or on any of the subgroups of children that may have particularly complex care needs (e.g., poor children, children who have chronic conditions). Managed care promises significant improvements over the fee-for-service system: care that is more coordinated, improved access to preventive services, and the prospect of more personalized relationships with health care practitioners. But these promises must be balanced against the perverse incentives built into capitated payment systems to limit services, to enroll only healthy children, and to avoid children with costly care needs.

To make managed care work, it will be necessary to know a lot more about the dynamics of various forms of managed care. Also necessary are better measures of children's health status, quality of care, and the long-term impact of health interventions. It is worth emphasizing that none of this information was available in the fee-for-service system; however, there the incentive was to provide too much care. The incentive to limit services in managed care arrangements is of greater concern, and makes the need for these kinds of measures and information all the more pressing.

Despite the murkiness of the general subject there are some bright spots around the country, examples where managed care plans are taking their community and public health responsibilities seriously, and conducting aggressive outreach, community education, and public health activities. Curiously, however, the evidence suggests that these activities are driven as much by public re-

lations considerations as by the conviction that investment in community health makes long-term economic sense.

The reality is that altruism has never been the guiding force in any business, and until the incentives are structured appropriately, there is a need for government regulation and intervention. In particular, in the near term, there is a need for precise articulation of expectations and standards in the contracts that states are executing with managed care plans to serve their Medicaid populations. Such precision is necessary to protect against the dangers of underservice, to make sure that children have access to appropriate pediatric subspecialists, and to make sure that children with special needs receive appropriate care using a child-specific standard of medical necessity. Without specific contract language, hard-won advances in the delivery of a higher standard of care to children are in jeopardy. With such assurances, managed care may indeed fulfill its promise.

9

Protecting Children: Defining, Measuring, and Enforcing Quality in Managed Care

Sara Rosenbaum

Introduction

IN THE UNITED STATES, health care is delivered within a complex legal framework that establishes the rights and duties of payers, health care providers, and individuals. The U.S. health care system is undergoing a transformation of nearly unprecedented importance, from one in which individual services and procedures are furnished on a fee-for-service basis by independent health care professionals and institutions to one in which large corporations sell medical care to purchasing groups for a preset, all-inclusive fee. The fundamental structural shift in health care financing and delivery will have an enormous impact on the relationships among the various parties within the system and will alter many previously established notions of accountability for both the cost and quality of health care.

This chapter explores the issue of quality of care measurement and the changing legal framework in which quality of care standards are established and enforced. It reviews quality of care standard setting and oversight in the traditional fee-for-service system. It then examines the extent to which the transformation to managed care is altering the traditional approach to quality measurement and specifically considers the role of contracts between public and private group purchasers and managed care organizations in quality of care standard setting and enforcement. The chapter concludes with some thoughts on the prospects for further shifts in the legal environment as managed care matures.

Techniques for Measuring Quality of Care

Quality of care measurement has been a matter of longstanding concern in U.S. health care. Americans are routinely reminded that they have the best quality medical care in the world, even as more than 17 percent of the nonelderly population and 14 percent of children remain uninsured. Moreover, despite these assertions, the nation's approach to measuring quality historically has been limited, although the transformation to an integrated system of financing and service delivery shows signs of changing this "handsoff" approach to quality measurement and enforcement.

Achieving quality in health care is a function of the *structure* of the delivery system, the *process* by which care is delivered, and the *outcomes* (both technical and patient-measured) that are achieved. Any system for measuring the quality of health care, whether furnished by physicians, hospitals, nursing homes, or managed care systems, uses one of these three basic measures of quality (Rosenblatt et al., 1997, ch. 3). A structural measure considers whether the organization and components of the health care entity whose care is being assessed are conducive to good health care outcomes. An example of a structural measure would be whether a hospital's emergency room is adequately equipped or staffed to deal with a full array of emergency conditions. A process of care measure considers whether the particular treatment or procedure is carried out in a manner consistent with accepted health care practice standards. Thus a determination of whether a provider begins treatment for pregnancy within two weeks of a request for an initial appointment would be a process of care measure. Another process of care measure would be one that considers whether children with asthma are treated with proper medication.

An outcome measure considers whether patient outcomes fall within an accepted range of adequacy. An example of an outcome measure would be the proportion of children who are fully immunized by age two. Another measure would be whether a patient reports being able to achieve a fuller range of motion following physical therapy. Developing outcome measures is exceedingly difficult for several reasons. First, except for very basic measures of care such as childhood immunizations, routine dental care, and certain preventive screening services, few patient outcomes are sufficiently documented in the literature to permit the articulation of an acceptable outcome standard. Second, unless measures are risk adjusted to take into account the severity of patients' illness or conditions, certain providers might be unfairly criticized for achieving poor outcomes. Reducing infant low birthweight rates to national norms might not be feasible for providers treating large numbers of African-American women, given the significantly higher incidence of low birthweight among babies born to these women. Such a measure could encourage providers to avoid treating large numbers of high-risk patients in order to maintain acceptable practice profiles. Similarly, using unadjusted mortality data to judge the performance of hospitals might unfairly classify as poor quality those hospitals treating large numbers of high-risk patients.

Third, outcome measures must be designed to measure an activity over which a provider has control and can directly affect through its action (National Committee for Quality Assurance, 1996). The purpose of outcome measures is to determine whether providers achieve certain types of results, whether they be the immunization of children or successful recovery from coronary artery bypass surgery. Accordingly the measure chosen must relate directly to the provider's conduct and cannot involve a measure (such as the proportion of smoking patients who quit) that depends to a significant degree on the actions of individuals or other factors and whose outcome therefore could be confounded by other events.

Finally, developing good outcome measures is complicated by the fact that in order for a measure to produce a reliable result, the universe of patients against which the measure is applied must be large enough to permit a fair and reliable assessment of outcome (National Committee for Quality Assurance, 1996). The lack of sufficient numbers can produce unreliable results, even for simple and accepted measures. The problem of small numbers also makes it very difficult to measure outcomes of interventions for low-prevalence health conditions, such as the quality of care furnished to children with cystic fibrosis. Assuming, for the moment, that appropriate outcome measures could be developed (and they no doubt can be), the number of children with the condition is so small that the use of outcome measures to gauge the performance of any single provider or health plan (or even a group of providers or plans) would be difficult. In the case of low-prevalence conditions, structural and process-of-care measures (including medical records reviews examining patient care practices against accepted processes of care) probably are the only realistic approach to measuring the quality of clinical care on a plan by plan basis.

The limitations on quality oversight are further exacerbated by serious data limitations. In order to evaluate performance, a great deal of data are needed. Much of the most important data for purposes of measuring process of care and outcomes are contained in medical records. Yet only a handful of providers and health plans at this point maintain electronic medical records systems that permit medical records data to be collected and easily aggregated within an administrative reporting system. The lack of electronic records seriously reduces the range of information available and forces quality assurance systems to rely on medical records reviews, a costly and time-consuming endeavor. The absence of data is even greater if purchasers do not require providers or plans to generate at least "dummy claims" to memorialize the provision of medical care within administrative systems, at least at the gross encounter level.

Measuring the Quality of Health Care in the Traditional Fee-for-Service System

To the extent that the quality of care was measured at all by either peer review or external reviewers, structure and process of care measures dominated the quality of care landscape in the traditional fee-for-service system. The primary tools for ensuring quality were health professions training and certification, licensure of individual health professionals, accreditation of institutions, and informal efforts by groups of health care professionals to prevent entry into practice of members of the profession deemed to be offering care of less than adequate quality (e.g., decisions by medical staff to deny admitting privileges to individual physicians). Peer review, accreditation, and other quality of care activities were confined to institutions and organized health settings. Office-based physicians and health professionals were virtually exempt from any peer review system (Rosenblatt et al., 1997, ch. 3).

For some time it has been evident that while essential, these tools alone are insufficient to ensure a basic level of quality in health care. The work of Wennberg and others helped draw national attention to the inadequacy of structural and process measures and enforcement tools in light of the enormous variation in health care practice styles within comparable communities, with few if any measurable differences in health care outcomes (Rosenblatt et al., 1997, ch. 3). Added to the variations in practice and outcomes documented by Wennberg are examples—far too numerous to mention—in which grossly substandard health care institutions and individual health care professionals have been permitted to remain in practice even in the face of extensive documentation of the poor quality of the care they furnished (Rosenblatt et al., 1997, ch. 3). In the absence of evidence of a systemic approach to holding health care professionals accountable for the quality of the care they furnish in a timely and definitive fashion, it should perhaps not be surprising that Americans have been loathe to relinquish their right to bring individual actions against health care professionals and institutions for breaching their duty to furnish care of reasonable quality.

Quality of Care Measurement in a Managed Care Environment

In order to understand how quality of care measurement changes in a managed care environment, it is first necessary to understand how managed care differs from fee-for-service medical care.

Managed Care Defined

There is no single definition of managed care (for an excellent typology of managed care systems, see Weiner and de Lissovoy, 1993). In this chapter, managed care is defined as any health insurance arrangement in which the functions of health insurance and health care delivery are carried out through an entity that

1. covers individuals for a defined set of benefits;
2. furnishes covered services to members through a network of participating providers selected by the entity and either under contract to, or employed by, the entity;
3. employs prospective utilization controls to manage service utilization; and
4. monitors the quality of care or services furnished to members as well as performing other administrative functions.

Managed care plans range from loosely to tightly structured plans, with the tightness of the structure tied to the degree of freedom on the members' part to use providers that are not affiliated with the plan network (Table 9.1). Tight plans include classic staff and group model health maintenance organizations (HMOs) that deliver all care through health care professionals under contract to the plan. Members are restricted to these providers and are uncovered when they obtain covered services (other than emergency care) from non-network providers. Loose models include preferred

Table 9.1
The Managed Care Spectrum

The affluent privately insured	Medicaid enrollees/traditional HMOs
Loose network structure	Tight network structure
Limited copayments for out-of-network use	No coverage for non-network care
Limited utilization controls	Strong utilization controls
Managed care functions as discounted insurance	Managed care functions as a health care system

provider organizations "point-of-service" HMOs that permit members relatively wide latitude in obtaining covered services; members have more freedom to select their primary care providers and for an added fee may use out-of-network providers for covered services. Because Medicaid agencies pay premiums that are low in relation to the health risks of their patients (Welch and Wade, 1995), Medicaid managed care plans are tightly constructed; that is, members are restricted to providers belonging to the plan network for covered care and are uncovered for care furnished out of network.

A key question is what makes a particular insurance product "managed care" as opposed to traditional insurance. Utilization controls alone do not provide the answer. For many years traditional insurers have used prospective utilization review to curtail consumption of services that are deemed either inappropriate or unnecessary (Rosenblatt et al., 1997, ch. 2). The notion of "participating providers" also does not distinguish managed care from other forms of health insurance; indeed, since its inception, the Blue Shield system (as well as Medicare, which was patterned after Blue Shield) has utilized providers who contract to furnish covered benefits to members on a direct-billed basis (at the option of the provider) (Law, 1976).

Two principal attributes appear to set managed care plans apart from other forms of health insurance, whether indemnity-style or "service benefit" plans. The first distinction lies in the expectation of managed care purchasers. In managed care, unlike traditional insurance, purchasers typically contract for *services*, not merely coverage. Buyers expect that plans will maintain a network of participating providers to furnish covered benefits;

these expectations are reflected in the service agreements between group sponsors and health plans, discussed at greater length below. This expectation of service is particularly strong in the case of Medicaid agency purchasers because of the closed nature of managed care plans. Indeed, Medicaid agencies' strong embrace of managed care arose in part from concerns over the access barriers traditionally faced by beneficiaries (National Academy for State Health Policy, 1990).

Private group purchasers also expect services rather than coverage; as noted, however, private purchasers tend to buy managed care products that are more loosely structured and that leave enrollees with greater flexibility and choice of providers (for which cost-sharing obligations are higher). Medicaid agencies, on the other hand, cannot rely on Medicaid beneficiaries to purchase any supplemental services given their poverty. The services that enrollees obtain from their Medicaid managed care plans constitute their only insured health care system, at least with respect to those services that are covered under the Medicaid agency's managed care service contract with participating health plans.

Second, and even more importantly, managed care can be distinguished from other forms of health insurance by the terms of the contractual relationship between the plan and its participating network of health care providers. In traditional forms of health insurance, health professionals (even if "participating") maintain their independent business status; physicians, hospitals, and other providers remain free to decide on an ad hoc basis whether to sell their services to any given enrollee. Managed care fundamentally changes the relationship between physicians and insurers on the one hand and physicians and individuals on the other. Because managed care plans create service systems as well as coverage arrangements, providers who are members of managed care networks must agree to serve members of the plans with which they are affiliated as a condition of participation. Thus, a typical participation contract for a managed care provider requires that unless the provider's practice is full and closed to all individuals, the provider must accept as a patient any member referred by the plan (Rosenbaum et al., 1995).

In effect, managed care participation agreements create among participating providers a contractual duty to serve individual enrollees. This duty is unprecedented in U.S. health law, which has always accorded health providers the basic right accorded any seller of goods and services, namely the right to select one's customers. Prior to managed care, the only exceptions to this "freedom of contract" were state and federal laws that created certain emergency care duties in hospitals with emergency facilities. While physicians had a duty to provide services of adequate quality to individuals whom they undertook to serve, they had no duty to care for any individual (Rosenblatt et al., 1997, ch. 3) except as a by-product of their membership on the staff of hospitals covered by emergency care laws.

It is this duty on the part of health professionals to care for members of a health plan, even when no direct patient relationship has yet been formed, that distinguishes physician participation in managed care from participation in other forms of coverage. This duty also helps explain why coverage determinations by health plans are viewed by patients and providers alike as health *care* decisions rather than simply health *coverage* decisions. In effect the plan has promised to serve enrollees, and has contracted with health care providers to serve enrollees on the plan's behalf; as a result, what might have been considered a coverage decision under traditional coverage becomes a decision not to provide care. Moreover, and of direct relevance to this chapter, because health plans assume a duty to serve, they also assume a direct duty to monitor the quality of care furnished by providers employed by or under contract to the plan in the discharge of its duty.

The transformation of the relationship between physicians and health plans under managed care thus creates a need for a comprehensive quality assurance program that is capable of measuring the adequacy of all aspects of the contracted health care system. In this highly integrated system connected by internal agreements and contracts, the task of measuring quality is more complex than previously, when each physician, hospital, and health care provider was an independent business whose services were not part of a larger enterprise. In managed care, the notion of quality extends to all health care providers under contract to the health plan. The plan is responsible for the quality of each service component within the system, as well as the quality of the system as a whole. Moreover, under managed care the locus of perceived responsibility for the quality of care shifts from individual health care providers to the prime contractor: the company that selects providers and controls providers' and patients' access to services, and monitors utilization and quality.

This changing vision of who bears the responsibility for quality in health care parallels the evolution of medical practice liability law among hospitals. In the first half of the century, hospitals were viewed simply as workplaces for physicians with no independent role in the provision of care or quality control. As hospitals grew into complex institutions with duties of their own, their independent role in monitoring and assuring quality of their staff and services became accepted.

The same is true with managed care plans. Managed care plans create the aura, if not always the reality, of health care service systems (indeed, many health plans use this expression to describe their programs). It is not surprising, therefore, that purchasers and consumers expect to base their purchasing decisions on measures of health care quality, not merely the extent of health care coverage. Moreover, the quality of care measures used in reporting systems such as the Health Plan Employer Data and Information Set (HEDIS) developed by the National Committee on Quality Assurance (1996) seek to measure the quality of the entire health care system, not just individual performers (e.g., doctors, hospitals) within the system. The image projected by managed care plans themselves leads the public to view plans as health care providers possessed of health care duties, not merely as insurance companies or loose federations of independent businesses. Consider this advice excerpted from a recent newspaper article (Auerbach, 1995) about choosing a managed care plan:

- Visit a plan's facilities to see how they treat patients in real life—not in television commercials—and whether you feel comfortable in that setting. See if they have evaluations by patients you can look at.
- Find out what provisions are made for after-hours and emergency care. . . .
- See if you have the right to change doctors at any time within the plan. And if you want to go outside the network for a specialist, find out if you can by paying a greater portion of the cost. . . .

This focus on the quality of the managed care plan's health care (rather than simply the extent of its coverage) was evident during a July 1995 meeting in Jackson Hole, Wyoming, attended by major purchasers of managed care representing 80 million covered individuals, at which the issue of quality measurement was discussed at length:

"Monitoring quality will be the next battlefield," said Tom J. Elkin, assistant executive director of the California Public Employees Retirement System. . . . He predicted that only health plans that demonstrated high quality would still be in existence by 2000. . . . "What we want to do," said [Dwight] McNeill [chosen by the group to head a new quality of care initiative], "is have information out there in the marketplace on performance and outcome measurements. If consumers and purchasers have information on both outcome and cost, it drives market share toward that vendor that has the best value, and surprisingly, we haven't got that as yet." (Noble, 1995)

Managed care in effect replaces a sovereign medical profession with companies whose "product" is a health care system for "covered lives" delivered through a network of providers employed by or under contract to a health plan. As a result, managed care changes both the concept and the reality of health care practice and decision making, alters the range and types of quality measurement tools that are needed, and inevitably appears to point in the direction of a fundamental restructuring of principles of legal liability for the quality of care, just as the advent of hospitals as institutions independent of the physicians who practiced in them ultimately altered concepts of hospital liability for the quality of physicians' care (Rosenblatt et al., 1997, ch. 3).

As difficult as defining and measuring quality may be in managed care generally, several factors make quality measurement even more difficult—and yet far more important—in the case of low-income managed care enrollees. First, as noted, unlike their more affluent counterparts, the poor who are members of managed care plans cannot afford to supplement the services their plans give them. They cannot pay higher cost sharing and go out-of-plan for needed care as can middle-income patients with point-of-service plan options, nor can Medicaid agencies afford to buy this type of access for them. Medicaid beneficiaries also frequently face serious shortages of physicians in the communities in which they live (Fossett and Perloff, 1995). These shortages can translate into serious access difficulties if individuals are enrolled in managed care systems that have insufficient primary and specialty care capacity.

Second, the lower premiums that Medicaid agencies pay for care may mean that plans must utilize more stringent networks and stricter access controls in order to stay within budget. Third, Medicaid beneficiaries may have less familiarity with managed care and less understanding of the systems in which they are enrolled or less ability to adapt to the demands that managed care places on patients. As a group, most Medicaid-eligible families with children are young and have limited education levels. For others, eligibility is directly related to the presence of a serious illness or disability that may hinder their ability to navigate managed care plans successfully (as of the end of 1996, 20 states and the District of Columbia had either indicated their plans to enroll some or all noninstitutionalized disabled persons into Medicaid managed care plans or were already on their way to doing so). Moreover, many beneficiaries face added challenges in using health care because of special language or cultural needs.

Fourth, the tasks of serving Medicaid beneficiaries in managed care systems and measuring the quality of care are hindered by the short duration of their enrollment. Approximately half of all Medicaid beneficiaries are continuously enrolled in a single managed care plan for less than one year (National Committee for Quality Assurance, 1996). Data on managed care disenrollment among Medicaid beneficiaries indicate that the overwhelming cause of disenrollment is not frequent plan switching on the part of beneficiaries but the loss of Medicaid coverage itself. Medicaid coverage is so short that it is difficult for patients to develop and sustain a relationship with their managed care plan providers before they lose coverage altogether. Most quality of care outcome measures depend for their reliability on the existence of a sufficiently large measurement group of individuals who have been continuously enrolled in a plan for a long enough period of time for the plan's care to be measurable in terms of health status changes. Short enrollment periods frequently make quality of care measures unworkable (National Committee for Quality Assurance, 1996).

Take for example the case of childhood immunizations. On the surface, measuring whether a plan's two-year-olds are sufficiently immunized would appear to be a straightforward matter. However, in order to judge any provider's performance, there must be a sufficient number of events to yield a reliable estimate. For childhood immunizations, the proper outcome measure is the number of children immunized in a timely fashion by their second birthday. For this measure to be a reliable test of plan performance, a child must be continuously enrolled in the plan from 45 days to two years of age (the period of time over which the plan's performance is to be measured). In the case of Medicaid enrolled children, however, discontinuous eligibility means that only a tiny fraction of all children are continuously enrolled for a sufficiently long period to permit accurate measurement of plan performance. As a result, plan performance would be measured against a mere handful of children rather than a large group, and the reliability of the measure would be open to question. To compensate for this problem, the HEDIS system uses a 10-month immunization catch-up outcome measure for Medicaid-enrolled children rather than the two-year-old full immunization measure that is used for the commercially insured population.

Finally, the brief enrollment problem is exacerbated by the fact that on average nearly half of all Medicaid managed care enrollees do not select their plans but are instead "auto-enrolled" into a health care system (unpublished data, Health Care Financing Administration, Washington, DC, 1996). Once plan auto-enrollment occurs, plans may further auto-assign individuals to primary care physicians. Little is known about the impact of auto-enrollment on quality of care, but it is known that auto-enrollees use less services. The cause of this lower utilization may be that persons who are auto-enrolled are low health care utilizers. It also may be that auto-enrolled persons are normal or even high users of care but use less care during their enrollment periods; this may be because they are unaware of the plan to which they have been assigned and leave the plan before they have had the opportunity to use its services.

The problem of how to ensure quality in Medicaid managed care plans is further complicated by the fact that Medicaid managed care products may differ significantly from those sold to private purchasers. These differences, which center on the size and scope of provider networks and the extent to which utilization controls are imposed on both beneficiaries and providers, help plans control costs; however, they also may have implications for the quality of care. Medicaid members may not have access to all providers that participate in the plan's network. A Medicaid contractor may restrict patients' access to certain network providers and may not permit patients to select other providers, as evidenced by recent data from a study of New York City's Medicaid managed care system (New York City Office of Consumer Affairs, 1995) as well as anecdotal evidence from Medicaid agencies throughout the country. These restrictions may be imposed to control costs, since larger networks may require more costly premiums, because they permit more ready access to both primary and specialty care and thus enhance the opportunities to utilize services. They also may be imposed in order to appease office-based physicians who do not wish to treat Medicaid patients (letter of the New York State Medical Society to HHS Secretary Donna Shalala, November 1996).

Medicaid network providers also may have less utilization discretion than that accorded to network providers serving privately insured members, whose premium payments are higher in relation to utilization. Approved drug formularies may be narrower. More services might require prior authorization by a plan before they may be furnished. Fewer treatment options might be available, and those that are might be more narrowly drawn. In the absence of any systematic study of the differences between commercial plan products and those offered to Medicaid patients, it is possible only to speculate on how lower premiums and sicker patients might affect the administration of a health plan open to both publicly and privately insured patients.

Thus, while there is a particularly great imperative to develop quality of care measures for Medicaid managed care enrollees, developing such measures may be quite difficult because of the attenuated relationship between Medicaid managed care enrollees and the health systems of which they are members.

Systems for Measuring the Quality of Managed Care

The large service contracts signed by a managed care group sponsor (in this example, a Medicaid agency) operate against a regulatory backdrop of federal and state Medicaid law, insurer and provider licensure laws, and other state laws (Table 9.2). Against this backdrop of laws the contracts seek to

- define the benefits that the contractor must furnish,
- describe the service system (with greater or lesser specificity) that the

Table 9.2
The Legal Framework for the Delivery of Health Care to Medicaid Beneficiaries

---

The Fee-for-Service System

The provider agreement: any willing provider, nominal participation requirements (except for institutional providers and agencies)
State Medicaid provider participation statutes and regulations
State provider licensure laws
The federal Medicaid statute: conditions of participation and state plan requirements
The procurement process in states using authority to selectively contract among willing providers for certain services

The Managed Care System

The service agreement (the contract) between the purchaser and the plan
State Medicaid provider participation statutes and regulations
State provider licensure laws, state insurance laws, state business laws
The federal Medicaid statute: conditions of participation and state plan requirements
The procurement process in states using authority to selectively contract among qualified providers for certain services

---

contractor must furnish to enrollees and how quality will be measured, and

- describe the contractor's relationship to the rest of the health care system (Table 9.3).

Purchasers' contracts (in this case, those of state Medicaid agencies) vary widely in the specificity with which they describe plans' coverage and service duties, as well as how they attempt to define quality measurement. For example, all states seek to collect encounter (i.e., process of care) data, but only a handful require plans to report outcomes measures (such measures are required by HCFA in all Section 1115 Medicaid managed care demonstrations and include prenatal care, immunizations, and pediatric hospitalization).

Extensive analysis of state Medicaid managed care contracts also reveals wide variations in the degree of specificity with respect to requirements for

Table 9.3
Categories of Issues Addressed in Managed Care Contracts

Enrollment

Coverage and Benefits
    Who is enrolled
    Enrollment procedures
    Disenrollment
    Information to enrollees

Service Duties
    Classes of covered services
    Limitations on covered services
    Medical necessity definition
    Process for determining service coverage

Public Health and Social Service Relationships
    Relationship between the plan and selected agencies furnishing or overseeing care
        for managed care enrollees

Quality Assurance, Data, and Reporting
    Quality assurance measurement tools
    Data to be reported

Business Terms
    Term and termination
    Disclosure and conflict of interest rules
    Payment terms

lead testing, a basic requirement of the Early and Periodic Screening, Diagnosis and Treatment (EPSDT) program. The terms of state contracts range from Massachusetts' highly specific provisions to Kansas's much less specific requirements (Table 9.4). Showing equal range are state approaches to the issue of obstetrical and pediatric care, with some states expressing a contractual expectation that pregnant women be treated by a designated maternity care provider holding obstetrical admitting privileges and others including no express requirement that each pregnant woman have an obstetrical provider. States also vary in the degree to which they specify standards for immunizations, pediatric developmental assessment, and pregnancy-related care. In many state contracts, the standard specified falls short of current federal coverage standards.

Beyond the purchaser's contract, there are several basic ways in which quality of care in managed care is measured:

• Health plans, as part of their accreditation standards and as a condition of participating in Medicare and Medicaid, must have procedures for measuring the quality of care. Quality of care measurement may also be a requirement for licensure as an HMO or other form of managed care organization in a state. Most quality of care measurement is done by plans themselves, since purchasers (whether private or governmental) do not have the personnel or resources to oversee each plan's performance in detail. This is true not only for managed care but for all forms of health care delivery where, traditionally, the public relies on providers to police themselves through accreditation and self-examination (Rosenblatt et al., 1997, ch. 3). Quality of care monitoring procedures include structure, process of care, and outcome standards, as well as consumer satisfaction studies, although these studies are still in their infancy. Measuring the satisfaction of parents with their children's care presents special challenges, as does measuring satisfaction in the case of low-income consumers. In a recent survey of consumer satisfaction in the Arizona mandatory Medicaid managed care demonstration conducted for the Flynn Foundation, researchers found that despite the fact that poor enrollees were significantly more likely to be denied coverage or face serious delays in the provision of care, they were as likely as their nonpoor counterparts to be satisfied with their health plans. This finding suggests that the poor may be less likely to find fault with the quality of health care than their nonpoor counterparts, even though they have dramatically less ability to do anything about inadequacies of care.

Table 9.4
Managed Care Contract Language Pertaining to Lead Testing

The following excerpts from two states' Medicaid managed care contracts demonstrate very different approaches. Unlike Kansas, Massachusetts has elected to be highly specific about lead blood testing; its contract provides plans with the standard of practice it expects companies to follow as a specific contractual matter. In both states' contracts, lead blood level testing would be covered, since the test involves both a health history and a blood test. However, Kansas has elected to provide no specific guidance on the issue of lead testing; in such a case, lead testing is not a specific contractual promise, and it would fall to the health plan, acting under reasonable standards of practice, to make decisions about how and when to test. The state would ultimately be accountable to beneficiaries for the reasonableness of the plan's conduct.

Kansas

The EPSDT screening provision of Kansas's contract provides as follows:

"The HMO shall ensure the completion of health screenings at the entrance to the program, and at specific intervals, which consist of a health history, developmental assessment, complete physical exam, vision screening, hearing test, urinalysis, blood test, immunizations, nutrition screen, anticipatory guidance and other tests as needed and referrals for treatment." **Kansas Contract**, page 12.

Massachusetts

Other diagnosis and treatment
***

(11)   Lead Toxicity Screening. The required screen for the presence of lead toxicity in children consists of two components: verbal risk assessment and blood lead testing.

(a)   Verbal Risk Assessment. The provider must perform a verbal risk assessment for lead toxicity at every periodic visit between the ages of six and 72 months as indicated on the Schedule. The verbal risk assessment includes, at a minimum, the following types of questions:

(i)   Does your child live in or regularly visit a house built before 1960? Does the house have peeling or chipping paint?

(ii)   Was your child's day care center/preschool/babysitter's home built before 1960? Does the house have chipping or peeling paint?

(iii)   Does your child live in a house built before 1960 with recent, ongoing, or planned renovation or remodeling?

(iv)   Have any of your children or their playmates had lead poisoning?

(v)   Does your child frequently come in contact with an adult who works with lead? Examples include construction, welding, pottery, or other trades practiced in your community.

(vi)   Does your child live near a lead smelter, battery recycling plant, or other industry likely to release lead, such as (give examples in your community)?

(vii)   Do you give your child home or folk remedies that may contain lead?

(viii)   Does your child live near a heavily traveled major highway where soil and dust may be contaminated with lead?

(ix)   Does your home's plumbing have lead pipes or copper pipes with lead solder joints?

A child's level of risk for exposure to lead depends upon the answers to the above questions. If the answers to all questions are negative, a child is considered at low risk for high doses of lead exposure.

If the answer to any question is affirmative, a child is considered at high risk for high doses of lead exposure. A child's risk category can change with each administration of the verbal risk assessment. . . .

(b)   Blood Lead Testing. Screening blood lead testing may be performed by either a capillary sample (fingerstick) or a venous sample. However, all elevated blood levels (equal to or greater than 10 micrograms per 1 deciliter) obtained through a capillary sample must be confirmed by a venous sample. The frequency with which the blood lead test is to be administered depends upon the results of the verbal risk assessment. For children determined to be at low risk for high doses of lead exposure, a screening blood lead test must be performed once between the ages of nine and 12 months, and annually thereafter until the age of 48 months. For children determined to be at high risk for high doses of lead exposure, a screening blood lead test must be performed at the time a child is determined to be a high risk beginning at six months of age. . . .

(i)   If the initial blood lead test results are less than 10 micrograms per deciliter, a screening blood lead test is required at every subsequent periodic visit through 72 months of age, unless the child has already received a blood lead test at the periodic visit within the last six months.

(ii)   If the child is found to have a blood lead level equal to or greater than 10 micrograms per deciliter, providers should use their professional judgment, in accordance with the CDC guidelines regarding patient management and treatment, as well as follow-up blood test and initiation of investigations, to determine the source of lead, where indicated.

(iii)   If a child between the ages of 24 months and 72 months has not received a screening blood lead test, the child must receive the blood lead test immediately, regardless of whether the child is determined to be a low or high risk according to the answers to the above-listed questions.
        Massachusetts contract, Appendix E, Section 1, unnumbered pages.

Source: Rosenbaum et al., 1995.

• Purchasers use external quality assurance monitoring systems to measure quality. These systems utilize the various structural, process of care, and outcome techniques used by plans themselves and may also incorporate other measures of quality in which a sponsor has a particular interest. An example of an external monitoring system is the Quality Assurance Reporting Initiative (QARI) developed by the Health Care Financing Administration for use by state Medicaid agencies in monitoring the quality of managed care systems. The QARI system incorporates many of the same procedures and standards used in internal review systems such as HEDIS and is intended to promote internal consistency among the states in managed care quality oversight. (For a comprehensive review of QARI, see Gold and Felt, 1995.)

In the case of contractual performance standards, even clear and specific standards may be of limited value unless the purchaser also identifies the data that must be furnished to document compliance and has the resources to monitor performance adequately. Increasingly, Medicaid beneficiaries themselves are now filing suit for redress of alleged quality violations, a phenomenon with direct parallels in the employer-insured population (Rosenblatt et al., 1997, ch. 2 and 3).

In developing contracts with managed care plans, purchasers (particularly public purchasers) must be explicit regarding the quality standards they expect contractors to meet, how performance will be measured, and what actions will be taken in the event that performance is substandard. As with all contracts, a managed care contract is an enforceable promise (in this case regarding what purchasers expect managed care systems to be able to do, how the buyer will measure the seller's performance, and the sanctions that the buyer will employ in the event that performance problems do arise). Once signed by both parties, the contract becomes the document that both parties, the intended beneficiaries of the agreement, and ultimately the courts will look to in determining if performance meets articulated standards. As a result, clarity and comprehensiveness in the development of a contract are of critical importance. Ironically, it is the very purchasers whose expectations must be the strongest (i.e., Medicaid agencies) who also may be in the weakest position to demand and enforce high-quality managed care because of the political weakness of agencies and their limited resources and low premiums they can afford to pay.

The need for clarity is particularly important for public agencies. Historically states have set forth their expectations for health care system performance in detailed rules. Under principles of administrative law, state regulations have the force and effect of law, and courts give great judicial deference to interpretations of duly promulgated regulations made by the agency that promulgated the rule. In the case of contracts, however, a state gives up its role of "sovereign" in exchange for a more flexible role of market purchaser. This process gives states more flexibility to negotiate performance standards. However, states also lose the judicial deference to their interpretation of the legal document that they had had with regulations. Indeed, under the doctrine of *contra proferentum*, a contract will be interpreted *against* the drafter (in this case, the state) on the grounds that the drafter knew what it wanted and had a corresponding duty to draft with clarity.

In sum, by integrating financing and service, managed care brings into sharp relief the need for quality of care measurement throughout all phases of the health care systems that are purchased. The transformation to managed care has occurred well in advance of the development of adequate tools for measuring quality. Moreover, a prime means for enforcement of quality of care expectations today—namely the service agreement—works to the disadvantage of purchasers, particularly public purchasers.

Prospects for the Future Regulation of Managed Care Quality
Inevitably the tools for measuring managed care quality will mature. Moreover, recent events suggest that as the managed care market matures, federal and state governments are increasingly willing to set relatively detailed performance standards, in recognition of the fact that it is not possible to rely on the private contracting process (or the self-policing process of industry accreditation and report cards) to promote the public's interest. This cycle of deregulation and reregulation should be familiar to any student of the U.S. health care system.

Recent State Efforts
During 1995 and 1996, as both public and private managed care enrollment exploded, state and federal governments increasingly began to step in to regulate the quality of managed care. In recent years states have grown increasingly active in the regulation of managed care arrangements. A study of state "any willing provider" statutes (laws requiring network insurers to allow membership to any provider willing to accept its terms and conditions) enacted through 1994 found that 28 states had passed any willing provider statutes of one type or another in order to curb efforts by plans to narrow their networks. Fifteen states specifically covered pharmacies under

their laws; a total of 15 states also covered all providers. In only six states did the any willing provider law apply to all types of health plans, including HMOs (Marstellar et al., 1995).

Similarly, as of 1996, 14 states had enacted legislation to curb certain managed care practices, such as the imposition of "gag clauses" in provider contracts, which prohibit communications between health care providers and plan members regarding treatment recommendations and options. As of September 1996, 29 states had enacted legislation restricting the right of managed care plans to discharge new mothers in less than 48 hours (GAO, 1996). Other states have passed legislation increasing consumer protections and the rights of providers not to be terminated from plan networks without a minimum level of due process.

An example of a particularly sweeping law regulating managed care is a 1996 New York law, enacted as part of comprehensive legislation repealing the state's rate-setting system. The managed care legislation restricts many of the practices of managed care organizations. The law requires full disclosure by the HMO to subscribers and potential subscribers of its utilization review policies, methodologies of reimbursement to health care providers, as well as affirmative notice that subscribers may seek care outside the network if the plan does not have an appropriate health care provider within the network and affirmative notice to enrollees that they may seek a specialist's care for a chronic illness or condition that requires such care. Likewise, the bill calls for adequate grievance procedures supported by adequate and affirmative notice of rights to subscribers. The law also includes provisions to limit at-will contracts between HMOs and network providers and to provide for due process in contracts. The legislation also prohibits the use of "gag clauses" by HMOs. Moreover, the legislation gives the state health commissioner access to patient-specific information for quality assurance review, and requires HMOs to participate in the quality assurance of its providers by mandating reporting of disciplinary actions and providing immunity for organizations that report in good faith. In addition, the legislation includes lengthy requirements for conducting utilization reviews that dictate, among other things, the makeup of a review panel, the procedures required, and the remedies available.

Federal Regulation: The 1996 Maternity Length of Stay Legislation

As noted above, the majority of states have enacted legislation to restrict the use of arbitrary upper limits on length of stay for maternity care. In 1996 President Clinton signed into law the Newborns' and Mothers' Health Protection Act of 1996 (PL. 104-130). The act establishes minimum requirements for various types of insurance and benefit plans, not merely those plans that are organized as managed care–style insurance arrangements (i.e., that deliver covered services through a network of professionals and institutions). While the law applies to both traditional and managed care–style insurance arrangements, the practice of limiting length of stay is most closely associated with managed care plans and the bill was perceived as a check on a specific type of managed care practice.

The law amends federal laws to prohibit all insurance carriers from restricting hospital lengths of stay for mothers and newborns to less than 48 hours in the case of a vaginal delivery and less than 96 hours in the case of a cesarean section. The act also denies plans the right to terminate or refuse to renew coverage solely in order to avoid the requirements of the act. The law also prohibits plans and insurers from offering mothers rebates or monetary payments in exchange for accepting less protection or from penalizing or limiting the reimbursement of a provider "because such provider provided care to an individual participant in accordance with this section." The law also prohibits plans from giving "incentives (monetary or otherwise) to an attending provider to induce such provider to provide care to an individual participant or beneficiary in a manner inconsistent with this section."

These legislative developments at the state and federal levels suggest that in the coming years, as the managed care market matures and as enrollment in plans becomes commonplace, state and federal lawmakers will begin to enact laws regulating the quality of care. These laws, along with judicial decisions allowing members to seek to hold plans liable for the quality of care their providers furnish (Rosenblatt et al., 1997), suggest that the legal framework for regulating the quality of managed care will grow over time beyond the contract itself, just as the traditional fee-for-service system came to be regulated in many areas over the 20th century.

References

Auerbach S. 1995 Nov. 7. Choosing a health plan. Washington Post, Health Section, p. 7.

Fossett J, Perloff J. 1995. The new health reform and access to care: The problem of the inner city. Washington: Kaiser Commission on the Future of Medicaid.

[GAO] General Accounting Office. 1996 September. Maternity care: Appropriate follow-up services critical with short hospital stays. HEHS-207. Washington: GAO.

Gold M, Felt S. 1995 Summer. Reconciling practice and theory: Challenges in monitoring Medicaid managed care quality. Health Care Financing Review 16(4):85–99.

Law S. 1976. Blue Cross: What went wrong? New Haven, CT: Yale University Press.

Marstellar J, et al. 1995. Managed care and the resurgence of any willing provider and freedom of choice state legislation, pp. 20–25. Washington: Urban Institute.

National Academy for State Health Policy. 1990. Medicaid managed care: State of the art. Portland, ME: NASHP.

National Committee for Quality Assurance. 1996. Medicaid HEDIS. Washington: NCQA.

New York City Office of Consumer Affairs. 1995. Unpublished manuscript.

Noble HB. 1995 July 3. Quality is focus for health plans. New York Times, p. A-1.

Perloff JD, Kletke P, Fossett JW. 1995. Which physicians limit their Medicaid participation, and why. Health Services Research 30(1):7–26.

Rosenbaum S, Serrano R, Wehr E, Spernak S. 1995. Negotiating the new health care system: An analysis of primary care provider participation contracts under managed care plans. Washington: Center for Health Policy Research, The George Washington University Medical Center.

Rosenbaum S, Shin P, Smith B, Wehr E, Borzi P, Zakheim M, Shaw K, Silver K. 1997. Negotiating the new health system: A nationwide study of Medicaid managed care contracts. Washington: Center for Health Policy Research, The George Washington University Medical Center.

Rosenblatt R, Law S, Rosenbaum S. 1997. Chapters 2 and 3. In: Law and the American health care system. Waterbury, NY: Foundation Press.

Weiner J, de Lissovoy G. 1993 Spring. Razing a Tower of Babel: A taxonomy for managed care and health insurance plans. Journal of Health Politics Policy and Law 18(1):76–103.

Welch WP, Wade M. 1995 Summer. The relative cost of Medicaid enrollees and commercially insured in HMOs. Health Affairs 14(2):212–25.

10

Opportunities and Challenges for Promoting Children's Health in Managed Care Organizations

Sheila Leatherman and Douglas McCarthy

MANAGED CARE is receiving widespread attention as a central mechanism by which the United States is transforming its health care system. As both private and public purchasers of health care move away from traditional fee-for-service arrangements, the number of children served by managed health care plans continues to increase. An estimated 16.7 million children, or 22 percent of Americans under 20 years of age, were enrolled in health maintenance organizations (HMOs) in 1994 (Table 10.1). Managed health care plans are increasingly blending elements of the traditional public health mission with competitive market-oriented approaches to the organization and financing of health care delivery. This fusion of historically distinct private-sector methods and quasi-governmental roles creates new opportunities as well as challenges for health plans serving children.

Well-designed managed care programs emphasize preventive health care, continuity of primary care, and timely coordination of other needed care in the most appropriate clinical setting. Achievement of these goals would greatly benefit children and improve upon suboptimal practices that characterize much of the U.S. health care system today. Managed care's ability to control growth in costs offers the potential to achieve two other

The authors are grateful to the following individuals for sharing their insights and comments: David Amerine, Marie Dotseth, Cathy Halverson, Richard Justman, MD, William Kincaid, MD, Luanne Nyberg, Charles Oberg, MD, Eileen Peterson, and Cheryl Rantala. The views expressed are those of the authors, and no endorsement by United HealthCare Corporation is intended or should be inferred.

Table 10.1
Children Enrolled in Health Maintenance Organizations
United States
1989–1994

	1989	1993	1994
Total Population (in thousands)			
Total HMO enrollment[a]	34,748	45,205	51,138
Total U.S. resident population[b]	246,819	257,783	260,341
Percent of U.S. population in HMOs[c]	14.1%	17.5%	19.6%
Children (in thousands)	(<15 years)	(<15 years)	(<20 years)
Number of children in HMOs[d]	9,278	11,799	16,671
Number of children in United States[e]	53,222	56,741	74,955
Percent of U.S. children in HMOs[f]	17.4%	20.8%	22.2%
Distribution	(<15 years)	(<15 years)	(<20 years)
Children as percent of HMO enrollment[g]	26.7%	26.1%	32.6%
Children as percent of U.S. population[h]	21.6%	22.0%	28.8%

Note: AAHP changed its survey methodology in 1994 to count HMO members under 20 years of age rather than under 15 years as in prior years. The 1993 data are shown for comparison. The U.S. Census count for children reflects the corresponding AAHP age definition in each year.
[a]Data from American Association of Health Plans, National Directory of HMOs.
[b]Data from U.S. Bureau of the Census, Current Population Reports.
[c]Calculated by dividing total HMO enrollment by total U.S. resident population.
[d]Calculated by multiplying total HMO enrollment by children by percent of HMO enrollment.
[e]Data from U.S. Bureau of the Census, Current Population Reports.
[f]Calculated by dividing number of children in HMOs by number of children in United States.
[g]Data from American Association of Health Plans, HMO Industry Survey.
[h]Calculated by dividing number of children in United States by total U.S. resident population.

important policy goals: preserving access to comprehensive health care benefits for children by halting or possibly even reversing the decline in employer-sponsored dependent coverage, and financing affordable coverage for uninsured children (GAO, 1996).

At the same time, there are legitimate questions about the role of health plans within an already fragmented infrastructure of public health and social services programs for children and their families. Children have unique and interwoven physical, emotional, and cognitive development needs that are met most effectively through a broad range of interventions encompassing but also transcending medical care (Halfon et al., 1996, pp. 229–231; Oberg et al., 1994, p. 52). In addition, publicly financed programs such as Medicaid present new issues for health plans that have traditionally covered privately insured individuals. Medicaid members often have lower educational levels and different cultural and linguistic backgrounds, and face other socioeconomic issues that may hinder access to appropriate medical care. As the nation moves to a market-oriented health care system, health plans must play a role in integrating health care within community health and social service strategies to promote the total well-being of children in society today (DeFino, 1995; NASHP, 1993).

Consumer advocates and commentators have expressed concerns that competitive market pressures to hold down premiums and maintain corporate profits could lead to overly aggressive managed care practices that limit children's access to medically necessary care. They cite a lack of adequate tools to compare health plan performance as an imperfection in the market that could allow less reputable firms to coexist alongside more responsible organizations (Angell and Kassirer, 1996; Finkelstein et al., 1995, p. 2). Other observers believe that information can be made available to purchasers and consumers so that competition favors health plans that satisfy patient needs through innovations in efficiency, quality, and accountability—encouraging other firms to "follow the leader" (Ellwood and Lundberg, 1996; Luft, 1996). This dynamic appears to be taking hold in health care markets; a recent federal study reports that "external pressures on plans are promoting more comprehensive and systematic approaches to quality improvement and performance reporting" (Hurley et al., 1996, p. xix).

To meet these dual community health and marketplace challenges, our country needs to define health plan accountabilities for performance in meeting children's needs. This chapter outlines the conceptual foundations to help health plan managers, purchasers, policymakers, and the public define health plan responsibilities for children in a way that will benefit society as a whole, including the constituencies to which health plans have fiduciary, contractual, and regulatory obligations. We briefly review the factors underlying the growth of managed health care plans and their potential to improve children's health care. We then propose a two-tiered framework of interrelated health plan operating responsibilities and com-

Table 10.2
Health Plan Responsibilities for Children

Responsibilities for Enrolled Children

1. Health plans should promote the integrity of relationships between patients and health care professionals.
2. Health plans should recognize the unique developmental needs of children in covering and coordinating appropriate care.
3. Health plans should help lower nonfinancial barriers to care through sensitivity to cultural, linguistic, socioeconomic, and familial support needs.
4. Health plans should work with health care professionals to improve the effectiveness of health care delivery for children.
5. Health plans should establish linkages with public health, educational, social service, and other community-based organizations to prevent child health problems.

Responsibilities to the Community

1. Health plans should participate in community-based prevention and intervention efforts to improve long-term health outcomes for children.
2. Health plans should be accountable for their performance in meeting children's health needs.
3. Health plans should recognize and respect ethical standards of conduct toward children and their families.
4. Health plans should support community health monitoring and health services research concerning the care of children, while protecting patient confidentiality.
5. Health plans should support reasonable public policy initiatives that advance children's health.

munity accountabilities for children (Table 10.2), and review exemplary practices from health plans that are meeting these challenges. These guidelines and illustrations may be useful in thinking about how to measure managed care performance and encourage continuing improvement in the organization of health care delivery for children in the United States.

Antecedents for Managed Care and Its Potential Benefits for Children
The growth of managed care from an alternative to a mainstream method of structuring the delivery of health care services is often characterized as the result of evolutionary forces that are transforming the health care system. These forces arise from the recognition that:

- the traditional open-ended fee-for-service reimbursement system—
  with its emphasis on choice of health care professionals—generally

lacks mechanisms to coordinate care, evaluate performance systematically, or encourage appropriate preventive and primary care (Booth et al., 1993);

- conventional approaches to controlling rising medical costs—such as reducing provider reimbursement—have had perverse effects such as limiting physician participation in Medicaid and encouraging routine use of hospital emergency rooms (Cohen, 1993; Reisinger et al., 1994); and
- unwarranted variation in clinical practices—as seen in divergent rates of hospitalization and surgery for children in different communities— indicates a need for information and methods to improve the scientific basis and consistency of medical decision making (Berwick, 1989; Perrin et al., 1989; Wennberg and Gittelsohn, 1973).

In the early 1970s, the federal government sought to address these concerns, and to halt double-digit medical inflation, by encouraging the creation of a competitive health care market based on HMOs. HMOs originated earlier in this century as prepaid group practices that integrated the financing and delivery of health care to provide workers with coordinated, predictably priced, comprehensive benefits. Today, there are many health plan models, including broad networks of contracted physicians in private practice.

Well-run managed care organizations have adopted many common techniques to help optimize health care delivery (Table 10.3). These methods are important because health care professionals generally do not change their practice behaviors without some type of intervention, and many physicians have never received objective information about how they practice medicine (Grimshaw and Russell, 1993). By partnering with health care professionals to share information and encourage population-based health promotion, managed care programs may help rationalize episodic personal care services. Such an approach is both cost-effective and attractive from the point of view of patient quality of life. Ideally, this focus should include primary prevention through well-child care and immunizations, secondary prevention through early identification and treatment of problems, and tertiary prevention to minimize long-term complications and improve outcomes.

A growing body of research indicates that HMOs are making progress toward these goals for their enrolled populations (this discussion focuses on HMOs since there has been less evaluation of other forms of managed care). For example, HMO members are more likely to receive preventive cancer

Table 10.3

Methods Used by Managed Care Organizations to Optimize Health Care Delivery

1. Covering comprehensive benefits, including preventive services, with minimal copayments as appropriate to encourage prevention and early treatment of health problems.

   Examples: covering well-child visits including immunizations, ancillary therapies, home care, and outpatient mental health care; waiving copayments for prenatal care, or for those who complete the entire series of prenatal care visits.

2. Providing member education to encourage responsible use of health care resources and other interventions to address non-financial barriers to care.

   Examples: offering pediatric asthma education programs to avoid hospitalization for acute attacks; providing 24-hour telephone access and coordinating transportation services to physician offices for low-income families to reduce nonurgent use of the emergency room.

3. Coordinating and reviewing the medical necessity of coverage to encourage the provision of effective care in the most appropriate care setting.

   Examples: substituting effective outpatient treatment or home visits for inpatient care; coordinating transplant treatment at experienced medical centers to achieve better outcomes; covering Mantoux (PPD) tests instead of multipuncture (tine) tests for tuberculosis screening in accordance with American Academy of Pediatrics and CDC guidelines.

4. Selectively contracting with an appropriate mix of qualified hospitals, physicians, and other health care providers to stimulate accountability and price competition.

   Examples: reviewing the credentials of health professionals before contracting with them to ensure they meet professional standards; using a variety of compensation methods (including salary, discounted fee-for-service, or prepayment) based on plan philosophy, research, customer input, and marketplace factors.

5. Sharing financial risk, performance feedback, and clinical guidelines with physicians to reduce idiosyncratic variation in care and encourage cost-effective practice improvements.

   Examples: profiling physician performance on factors such as resource use, quality of care, and patient satisfaction compared to standards and/or peer-group norms; sharing data showing the benefit of administering antenatal corticosteroids to women in preterm labor (e.g., improved infant health outcomes and survival).

screening and participate in health promotion programs such as prenatal smoking counseling, elderly HMO members are more likely to visit their physician for a check-up and have cancer diagnosed at an earlier stage, and appendicitis patients in California HMOs are less likely to experience a ruptured appendix than fee-for-service patients (Braveman et al., 1994; Ershoff et al., 1990; Makuc et al., 1994; Miller and Luft, 1994; Riley et al., 1994).

Evidence on the Effectiveness of Managed Care for Children
It is helpful to review the research on managed care to identify the gaps in performance as well as in our empirical knowledge. More than 80 peer-reviewed studies and government-sponsored evaluations of managed care have been published since 1980, but these findings must be interpreted with caution given the infant state of measurement tools and limitations in study size and time frame, especially for children (Miller and Luft, 1994). Only a few studies focus on children, and studies of adults may or may not represent children's experiences in managed care. While studies of Medicaid managed care generally focus on women and children, administrative and population attributes of the Medicaid program may not be representative of private insurance coverage. Even where studies make use of a control group, there is little evidence that traditional coverage arrangements represent an adequate standard for comparison. In addition, rapid market changes and health plan development make it difficult to extrapolate from past to current performance. Descriptive articles indicate that health plans are undertaking a wide variety of initiatives to improve population health that are beginning to yield results. One example is an industrywide collaborative project with the Centers for Disease Control and Prevention (CDC) to increase pediatric immunization rates (CDC, 1995; Coffey, 1996).

Preventive and Primary Care
Some early Medicaid managed care demonstrations achieved little improvement in preventive care compared to traditional Medicaid (Carey et al., 1990). More recent studies have found increases in rates of pediatric immunization and other screening tests, the frequency and completeness of checkup visits, and the percentage of children who visit a primary care physician for allergy care and other treatment in managed care plans compared to traditional coverage (Balaban et al., 1994; Godfrey and Christiansen, 1995; Mustin et al., 1994; Szilagyi et al., 1992; Valdez et al., 1989). Controlled studies of payment methods have found no decline in primary care office visits

for Medicaid-insured children treated by prepaid (capitated) physicians. The frequency of primary care visits increased among physicians who received higher fee-for-service payments rather than the traditional Medicaid reim-bursement rates (Davidson et al., 1992; Hohlen et al., 1990). Another study of Medicaid found that the frequency of primary care visits was higher, and emergency room use lower, when patients selected plans that included their regular source of medical care (Hurley and Freund, 1989).

Emergent and Acute Care

Most studies of Medicaid managed care programs report declines in the use of emergency rooms for nonurgent care. While there is some evidence that HMOs can reduce inappropriate hospital use for children, results are not consistent in studies of Medicaid managed care. Children generally use the hospital less than adults, so reduction in rates of inappropriate hospital use may be limited primarily to those cases in which a child has a chronic con-dition that is responsive to improvements in access to ambulatory care (Bindman et al., 1995; Freund and Lewit, 1993). There were no observable short-term adverse outcomes associated with reduced hospital use for adults enrolled in one HMO (Siu et al., 1988). Newborns enrolled in the managed care plans of one national insurer had shorter hospital stays but no signifi-cant difference in readmission rates compared to those covered by tradi-tional insurance (Gazmararian and Koplan, 1996). Birth outcomes in two Medicaid managed care demonstration plans were similar to those in tradi-tional Medicaid (Carey et al., 1991). Noncontrolled studies of HMOs have reported low-birthweight rates better than the national average (rates were not adjusted for differences in patient characteristics) (Murata et al., 1994; NCQA, 1995).

Chronic/Specialty Care

One observational survey found that HMOs offer several advantages to children with special needs, such as more comprehensive benefits and med-ical case management. On the other hand, researchers interpreted some benefit limits and network and referral arrangements as potentially prob-lematic for children with chronic conditions (Fox et al., 1993). Rates of re-ferral to specialists are generally lower in managed care compared to traditional arrangements; more research is needed to judge whether this finding reflects improvement in continuity of primary care or inappropri-ate limitations on access to specialty care (Freund and Lewitt, 1993). Some pediatricians have reported perceived obstacles to specialty referral in health plans; clinical appropriateness of care was not evaluated in this survey (Cartland and Yridkonsky, 1993). In contrast, one study found that an HMO appropriately targeted needed services to low-income children with chronic conditions such as diabetes and allergies (Mauldon et al., 1994). The Medical Outcomes Study found no significant difference in outcomes between adults with mild to moderate chronic illness treated by HMO clinicians compared to those treated by fee-for-service practitioners; however, a subgroup of low-income patients did not fare as well in HMOs as in traditional care (Greenfield et al., 1995; Ware et al., 1996).

Mental Health Care

Prepaid coverage of mental health services for adults appears to achieve cost savings with little difference in outcomes for the average patient, though patients with more severe forms of mental illness fared less well over time compared to those with fee-for-service coverage. On the other hand, the quality of traditional mental health care was not appreciably better despite its much higher costs (Mechanic et al., 1995; Wells and Sturm, 1995). An early evaluation of Medicaid-insured children enrolled in a mental health preferred provider organization in Massachusetts found an increase in hospital readmissions, possibly due to problems with the clinical review process (Callahan et al., 1994). Another study found that managed care review programs were not associated with shorter hospital length of stay or with adverse clinical outcomes for children hospitalized in specialty mental health facilities (Eisen et al., 1995).

Satisfaction and Access

Adult family members generally assess satisfaction on behalf of children. In several studies overall satisfaction is similar or higher in managed care plans, while in some other studies it is higher in traditional arrangements; the vast majority of patients are generally satisfied regardless of type of coverage. Managed care enrollees tend to be more satisfied with plan cost and benefits and, in some studies, somewhat less satisfied with perceived access to, or choice of, physician (Allen et al., 1994; Davis et al., 1995; Donelan et al., 1996; Freund et al., 1989; MHDI, 1996; Safran et al., 1994; Sisk et al., 1996; Tempkin-Greener and Winchell, 1991). In several studies of perceived access, those in managed care plans were more likely to report that they had a medical visit or a usual source of care, greater overall and after-hours availability of health services, and shorter waiting times compared to those covered by traditional insurance or Medicaid. However, in one study, managed care participants were slightly more likely to say that they had an unmet medical need compared to similar people with traditional coverage (Freund et al., 1989; Mark and Mueller, 1996; Sisk et al., 1996).

Higher patient satisfaction is associated with length of enrollment and the ability to maintain one's regular source of care when switching to a managed care plan (Hurley et al., 1991). Hence, in states that require Medicaid beneficiaries to enroll in one of several HMOs (mandatory enrollment), health plans may face challenges to member satisfaction and retention, especially for families who fail to choose a plan on their own and are automatically assigned to one by the state. On the other hand, mandatory enrollment also can have positive benefits by reducing the potential for biased selection of healthy members that may occur in voluntary programs, increasing the average length of enrollment in plans, and encouraging more health plans to participate in serving Medicaid beneficiaries (Welch, 1988; West et al., 1996). Higher HMO enrollment in an area is associated with greater physician participation in Medicaid HMO networks, which leads to increased patient choice (Welch and Miller, 1988).

Cost Savings

Areas with higher HMO enrollment and hence a higher level of market competition experience a lower rate of increase in overall hospital and Medicare costs and commercial insurance premiums compared to markets with less competition (Robinson, 1996; Welch, 1994; Wickizer and Feldstein, 1995). Health care spending increased substantially less in California—where health plans selectively contract and negotiate payment with hospitals—than in states such as Maryland where the government regulates hospital rates (Melnick and Zwanziger, 1995). An evaluation of Medicaid managed care programs found cost savings ranging from 5 to 15 percent per beneficiary (Hurley et al., 1993, p. 102). States such as Arizona that require Medicaid beneficiaries to enroll in one of several HMOs have reduced the rate of growth in Medicaid spending over time to levels below the rate of growth in comparable traditional Medicaid programs (McCall et al., 1994).

Conclusion

The preponderance of available research indicates that most HMO members achieve similar health outcomes while receiving less intensive services than those covered through traditional arrangements (Brown et al., 1993; Freund et al., 1989; Miller and Luft, 1994). Because of the historic lack of methods to evaluate quality in health care, particularly for children, health plans have developed systems for measuring quality of care and patient satisfaction; however, more work is needed to refine and validate these tools (Gold et al., 1995b; Leatherman et al., 1991). Quality of care should continue to receive diligent study by impartial experts, and by health plans themselves, to detect areas for improvement in both managed care and traditional coverage arrangements.

Responsibilities for Enrolled Children

A health plan is operationally responsible to meet the medical needs of its enrolled patients, taking into account other environmental factors that may affect that goal. Children now represent an estimated one-third of the total membership in HMOs, a larger proportion than in the population generally (Table 10.1). Effective management of this age group is thus critical to the success of health plans. Only by successfully serving their members can health plans continue to provide benefit to the community at large.

The following responsibilities represent possible, but not necessarily exhaustive, general guidelines of conduct for health plans serving children. These goals are meant to build on the strengths of managed care and improve its performance, based on research findings described previously, and on our own vantage point within a managed care organization. To illustrate the current practices of some leading health plans in achieving these principles, we offer examples taken from published articles, industry reports, and the experience of health plans affiliated with United HealthCare Corporation, representing efforts of both nonprofit and for-profit organizations. These examples should not be regarded as rigid prescriptions for action, since health plans will continue to adopt innovative approaches to achieve these goals and to assess the effectiveness of their initiatives over time.

1. *Health plans should promote the integrity of relationships between patients and health care professionals.* Health care is not a business like any other, but involves a personal relationship between a child, a child's parent as appropriate, and the child's health care professional. Trust and open communication are key factors in patients' adherence to their physician's advice, satisfaction with their physician, and improved health status (Koehler et al., 1992; Safran et al., 1996). Physicians and other health care

professionals who provide medical care to children also act in a broader role as advocates for children, and can, if adequately trained and informed, screen for, and refer needs to, the social service system.

Health plan administrative processes should be structured to support health care professionals in improving their practices while avoiding unwarranted intrusion in professionals' relationships with patients. Likewise, medical guidelines should be viewed as augmenting physicians' training and experience, not replacing their judgment. For example, some health plans do not retrospectively review the appropriateness of coverage for ambulatory services performed by physicians whose overall practice style is consistent with health plan standards. Other plans use their information systems to generate immunization reminder letters for physicians, who in turn send them on to parents.

2. *Health plans should recognize the unique developmental needs of children in covering and coordinating appropriate care.* Health plans should evaluate and adapt their basic managed care approaches to address children's unique developmental vulnerabilities and age-specific characteristics in the epidemiology and management of disease (Halfon et al., 1996, p. 231; Newacheck and Taylor, 1992). This effort encompasses a plan's covered benefits, coordination of care, provider networks, payment mechanisms, and member education programs.

Covered Benefits.   Health plans act as the agents of purchasers in arranging for benefits specified in coverage contracts. Health plans should define and educate purchasers as needed on what is considered appropriate and cost-effective care for children based on scientifically valid evidence whenever available (Wagner et al., 1989). Benefits and clinical review criteria can then be tailored to account for the range of services needed to prevent and treat childhood health problems. Children with special needs may require rehabilitative and social support benefits that are broader than those typically covered under a traditional medical care model. Health plans should have mechanisms (such as case management) to offer a flexible assortment of benefits to enable intelligent and effective substitutes for more costly care (Mechanic et al., 1995).

Copayment levels should encourage responsible use of services without discouraging needed care. Research indicates that a nominal office visit copayment did not act as a barrier to immunization in one employer-insured population (Cherkin et al., 1990). Cost-sharing requirements generally should be reduced or waived for low-income families, for whom they are more likely to act as a financial barrier (Ching, 1995; Newacheck and Halfon, 1986a). Some health plans offer positive incentives to encourage preventive care, such as a coupon for diapers or groceries for families who complete their child's immunization series (Zablocki, 1995). Similarly, coverage of peak flow meters for children with asthma may encourage their use in adjusting medication and may promote communication with physicians to avoid acute asthma attacks.

Provider Networks. Health plans need to contract with geographically accessible primary care professionals and with an appropriate number and mix of specialists who are trained to address children's needs. Certain subspecialty care should almost always be provided in a tertiary care facility specially equipped to serve children (e.g., pediatric cardiology and neurosurgical services), while other services may be well managed in community facilities that provide medical-surgical care to both adults and children (e.g., routine ear, nose, and throat procedures). Health plans should evaluate whether children with severe mental illness or physical disabilities are best served through a specialized provider network that offers multidisciplinary expertise and community linkages to assure quality across a range of care needs. For example, one Ohio health plan contracts with an academic medical center for care of disabled patients (Ludden and Shusterman, 1995; Mechanic et al., 1995, p. 44; Master et al., 1996; Neff and Anderson, 1995).

Health plans are increasingly establishing contractual partnerships with inner-city hospitals and community health centers that are experienced and conveniently located to serve low-income children (Cisneros, 1996). Inner-city hospitals with affiliated primary care clinics can easily refer families who present at the emergency room with nonurgent symptoms. Health plans report that many community health centers can provide cost-effective, culturally sensitive services and share common goals emphasizing prevention and primary care (Abrams et al., 1995). Community health clinics can help health plan managers better understand the needs of underserved populations, and health plans can help selected clinics adapt to the business requirements of a managed care environment.

Coordination of Care. Research indicates that adequate primary care is the single most important aspect of a health care system associated with improved health and life expectancy overall (Starfield, 1994). Mental health and other chronic health problems are often encountered by primary care clinicians, who may need education and other support to help detect and treat these conditions, and to judge when they should seek consultation with, or referral to, specialists (AHCPR, 1993, p. iii). To assist in this effort, health plans should evaluate and share data describing the conditions under which the best processes and outcomes of care are achieved through primary or specialty care treatment, or through multidisciplinary teams of professionals. Current scientific knowledge in this area is often limited, and much more research is needed (McManus and Fox, 1996; Schwartz and Hillman, 1996).

Health plans with "gatekeepers" require that primary care physicians make all referrals to specialist physicians. Under this system, the primary care and specialty physicians should be able to arrange treatment plans allowing children with special needs to access specified services or see the specialist without getting repeated referrals. Some plans that review and approve specialist referrals are simplifying their systems to approve multiple visits rapidly based on diagnosis, or exempting most referrals from preauthorization requirements. A growing number of health plans allow patients to visit any provider in the network without getting a referral—a model likely to be attractive to families of children with special needs. Still other health plans allow a specialist to serve as a primary care provider for children with severe chronic illnesses; however, in these cases, the specialist must be willing and capable of coordinating the child's total care needs (Baldassano, 1996; Bilodeau, 1996).

Payment Mechanisms.   Health plans can support research and demonstration initiatives to analyze the effect of various payment methods on the delivery system. Under current market mechanisms, health plans and providers that are capitated may suffer losses if they attract a disproportionate number of individuals with conditions that are especially costly to treat (a situation known as "adverse risk selection"). In response, several states and other purchaser groups are working with health plans to study and test methods of risk-adjusting payment to account for high-cost conditions and care for severely disabled enrollees. Properly structured risk adjustment would provide incentives for health plans to contract with specialized providers and develop programs to serve children with special needs (Anonymous, 1996a; Master et al., 1996; Shewry et al., 1996).

Other prudent and innovative approaches are needed to address the growing budgetary limitations of the Medicaid program. For example, health plans are using savings achieved from reducing inappropriate hospital use (through better primary care management) to fund provider fee enhancements and improve provider participation rates, thus increasing choice of provider for low-income families with children. Some health plans also have designed incentives to encourage the provision of preventive care, such as paying an additional fee to capitated physicians when they submit timely reporting data after administering immunizations or Medicaid Early and Periodic Screening, Diagnosis and Treatment (EPSDT) exams (Zablocki, 1995).

Member Education. Families of children can benefit from age-specific education designed to improve quality of life and encourage appropriate use of health care resources. Member education is particularly important for children in low-income families headed by one parent, who are at greater risk for underusing primary and preventive care (Cunningham and Hahn, 1994). Many health plans offer 24-hour access to telephonic nurselines for education on self-care needs and help in navigating the health care system. This service can be helpful to families with children, especially in rural areas where after-hours access is limited. Pregnant and parenting adolescents have a unique combination of maternal and child health needs. A Massachusetts health plan teams high-risk pregnant teenagers with local medical students, who act as patient advocates and mentors to help teens obtain adequate prenatal and postnatal care (Packer-Tursman, 1996).

Education on plan procedures demonstrates a commitment to consumer protection and helps establish rapport, which may lead to greater patient satisfaction and retention. Some health plans offer parent support groups, resource centers, and consumer advisory committees to help identify and address gaps in performance (Anderson, 1996). Some make a personal "welcome call" to newly enrolled families (via telephone or home visit) to inform them about the plan and conduct a baseline health assessment at this time. Other plans arrange for a health plan nurse to visit mothers of newborns in the hospital to explain the importance of well-child care and help them choose a pediatrician (DeFino, 1995).

Since the care-seeking behavior of parents largely determines health care access for children, member education should emphasize the family's responsibility for the "self-care" of young children. Education programs should address unique child health beliefs and the benefits of parental involvement in child health promotion (Bush and Ianotti, 1990; Newacheck and Halfon, 1986b; Perry et al., 1989). Health plans serving children with special needs will find it important to involve families in defining goals for health achievement. Plans may need to designate specially educated member services staff or case management teams to answer complex questions and coordinate access to medical and social services. For example, disabled patients (or their parents) in an Ohio health plan are full participants on a treatment planning team that includes their primary care physician, nurse case manager, and social worker (see chapter 16 for a full description of this program) (Anderson, 1996; Master et al., 1996).

An emphasis on primary care prevention and counseling can make a difference in children's attempts to make health behavior changes (Gemson et al., 1995). Teenagers especially may benefit from confidential counseling on topics including pregnancy prevention, sexually transmitted diseases, proper nutrition, and use of tobacco or alcohol. For example, teenagers in one HMO reduced their alcohol consumption as a result of a comprehensive chemical dependency treatment program (Freeborn et al., 1991). Health professionals may benefit from education about effective methods of counseling adolescents; many physicians in one group practice rated their competence in some areas of adolescent care as "less than desirable" (Klitsner et al., 1992).

3. *Health plans should help lower nonfinancial barriers to care through sensitivity to cultural, linguistic, socioeconomic, and familial support needs.* Research indicates that providing financial access is not sufficient to induce improvements in care-seeking behaviors (Halfon et al., 1995). For example, overuse of the emergency room is often a convenience issue for low-income parents who have difficulty negotiating public transportation with infants and children. In response, several health plans serving Medicaid beneficiaries are coordinating transportation and child care services and developing reminder systems to help parents keep scheduled office appointments (NASHP, 1993).

To overcome communications barriers, health plans are paying for interpreter services, hiring multicultural and multilingual member services staff, and helping low-income members establish phone service. Member education materials should be presented at a comprehension and cultural level appropriate to the intended audience and primary language spoken, and explain the consequences of noncompliance on health. One Medicaid health plan employs community residents as lay home health education visitors to reinforce preventive messages under the supervision of a visiting nurse who administers immunizations (DeFino, 1995).

Provider education and support can be important to help contracted health care professionals interact successfully with patients who do not share common backgrounds. A Minnesota health plan worked with the local health department to help health care professionals understand ethnically related care-seeking expectations of Medicaid-insured refugees in their service area. The setting for health visits and other contacts may be an important means of gaining trust and assuring confidentiality. A California health plan has created special teen clinics where adolescents can make private appointments to see a member of a multidisciplinary staff that includes physicians, nurse practitioners, social workers, psychologists, and nutritionists (AAHP, 1996b). A Rhode Island plan houses its Medicaid administrative staff at an inner-city hospital where members can drop in for information on benefits and services.

4. *Health plans should work with health professionals to improve the effectiveness of health care delivery for children.* A commitment to continuous improvement offers a mechanism for identifying and systematically correcting weaknesses in the health care system. Because health plans enroll defined populations, they are able to adopt epidemiological approaches such as using clinical information systems for data analysis of practice patterns, designing and implementing interventions at the level of the individual health professional or patient, and evaluating program effectiveness over time. Ideally, such a process will create a collaborative effort among health plans, families, and health professionals, who will work together to understand and lower barriers to effective care (Wagner, 1995).

For example, some health plan quality improvement projects have analyzed health plan data and surveyed physicians to understand the reasons for inadequate immunization rates. A common finding is that the majority of children with incomplete immunizations are in their physician's office near the immunization due date. Typical interventions include educating physicians about which contraindications are valid and which are not, according to the CDC; improving office-based reminder systems; and notifying parents of overdue immunizations. These efforts have improved completion rates by 30 percentage points or more in these managed care organizations (Cleary, 1995; Leatherman et al., 1995; Lieu et al., 1994; McPhillips et al., 1996).

Follow-up care of low-birthweight infants is another important area of inquiry, where research has shown that a supportive environment can improve outcomes such as intelligence quotient (IQ) and behavior-problem scores (Infant Health and Development Program, 1990). Using clinical data on preterm births, a Massachusetts HMO was able to design a developmental monitoring program of home education visits and telephone follow-up during the two years following birth. The goal is to improve family coping and quality of life, prevent adverse outcomes, and reduce a high rate of office visits (Ladden, 1996).

To reduce high rates of asthma-related emergency department visits and hospital admissions, a number of health plans have developed asthma management programs centered on a home visit by a nurse. Education in the home facilitates the identification of stressors and allergens in the day-to-day environment, the discussion of proper medication use, and the demonstration of routine monitoring with a peak flow meter. Other program components may include developing an action plan in conjunction with the child's physician, conducting follow-up phone calls to reinforce education and identify problems, establishing linkages to community-based organizations and schools, and measuring changes in functional status over time (Hanchak et al., 1996; Heinen et al., 1993; Plaut et al., 1996).

5. *Health plans should establish linkages with public health, educational, social service, and other community-based agencies to prevent child health problems.* Health status is influenced by a continuum of biologic, behavioral, environmental, and social determinants. Nonmedical needs that affect health include personal safety, nutrition, shelter, education, and family security (Oberg et al., 1994, p. 6). Through coordinated efforts with government, charitable, and advocacy groups, health plans can identify root causes of health problems and design programs to improve health outcomes considering medical and other factors. For example, health-related needs may be identified in nontraditional settings, such as schools, where opportunities for more frequent contacts can enhance prevention efforts. In recognition of this fact, some health plans are designating school-based clinics as network providers for screening, prevention, and counseling services (AAHP, 1996b; Brindis, 1995).

Health plans may need to collaborate with social service programs to arrange for education and information to support health professionals in screening for developmental deficits and making referrals to community services, since health professionals may not be aware of the full range of resources. Government programs such as the state's Title V Children with

Special Health Needs program office may provide assistance in this regard. To create such linkages, two health plans in Minnesota employ social workers to help assess family needs and make referrals to appropriate community programs (DeFino, 1995). Other health plans are contracting with local public health agencies and voluntary nursing associations to provide outreach and case management services (Cunningham, 1996). Cooperative efforts can have clear benefits for health plans. For example, referring the mother of a hungry child to apply for food supplements under the federal Special Supplemental Food Program for Women, Infants and Children (WIC) can reduce medical costs for treating the complications of malnutrition, estimated at $3 saved for every $1 of WIC benefits received (Oberg et al., 1994, p. 52).

Responsibilities to the Community
Templeton prize-winner Michael Novak argues that free enterprise serves an important democratic role as a counterbalance to government in a republic such as ours. He argues that every business has a duty to "protect the moral ecology of freedom" on which its existence as a private institution depends. It does this through right conduct and by exerting leadership with other private institutions to strengthen civil society and the welfare of the community at large. This imperative to uphold the right of private initiative transcends profit/nonprofit distinctions and differences in health plan tax status. Market incentive to maintain operating reserves or to create profit produces incidental social benefits—such as economically productive job creation and an inspiration for inventiveness—important to children's future economic opportunity (Novak, 1996).

All health plans benefit from the publicly funded medical, public health, and social service infrastructure in fulfilling their private duties to enrolled populations (Showstack et al., 1996). Health plans are not welfare agencies, but—through cooperative effort and moral encouragement of these institutions—they can support the goals of public health, defined by the Institute of Medicine as ". . . fulfilling society's interest in assuring conditions in which people can be healthy" (Breslow, 1996). For example, health plans serving the Medicaid population have an incentive to cultivate grassroots community linkages that build trust and essential "word-of-mouth" reputation. This civic interest can benefit the health plan's entire child-age population and make the plan a more responsible participant in the community. As health plans assume responsibility for safety-net medical care, public health agencies can focus on their core function—community-wide health surveillance and prevention—that in turn supports individual health plan efforts (Baker et al., 1994).

While many of the guidelines outlined next will benefit a health plan's enrolled children, they also have wider social benefit to the community at large.

1. *Health plans should participate in community-based prevention and intervention efforts to improve long-term health outcomes for children.* There is wide agreement that society—through both government and private institutions—owes a special obligation to assist families in helping children at risk for developmental deficits. Children are increasingly at risk from a new set of social "morbidities"—such as drug and alcohol abuse, violence, sexually transmitted diseases, and teen pregnancy—that affect health but cannot be treated as purely medical problems. Recent research has found that multilevel educational efforts linked to schools, families, and the community may achieve the best results in preventing the social "vectors" underlying these behaviors (Perry et al., 1996). These programs may be cost-effective from a societal standpoint, but not necessarily when considering only medical costs (Olds et al., 1993).

Managed care by definition encourages a public health focus on maintaining and improving the health of enrolled populations. Yet annual turnover in enrollment within managed care plans may weaken the incentive for certain prevention efforts that offer only long-term benefits. In response, one HMO medical director argues that health plans must take a broader perspective of the community as a pool of potential future enrollees (Anonymous, 1996b). An understanding of the wider social and environmental etiology of medical problems will help health plan managers recognize that collaborative public health initiatives promise greater collective gains in outcome for their enrolled populations than individual plans could achieve acting independently.

There are many promising examples of such public-private collaboration taking place today (AAHP, 1996b; Anonymous, 1996b; Thompson et al., 1995):

- Georgia HMOs are jointly building bridges with community public health services through the Atlanta Community Partnership Program to reduce avoidable problems associated with childhood asthma.

- Several health plans throughout the country are collaborating with the public schools to sponsor health and prevention education and immunization programs for students.
- One Ohio health plan partners with the county health department to offer a free community immunization clinic one Saturday each month; the county supplies the vaccine and the health plan provides nursing staff.
- In Minnesota, health plans are participating on a statewide task force to identify cooperative mechanisms for reducing community violence.
- A Washington State health plan collaborated in a community-wide program to increase the use of bicycle safety helmets, with corresponding reductions in bicycle-related head injuries among member children.

To ensure that community collaboration is an integral part of the health care market, community leaders must work with health plans, purchasers, providers, public health agencies, and community-based organizations to build such linkages—an approach bearing fruit in Kingsport, Tennessee (McLaughlin, 1995). However, current community health efforts may be more likely to occur in mature markets with higher levels of managed care penetration. One evaluation found that public health activities undertaken by health plans were motivated primarily by charitable considerations at the periphery of their operations (Chapel, 1996). To address these issues, purchasers such as business coalitions and state Medicaid agencies must create market norms so that health plans perceive communitywide prevention initiatives as business goals that are critical to their success—in effect, making these efforts an implicit part of the defined benefits package. Purchasers should find value in a health plan's participation in community-based efforts leading to a healthier labor pool, reduced absenteeism from school, and fewer lost workdays for parents (Anonymous, 1996b; Cunningham, 1996; Weitzman, 1986).

If voluntary effort to create a community-oriented market is not successful, legislators may feel compelled to mandate such a goal. The banking industry provides a useful analogy. Evidence that banks were failing to serve disadvantaged neighborhoods adequately led Congress to pass the Community Reinvestment Act requiring banking institutions to make credit available in all areas of the community, including low- and moderate-income areas. The Act does not specify numeric loan targets, but requires federal regulatory agencies to evaluate how well each institution meets its community obligations; such evaluations are publicly disclosed and considered in approving bank expansions (FFIEC, 1990). This kind of regulatory approach may encourage more uniform community responsibility across health plans, but also may pose drawbacks such as potential inflexibility in meeting local needs, disrupting existing voluntary arrangements, or giving market advantage to firms that have greater monetary resources to support collaboration.

2. *Health plans should be accountable for their performance in meeting children's health needs.* Health plans collectively benefit society by defining distinct goals to which they can be held accountable by their boards, consumers, purchasers, stockholders, and the public. All health plans have contractual obligations to health care purchasers and/or parents of covered children. Large employers and purchasing coalitions such as the Pacific Business Group on Health have created population-oriented contractual standards and premium rewards for health plans that meet agreed-upon patient satisfaction, preventive care, and performance reporting goals. These purchasers are collaborating with health plans to identify information that is meaningful to consumers in comparing the value of different plans (Hoy et al., 1996; Schaffler and Rodriguez, 1996). As government finances a growing share of total health care spending, its contractual role as purchaser may be its most effective means of holding plans accountable for meeting the needs of children. For example, Arizona's bidding process for Medicaid contracts places more weight on access and quality of care factors than on cost (GAO, 1995c). States should avoid micromanaging health plans through excessive contractual requirements, but set reasonably specific performance goals and allow health plans to innovate to achieve them (England and Cole, 1995).

Where there is variability in performance within a market-based system, purchasers and consumers must be educated and given information so that they can make informed choices leading to effective market norms. For example, consumers may have varying preferences for different health plan networks based on the type of professional practice (e.g., clinics or private offices) and geographic accessibility of providers. At the same time, they must be able to identify and express a preference for specific attributes of plan performance that they find important and relevant to their own unique situation, such as quality of doctors, courtesy of interactions with physicians and health plan staff, the range of services covered, and cost.

More research is needed on the amount and format of information that consumers understand and find useful in making actual decisions (Edgman-Levitan and Cleary, 1996; Isaacs, 1996). Since the average consumer may not be able to discern when trade-offs between costs and benefits might adversely affect children, this information (as well as the benefit plan design) must be structured to facilitate reasonable choices. In addition, health plans and purchasers should share information so that payment is not negotiated to the point of sacrificing quality or benefits that are essential to effective care of children.

To provide a structure for accountability, health plans should support the continuing development of community and industry standards to measure performance for reporting and accreditation purposes. Much work already has been done in this area through standard-setting bodies, such as the National Committee on Quality Assurance (NCQA) and the Joint Commission on Accreditation of Healthcare Organizations (JCAHO), among others (Corrigan and Nielsen, 1994; Iglehart, 1996). Additional work is currently underway to define new measures that adequately describe the full range of children's health issues meaningful to clinicians, health plans, and purchasers (McGlynn et al., 1996). More research is needed to identify the linkages between process and outcomes of care so that clinicians and health plans can identify actions to improve quality as a result of performance findings (Hammermeister et al., 1995). Where cost or data limitations make collecting outcomes indicators unfeasible, measuring compliance to process-of-care guidelines may represent the most practical (in some cases, the only) approach to performance reporting. National goals—such as the *Healthy People 2000* objectives—and other collaborative initiatives can help to ensure that individual health plan efforts to improve quality of care for defined populations make a difference in the broader national population.

Concern about public image and legal liability also plays a role in influencing the social accountability of health plans. Health plans must bear the burden for explaining the basis for their coverage decisions, and the fear of adverse publicity can play a constructive role in preventing unreasonable practices. However, in cases involving complex medical failures, it is difficult for the public to fix the proper locus for accountability. Health plans—as the visible agent organizing networks of physicians—may be implicated as culprits in cases of physician negligence. Health plans should be held accountable for establishing reasonable processes for assessing the credentials of physicians participating in their networks, and for objectively considering appeals of benefits coverage decisions from patients and physicians. However, holding health plans responsible in professional malpractice cases might cause plans to become more directive in medical care as they seek to control their exposure to liability—with negative consequences for physician autonomy. This is a thorny area for the legal system and for society as the promise of managed care raises performance expectations, and as anecdotal cases are used as ammunition in ideological debates about the motives of health plans (Boyd and Kelley, 1996; Zelman, 1996, p. 304).

3. *Health plans should recognize and respect ethical standards of conduct toward children and their families.* Health care is widely regarded as a fundamental human need, the provision of which differs qualitatively from typical business transactions. Arranging insurance coverage for such a socially valued need implies a duty of ethical behavior to the purchaser, the individual insured, and society at large. Such ethical duties include communicating honestly and fully with prospective enrollees and enrolled families of children, engaging in honest marketing practices, sponsoring responsible advertising, and so on (Novak, 1996). For example, health plans marketing to Medicaid-eligible families would do well to use health-related messages— such as a preventive-care display at a health fair—rather than token gifts to raise awareness in the community. Health plans can reinforce an ethical culture by establishing a "zero-tolerance" policy for violations of defined marketing standards, and set compensation for marketing representatives to reward retention of members rather than just initial enrollment (IAHMO, 1996).

4. *Health plans should support community health monitoring and health services research concerning the care of children, while protecting patient confidentiality.* Health plans routinely collect data for claims payment and administrative purposes, and use these data to monitor cost and quality issues for their defined populations. Combining these data (in aggregate or encrypted format to protect patient confidentiality) could facilitate comprehensive community health monitoring efforts, such as evaluating the impact of community-wide prevention efforts on aggregate medical care use. A voluntary public-private partnership can provide a flexible approach to creating shared goals and benefits. Objectives must be clearly defined, cost-beneficial, and feasible. For example, consider that vaccination records

are often fragmented among multiple physician offices and clinics that children visit over time. Creating a community-wide immunization registry would make vaccination information portable as children move between different providers and health plans.

Several managed care organizations have developed health services research expertise to study broader questions concerning medical and managed care practices and effectiveness, often in collaboration with external government, academic, and research institutions.* For example, several organizations are assisting the CDC in studies of prevention effectiveness. One such cooperative effort at United HealthCare involves studying treatment of acute otitis media (middle ear infection), a common problem affecting children. Such studies demonstrate the usefulness of health plan data for monitoring specific therapeutic approaches in disease management and changes in those patterns over time (Bernstein et al., 1996; CDC, 1996; Peterson et al., 1996).

5. Health plans should support reasonable public policy initiatives that advance children's health. Health plans have supported incremental federal portability standards, which will help ensure that children who have chronic illnesses do not lose access to employer-sponsored coverage when their parents change jobs or health plans. As a next step, health plans can exert leadership to help identify equitable broad-based funding mechanisms for uncompensated care, and solutions to increase coverage for uninsured children.

Health plans should recognize that reasonably balanced regulatory standards may be needed to protect the interests of vulnerable citizens—such as children—who lack economic clout in the marketplace. Federal and state legislation should complement but not substitute for market-based reforms, unless the market fails to produce desired outcomes or the risk of market failure is too great. Regulation should not stifle constructive innovation in health care delivery models or codify standards of care that restrict physicians' exercise of medical judgment.

---

*A partial list includes Aetna/U.S. Healthcare, Group Health Cooperative of Puget Sound, Fallon Community Health Plan, Harvard Pilgrim Health Care, Health Insurance Plan of Greater New York, Henry Ford Health System, Kaiser Permanente, Lovelace Health System (CIGNA), Prudential Healthcare, and United HealthCare.

Conclusion and Implications for Future Policy

As we think about the future, we should not presume that current forms of managed care necessarily represent an ideal, or that managed care is a panacea for solving all our nation's health care problems. One of the most important attributes of market-based managed care is its flexibility to evolve in response to consumer needs and purchaser demands, as well as to public policy challenges. Evidence can be found in efforts by health plans to ease access to specialists in response to market demand, and in recent announcements by the American Association of Health Plans that member organizations will share more detailed information with consumers and physicians on plan coverage procedures (AAHP, 1996a). Likewise, the recent maternity discharge issue offers an important lesson for health plans to design their coverage policies in careful consideration of physician discretion and patient quality of life. Health plans and purchasers must continue to share information so that consumer preferences become increasingly salient in defining market competition on the basis of performance improvement (Hoy et al., 1996).

Some may fear that evolutionary market improvement is too risky an undertaking where children's health is concerned. However, the alternative—a government single-payer program—would not necessarily guarantee access to high-quality care for children in this country. Today Canadians find their health system increasingly underfunded, and are discussing the need for a supplemental private system to address a lack of resources and common delays in treatment (BNA, 1996). The current funding crisis in the U.S. Medicare program stems in part from demographics, but also from a lack of accountability (GAO, 1995a,b). Nevertheless, the specter of a nationalized health system can make managed care organizations collectively more responsive to improvement over time. In turn, the effects of positive managed care practices—such as those illustrated in this chapter—may spill over to traditional coverage arrangements as health plans enroll and contract with an increasing proportion of patients and health care providers.

Underlying this chapter is a recognition that Americans tend to prefer a market-oriented allocation of resources to meet individual needs, but they still believe in a basic safety net so that everyone has an equal opportunity to succeed (Times Mirror Center for The People and The Press, 1995). In this light, cost-containment is not the end-goal of the health care system, but rather a necessary strategic objective to preserve and expand coverage for children and others. Cost-effective managed care practices enable health plans to cover comprehensive benefits, and have helped states such as Oregon and Tennessee subsidize coverage for thousands of previously uninsured individuals (Gold et al., 1995a). (While these programs have experienced some initial implementation problems, the potential benefits of expanded coverage should not be discounted.) Managed care savings alone are not enough to fund coverage for all uninsured children, but can assist in reaching that goal.

The challenge ahead is to provide all children with access to effective medical care that is well integrated within the continuum of services needed to improve health, both individually and collectively. This goal may require a reordering in our thinking about market-based health care delivery. Both the personal health care system and the free market system in the United States reflect deeply rooted notions of individual freedom and autonomy inherent in the American psychology. As a society, we benefit from a rich heritage of rights and justice that flow from this paradigm. Yet we may experience a cultural "downside" in the often-fragmented way that health services are delivered and a lack of coordination with and among public health and social services. Growing awareness of the benefit and need for communitywide prevention efforts provides an opportunity to engage the public in collaboration with all participants in the health and welfare system (Fielding and Halfon, 1994).

The guidelines elaborated in this chapter may provide a good starting point for health plan involvement in the community. Given a realistic appraisal of human nature and society, we should not expect health plans to actively pursue these goals if the market is not structured to reward such desired behavior. Purchasers, health plans, policymakers, parents, and the public must work in good faith to create market incentives so that accountability for long-term population health improvement (primarily for enrolled populations and secondarily in the community) is a key factor in competitive success for health plans. Enlightened by the knowledge that our collective future resides in the well-being of our children, our efforts should be guided by a vision of a community-oriented market that achieves the best possible outcomes for children in society.

References

[AAHP] American Association of Health Plans. 1996a Dec. 17. Health plans address patients' need for better information. Washington: AAHP.

[AAHP] American Association of Health Plans. 1996b. Health plans with infant and children's programs: Examples. Washington: AAHP.

Abrams R, Savela T, Trinity MT, et al. 1995. Performance of community health centers under managed care. Journal of Ambulatory Care Management 18(3):77–88.

[AHCPR] Agency for Health Care Policy and Research. 1993. Depression in primary care: Clinical practice guideline. Rockville, MD: U.S. Public Health Service.

Allen HM, Darling H, McNeill DN, et al. 1994 Fall. The employee health care value survey: Round one. Health Affairs 13:25–41.

Anderson B. 1996. Caring for children with special needs in HMOs: The consumer's perspective. Managed Care Quarterly 4(3):36–40.

Angell M, Kassirer JP. 1996. Quality and the medical marketplace—following elephants. The New England Journal of Medicine 335:883–5.

[Anonymous]. 1996a July. Risk adjustment: What is its real potential for reducing risk selection? In: Health care financing and organization news and progress, pp. 1–3. Washington: The Alpha Center.

[Anonymous] 1996b May–June. Public health and managed care organizations—a new era of collaboration? In: State initiatives in health care reform, pp. 2–4, 10. Washington: The Alpha Center.

Baker EL, Melton RJ, Strange PV, et al. 1994. Health reform and the health of the public. Journal of the American Medical Association 272:1276–82.

Balaban D, McCall N, Bauder EJ. 1994. Quality of Medicaid managed care: An evaluation of the Arizona health care cost containment system. Discussion Paper 94-2. San Francisco: Laguna Research Associates.

Baldassano V. 1996 Aug. 7. Member complaints push HMOs to streamline referrals to specialists. Managed Care Reporter, pp. 758–60.

Bernstein J, Bernstein AB, Shannon T, editors. 1966 March. Building bridges between the HMO and health services research communities. Medical Care Research and Review 53(special suppl.).

Berwick DM. 1989. Continuous improvements as an ideal in health care. New England Journal of Medicine 320:53.

Bilodeau JA. 1996 April. Trying out alternatives to the "gatekeeper" system. Managed Care, pp. 18–20.

Bindman AG, Grumback K, Osmond D, et al. 1995. Preventable hospitalizations and access to health care. Journal of the American Medical Association 274:305–11.

[BNA] Bureau of National Affairs. 1996 Aug. 26. Canadian doctors vote to reject two-tiered health care system. Health Care Policy Report, pp. 1372–3.

Booth M, Coburn A, Riley T. 1993. Improving access and quality of care under Medicaid managed care: Proposals for reform. Portland, ME: The National Academy for State Health Policy.

Boyd J, Kelley L. 1996 Fall. Health Law 2000: Regulation, litigation, or strangulation? Health Affairs 15:31–4.

Braveman P, Schaaf VM, Egerter S, et al. 1994. Insurance-related differences in the risk of ruptured appendix. New England Journal of Medicine 331:444–9.

Breslow L. 1996 Spring. Public health and managed care: A California perspective. Health Affairs 15:92.

Brindis C. 1995. Promising approaches for adolescent reproductive health service delivery: The role of school-based health centers in a managed care environment. Western Journal of Medicine 163(suppl.):50–6.

Brown RS, Bergeron J, Clement DG, et al. 1993 Feb. The Medicare risk program for HMOs: Final summary report on findings from the evaluation. Princeton, NJ: Mathematica Policy Research, Inc.

Bush PJ, Ianotti RJ. 1990. A children's health belief model. Medical Care 28:69–86.

Callahan JJ, Shepard DS, Beinecke RH, et al. 1994. Evaluation of the Massachusetts Medicaid mental health/substance abuse program. Waltham, MA: Heller School for Advanced Studies in Social Welfare.

Carey TS, Weis KS, Homer C. 1990. Prepaid versus traditional Medicaid plans: Effects on preventive health care. Journal of Clinical Epidemiology 43:1213–20.

Carey TS, Weis K, Homer C. 1991. Prepaid versus traditional Medicaid plans: Lack of effect on pregnancy outcomes and prenatal care. Health Services Research 26:165–81.

Cartland JDC, Yridkonsky YB. 1993. Barriers to pediatric referral in managed care. Pediatrics 89:183–92.

[CDC] Centers for Disease Control and Prevention. 1995. Prevention and managed care: Opportunities for managed care organizations, purchasers of health care, and public health agencies. Morbidity and Mortality Weekly Report 44:RR-14:5–6.

[CDC] Centers for Disease Control and Prevention. 1966 May. Inventory of managed care related projects: 1995–1996. Atlanta, GA: Public Health Service.

Chapel T. 1996 March. Private sector health care organizations and public health. Prepared for the Centers for Disease Control and Prevention. Atlanta, GA: Macro International.

Cherkin DC, Grothaus L, Wagner EH. 1990. The effect of office visit co-payments on preventive care services in an HMO. Inquiry 27:24–38.

Ching P. 1995. User fees, demand for children's health care and access across income groups: The Philippine case. Social Science and Medicine 41:37–46.

Cisneros RJ. 1996. U.S. hospitals and the future of health care: A continuing opinion survey. 6th ed., 1996. Philadelphia: Deloitte & Touche.

Cleary K. 1995. Using claims data to measure and improve the MMR immunization rate in an HMO. Joint Commission Journal on Quality Improvement 21:211–7.

Coffey LP. 1996 May–June. Care for children. HMO Magazine 37:86–93.

Cohen JW. 1993 Fall. Medicaid physician fees and use of physician and hospital services. Inquiry 30:281–92.

Corrigan JM, Nielsen DM. 1994. Toward the development of uniform reporting standards for managed care organizations: The health plan employer data and information set. Joint Commission Journal on Quality Improvement 19:566–75.

Cunningham PJ, Hahn BA. 1994 Winter. The changing American family: Implications for children's health insurance coverage and the use of ambulatory care services. The Future of Children 4:23–42.

Cunningham R. 1996 Aug. 5. Renegotiating the social contract in public health. Medicine and Health Perspectives. Washington: Faulkner & Gray, Inc.

Davidson SM, Manheim LM, Werner SM, et al., 1992. Prepayment with office-based physicians in publicly funded programs: Results from the children's Medicaid program. Pediatrics 89:761–7.

Davis K, Collins KS, Schoen C, et al. 1995 Summer. Choice matters for consumers. Health Affairs 14:99–112.

DeFino T. 1995 Sept.–Oct. Keeping the promise. HMO Magazine 36:46–51.

Donelan K, Blendon RJ, Benson J, et al. 1996 Summer. All payer, single payer, managed care, no payer: Patients' perspectives in three nations. Health Affairs 15:254–65.

Edgman-Levitan S, Cleary PD. 1996 Winter. What information do consumers want and need? Health Affairs 15:42–56.

Eisen V, Griffin M, Sederer LI, et al. 1995. The impact of preadmission approval and continued stay review on hospital stay and outcome among children and adolescents. Journal of Mental Health Administration 22:270–7.

Ellwood PM, Lundberg GD. 1996. Managed care: A work in progress. Journal of the American Medical Association 276:1083–6.

England MJ, Cole RF. 1995 Fall. Children and mental health: How can the system be improved? Health Affairs 14:131–8.

Ershoff DH, Quinn VP, Mullen PD, et al. 1990. Pregnancy and medical cost outcomes for a self-help prenatal smoking cessation program in a HMO. Public Health Reporter 105:340–7.

[FFIEC] Federal Financial Institutions Examination Council. 1990 Sept. Community Reinvestment Act: Performance evaluations. Washington: FFIEC.

Fielding J, Halfon N. 1994. Where is the health in health system reform? Journal of the American Medical Association 272:1292–6.

Finkelstein R, Hurwit C, Kirsch R. 1995 Oct. The managed care consumers' bill of rights: A health policy guide for consumer advocates. New York: The Public Policy and Education Fund of New York.

Fox HB, Wicks LB, Newacheck PW. 1993. Health maintenance organizations and children with special health care needs: A suitable match? American Journal of Disability in Children 147:546–52.

Freeborn DK, Beaudet MP, Mullooly JP, et al. 1991 March–April. Adolescent chemical dependency treatment in HMO. HMO Practice 4:44–50.

Freund DA, Lewitt EM. 1993 Summer–Fall. Managed care for children and pregnant women: Promises and pitfalls. Future of Children 3:92–122.

Freund DA, Rossiter LF, Fox PD, et al. 1989. Evaluation of the Medicaid competition demonstrations. Health Care Financing Review 11:81–97.

[GAO] General Accounting Office. 1995a March 22. Medicare and Medicaid: Opportunities to save program dollars by reducing fraud and abuse (testimony of S. F. Jagger). GAO/HEHS-95-110. Washington: U.S. Government Printing Office.

[GAO] General Accounting Office. 1995b Sept. Medicare spending: Modern management strategies needed to curb billions in wasteful spending. GAO/HEHS-95-210. Washington: U.S. Government Printing Office.

[GAO] General Accounting Office. 1995c Oct. Arizona Medicaid: Competition among managed care plans lowers program costs. GAO/HEHS-96-2. Washington: U.S. Government Printing Office.

[GAO] General Accounting Office. 1996 June. Health insurance for children: Private insurance coverage continues to deteriorate. GAO/HEHS-96-129. Washington: U.S. Government Printing Office.

Gazmararian JA, Koplan JP. 1996 Winter. Length-of-stay after delivery: Managed care versus fee-for-service. Health Affairs 15:74–80.

Gemson DH, Ashford AR, Dickey LL, et al. 1995. Putting prevention into practice: Impact of a multifaceted physician education program on prevention services in an inner city. Archives of Internal Medicine 155: 2210–6.

Godfrey L, Christiansen B. 1995. Wisconsin Medicaid program: HMO/fee-for-service comparison report: 1993–94. Madison, WI: Bureau of Health Care Financing.

Gold M, Frazer H, Schoen C, et al. 1995a July. Managed care and low-income populations: A case study of managed care in Oregon; A case study of managed care in Tennessee. Menlo Park, CA: The Henry J. Kaiser Family Foundation.

Gold MR, Hurley R, Lake T, et al. 1995b. A national survey of the arrangements managed care plans make with physicians. New England Journal of Medicine 333:1678–83.

Greenfield S, Rogers W, Mangotich M, et al. 1995. Outcomes of patients with hypertension and non-insulin-dependent diabetes mellitus treated by different systems and specialties: Results from the medical outcomes study. Journal of the American Medical Association 274:1436–44.

Grimshaw JM, Russell IT. 1993. Effect of clinical guidelines on medical practice: A systematic review of the rigorous evaluations. The Lancet 342:1317–22.

Halfon N, Inkelas M, Wood D. 1995. Nonfinancial barriers to care for children and youth. Annual Review of Public Health 16:447–72.

Halfon N, Inkelas M, Wood DL, et al. 1996. Refinancing and restructuring the U.S. child health system. In: Andersen RM, Rice TH, Kominski GF, editors. 1996. Changing the U.S. health care system, pp. 227–54. San Francisco: Jossey-Bass.

Hammermeister KE, Shroyer AL, Sethi GK, et al. 1995. Why it is important to demonstrate linkages between outcomes of care and processes and structures of care. Medical Care 22:OS5–16.

Hanchak NA, Murray JF, Arkans H, et al. 1996. Improved outcomes of an outpatient pediatric asthma patient management program in an IPA HMO. The American Journal of Managed Care 2:387–92.

Heinen L, Peterson E, Pion K. 1993. Quality evaluation in a managed care system: Comparative data to assess health plan performance. Managed Care Quarterly 1:62–76.

Hohlen MM, Manheim LM, Fleming GV, et al. 1990. Access to office-based physicians under capitation reimbursement and Medicaid case management: Findings from the children's Medicaid program. Medical Care 28:59–68.

Hoy EJ, Wicks EK, Forland RA. 1996 Winter. A guide to facilitating consumer choice. Health Affairs 15:9–30.

Hurley RE, Freund DA. 1989. Gatekeeping the emergency department: Impact of a Medicaid primary care case management program. Health Care Management Review 14:63–71.

Hurley RE, Gage, BJ, Freund DA. 1991. Rollover effects in gatekeeper programs: Cushioning the impact of restricted choice. Inquiry 28:375–84.

Hurley RE, Freund DA, Paul JE. 1993. Managed care in Medicaid: Lessons for policy and program design. Ann Arbor, MI: Health Administration Press.

Hurley R, Lake T, Gold M, et al. 1996. Arrangements between managed care plans and physicians II: A follow-up on the analysis of 1994 survey data and site visit information. Washington: Physician Payment Review Commission.

[IAHMO] Illinois Association of Health Maintenance Organizations. 1996 June. HMOs aggressively address marketing concerns in Medicaid—announce tougher standards and zero tolerance policy toward offenders. Chicago: IAHMO.

Iglehart JK. 1996. Health policy report: The national committee for quality assurance. New England Journal of Medicine 335:995–9.

Infant Health and Development Program. 1990. Enhancing the outcomes of low-birth-weight, premature infants. Journal of the American Medical Association 263:3035–42.

Isaacs SL. 1996 Winter. Consumers' information needs: Results of a national survey. Health Affairs 15:31–41.

Klitsner IN, Borok GM, Neinstein L, et al. 1992. Adolescent health care in a large multispecialty prepaid group practice: Who provides it and how well are they doing? Western Journal of Medicine 156:628–33.

Koehler WF, Fottler MD, Swan JE. 1992 Winter. Physician-patient satisfaction: Equity in the health services encounter. Medical Care Review 49:455–84.

Ladden M. 1996. Using clinical data in program design: A family support program for families with preterm births. Managed Care Quarterly 4(3): 30–5.

Leatherman S, Peterson E, Heinen L, et al. 1991. Quality screening and management using claims data in a managed care setting. Quality Review Bulletin 17:349–59.

Leatherman S, Venus P, Smalley MA, et al. 1995. Population health surveillance in a managed care setting: A continuous quality improvement project to increase pediatric immunization rates. Minneapolis, MN: United HealthCare Corporation.

Lieu TA, Black SB, Ray P. 1994. Risk factors for delayed immunization among children in an HMO. American Journal of Public Health 84: 1621–5.

Ludden J, Shusterman A. 1995 March–April. To carve out or not to carve out? HMO Magazine 36(2):50–5.

Luft HS. 1996 Spring. Modifying managed competition to address cost and quality. Health Affairs 15:23–38.

Makuc DM, Fried VM, Parsons PE. 1994. Health insurance and cancer screening among women. Advance Data No. 254. Washington: Centers for Disease Control and Prevention.

Mark T, Mueller C. 1996 Winter. Access to care in HMOs and traditional insurance plans. Health Affairs 15:81–7.

Master RJ, Connors S, Kronick R, et al. 1996. Medicaid working group project summary: Managed care for the severely disabled and chronically ill. In: Medicaid managed care sourcebook, pp. D31–42. New York: Faulkner & Gray.

Mauldon J, Leibowitz A, Buchanan JL, et al. 1994. Rationing or rationalizing children's medical care: Comparison of a Medicaid HMO with fee-for-service care. American Journal of Public Health 84:899–904.

McCall N, Wrightson CW, Paringer L. 1994 Spring. Managed Medicaid cost savings: The Arizona experience. Health Affairs 13:234–45.

McGlynn EA, Schuster M, Halfon N. 1996 June. State of the art in assessing quality of care for children. Presentation at the Association of Health Services Research 13th annual meeting, Atlanta, GA.

McLaughlin CP. 1995. Balancing collaboration and competition: The Kingsport, Tennessee experience. Joint Commission Journal on Quality Improvement 21:646–55.

McManus MA, Fox HB. 1996. Enhancing preventive and primary care for children with chronic or disabling conditions served in health maintenance organizations. Managed Care Quarterly 4(3):19–29.

McPhillips-Tangum CA, Lewis NA, Coleman CW, et al. 1996 March 8. Use of a data-based approach by an HMO to identify and address physician barriers to pediatric vaccination—California, 1995. Morbidity and Mortality Weekly Report.

Mechanic D, Schlesinger M, McAlpine DD. 1995. Management of mental health and substance abuse: State of the art and early results. The Millbank Quarterly 73:19–55.

Melnick GA, Zwanziger J. 1995. State health care expenditures under competition and regulation: 1980 through 1991. American Journal of Public Health 85:1391–6.

[MHDI] Minnesota Health Data Institute. 1996. Consumer survey: Summary report of health plan category comparisons. St. Paul, MN: MHDI.

Miller RH, Luft HS. 1994. Managed care plan performance since 1980: A literature review. Journal of the American Medical Association 271:1512–19.

Murata PJ, McGlynn EA, Siu AL, et al. 1994. Quality measures for prenatal care. Archives of Family Medicine 3:41–9.

Mustin HD, Holt VL, Connell FA. 1994. Adequacy of well-child care and immunizations in US infants born in 1988. Journal of the American Medical Association 272:1111–5.

[NASHP] National Academy of State Health Policy. 1993 April. Proceedings of the national conference on managed care systems for mothers and young children. Portland, ME: NASHP.

[NCQA] National Committee for Quality Assurance. 1995. Report card pilot project, technical report. Washington: NCQA.

Neff JM, Anderson G. 1995. Protecting children with chronic illness in a competitive marketplace. Journal of the American Medical Association 274:1866–9.

Newacheck PW, Halfon N. 1986a. The financial burden of medical care expenses for children. Medical Care 24:1110–7.

Newacheck PW, Halfon N. 1986b. The association between mother's and children's use of physician services. Medical Care 24:30.

Newacheck PW, Taylor WR. 1992. Childhood chronic illness: Prevalence, severity, and impact. American Journal of Public Health 82:364–71.

Novak M. 1996 May–June. Profits with honor. Policy Review 77:50–6.

Oberg CN, Bryant NA, Bach ML. 1994. America's children: Triumph or tragedy? Washington: American Public Health Association.

Olds DL, Henderson CR, Phelps C, et al. 1993. Effect of prenatal and infancy nurse home visitation on government spending. Medical Care 31:155–74.

Packer-Tursman J. 1996. The future of the safety net. In: 1996 Medicaid managed care sourcebook, pp. D24–5. New York: Faulkner & Gray, Inc.

Perrin JM, Homer CJ, Berwick DM, et al. 1989. Variations in rates of hospitalizations of children in three urban communities. New England Journal of Medicine 329:1183–7.

Perry CL, Juepker RV, Murray DM, et al. 1989. Parent involvement with children's health promotion: A one-year follow-up of the Minnesota home team. Health Education Quarterly 16:171–80.

Perry CL, Williams CL, Veblen-Mortenson S, et al. 1996. Project Northland: Outcomes of a communitywide alcohol use prevention program during early adolescence. American Journal of Public Health 86:956–65.

Peterson E, Shatin D, McCarthy D. 1996 March. Health Services research at United HealthCare Corporation. Medical Care Research and Review 53:S65–76.

Plaut TF, Howell T, Walsh S, et al. 1996. A systems approach to asthma care. Managed Care Quarterly 4(3):6–18.

Reisinger AL, Colby DC, Schwartz A. 1994. Medicaid physician payment reform: Using the Medicare fee schedule for Medicaid payments. American Journal of Public Health 84:553–60.

Riley GF, Potosky AL, Lubitz JD, et al. 1994. Stage of cancer and diagnosis for Medicare HMO and fee-for-service enrollees. American Journal of Public Health 84:1598–1604.

Robinson JC. 1996. Decline in hospital utilization and cost inflation under managed care in California. Journal of the American Medical Association 276:1060–4.

Safran DG, Tarlov AR, Rogers WH. 1994. Primary care performance in fee-for-service and prepaid health care systems: Results from the medical outcomes study. Journal of the American Medical Association 271:1579–86.

Safran DG, Tarlov AR, Rogers WH, et al. 1996 June. Linking primary care performance to valued outcomes of care. Paper presented at the Association for Health Services Research 13th annual meeting, Atlanta. Boston: New England Medical Center.

Schaffler HH, Rodriguez T. 1996 Spring. Exercising purchasing power for preventive care. Health Affairs 15:73–85.

Schwartz JS, Hillman A. 1996. The gatekeeper in managed care: Too much of a good thing? The American Journal of Managed Care 2:925–7.

Shewry S, Hunt S, Ramey J, et al. 1996 Spring. Risk adjustment: The missing piece of market competition. Health Affairs 15:171–81.

Showstack J, Lurie N, Leatherman S, et al. 1996. Health of the public: The private sector challenge. Journal of the American Medical Association 276:1071–4.

Sisk JE, Gorman SA, Reisinger AL, et al. 1996. Evaluation of Medicaid managed care: Satisfaction and access in New York City. Journal of the American Medical Association 276:50–55.

Siu AL, Leibowitz A, Brook RH, et al. 1988. Use of the hospital in a randomized trial of prepaid care. Journal of the American Medical Association 259:1343–6.

Starfield B. 1994. Is primary care essential? Lancet 344:1129–33.

Szilagyi PG, Roghmann KJ, Foye HR, et al. 1992. Increased ambulatory utilization in IPA plans among children receiving hyposensitization. Inquiry 29:467–75.

Tempkin-Greener H, Winchell M. 1991. Medicaid beneficiaries under managed care: Provider choice and satisfaction. Health Services Research 26:509–29.

The Times Mirror Center for The People and The Press. 1995 Feb. The new American electorate and health care reform. Menlo Park, CA: The Henry J. Kaiser Family Foundation.

Thompson RS, Taplin SH, McAfee TA, et al. 1995. Primary and secondary prevention services in clinical practice: Twenty years' experience in development, implementation, and evaluation. Journal of the American Medical Association 273:1130–5.

Valdez RB, Ware J, Manning W, et al. 1989. Prepaid group practice effects on the utilization of medical services and health outcomes for children: Results from a controlled trial. Pediatrics 83:168–90.

Wagner EH. 1995. Population-based management of diabetes care. Patient Education and Counseling 26:225–30.

Wagner JL, Herdman RC, Alberts DW. 1989 Fall. Well-child care: How much is enough? Health Affairs 8:145–57.

Ware Jr. JE, Bayliss MS, Rogers WH, et al. 1996. Differences in 4-year health outcomes for elderly and poor, chronically ill patients treated in HMOs and fee-for-service systems: Results from the medical outcomes study. Journal of the American Medical Association 276:1039–47.

Weitzman M. 1986. School absence rates as outcome measures in studies of children with chronic illness. Journal of Chronic Disability 39: 799–808.

Welch WP. 1988. HMO Enrollment and Medicaid. Medical Care 26:45–52.

Welch WP. 1994. HMO market share and its effects on local Medicare costs. In: Luft H, editor. HMOs and the elderly, pp. 231–49. Ann Arbor, MI: Health Administration Press.

Welch WP, Miller RE. 1988. Mandatory HMO enrollment in Medicaid: The issue of freedom of choice. Millbank Quarterly 66:618–39.

Wells KB, Sturm R. 1995 Fall. Care for depression in a changing environment. Health Affairs 14:78–89.

Wennberg JE, Gittelsohn A. 1973. Small area variations in health care delivery. Science 182:1102–8.

West DW, Stuart ME, Duggan AK, et al. 1996. Evidence for selective health maintenance organization enrollment among children and adolescents covered by Medicaid. Archives of Pediatrics and Adolescent Medicine 150:503–7.

Wickizer TM, Feldstein PJ. 1995 Fall. The impact of HMO competition on private health insurance premiums: 1985–1992. Inquiry 32:241–51.

Zablocki E. 1995 March–April. Taking aim at childhood illness. HMO Magazine 36:29–35.

Zelman WA. 1996. The changing health care marketplace. San Francisco: Jossey-Bass.

11

Doing the Right Thing: The Role of Market Forces and Public Policy in Managed Care Organizations' Performance on Child Health

Debra J. Lipson and Amy B. Bernstein

Introduction

THE INCENTIVES EMBODIED in traditionally defined managed care hold great promise for improvements in children's health. Capitation theoretically constitutes a financial incentive to keep children healthy so that they do not require costly medical care for conditions that could have been easily and inexpensively prevented. Similarly, managed care's vertically integrated systems theoretically make it possible for practitioners to provide coordinated care to children who need services in a variety of settings or from various specialists.

In some cases, these dual promises of more effective preventive services and more coordinated care have been fulfilled. Some studies have shown that compared to children with fee-for-service coverage, children enrolled in health maintenance organizations (HMOs) had better rates of preventive visits and better access to care. But other studies have shown that relative to their counterparts in fee-for-service care, children in HMOs had fewer preventive visits and worse access to specialty care.

Some of these contradictory results may be ascribed to shortcomings or inconsistencies in the studies, but this chapter contends that such findings may be inevitable, for despite the theoretical incentives, there is nothing inherent in managed care organizations' operations that will produce better health outcomes for children, without clear marketplace or public policy incentives. After reviewing the study findings on the subject in more detail, the chapter assesses the impact of market forces on the quality of care and child health outcomes in managed care organizations. It then reviews a number of public policy strategies or interventions that have been used, or could be adopted, to increase the likelihood that children's health goals are met by managed care organizations.

Performance in Children's Health

In 1992, about 27 percent of children under 18 years of age were enrolled in HMOs of all types (National Health Interview Survey 1993, unpublished data computed by the Alpha Center). Methodologically sound studies that examine how children fare in various types of managed care delivery systems are relatively rare, usually limited in scope to one or two organizations, and for the most part out-of-date. The paucity of studies is due in part to the difficulties of defining different types of managed care organizations and in part to the absence of nationally representative data sets that include information on utilization, detailed health status measures, place of care, and payer.

Managed care organizations differ in the care they provide, just as individual physicians differ in practice styles and even relative competence. Miller and Luft (1994) examined methodologically sound studies through 1994 on various aspects of HMO performance. (The literature on the performance of other types of managed care organizations is virtually nonexistent.) They found that compared to those in indemnity plans, those enrolled in HMOs had on average somewhat lower hospital admission rates and shorter hospital lengths of stay. They had the same or more physician office visits per person than fee-for-service members, less use of expensive procedures and tests, greater use of preventive services, and mixed results on the outcomes of care. HMO members expressed somewhat lower satisfaction with the services they received, but greater satisfaction with the cost of care and comprehensiveness of benefits. Very few of the articles reviewed by Miller and Luft, however, focused on children's experiences in managed care.

Previous studies of children's experience in managed care tended to look at whether children in a specific care setting received one or more specific services at the same rate as they did prior to entering that setting, or as compared to children in another setting. But these studies are not very generalizable from one managed care organization to another, state to state, population to population, or time period to another.

Children, as a group, do not consume a large proportion of health care resources. Approximately 70 percent of children are generally healthy (Evans and Friedland, 1994). Children as a group have on average about two physician office visits per year, compared to about five physician visits per year for the elderly. Annual health care expenditures averaged $505 per person under 25 in 1994, compared to $1,086 per person aged 25 to 34 years, and $2,144 per person aged 55 to 64 years. Thus, initiatives to control aggregate health expenditures by focusing on care for children are probably ill-advised.

Only 4.6 percent (about 3.1 million) of children under age 18 had a "limitation in their major activity" in 1993 (Mashaw et al., 1996), but these children consume the vast proportion of resources. It has been estimated that healthy children incur less than 10 percent of the medical expenditures used to treat all children (Neff and Anderson, 1995). Therefore, we can divide children into two distinct groups—those needing primary and well-child care, and those needing these as well as other special services. We first examine the literature on the question of whether managed care increases children's use of preventive services. Then we examine how managed care organizations could help or hinder access to special care needed by chronically and extremely ill children.

Children and Preventive Care

Most of the research on how managed care affects children's use of preventive services is based on their experiences under the Medicaid program because the focus of most Medicaid managed care programs to date has been the population of those receiving Aid to Families with Dependent Children (AFDC), which includes a high percentage of children. Moreover, the federal government and states fund the Medicaid program and have invested in evaluations of these programs. Freund and Lewit (1993) reviewed the literature as of 1993 on how children fare in Medicaid managed care compared to Medicaid fee-for-service. Another study (Hurley et al., 1993) reviewed 25 of the soundest evaluations of Medicaid managed care as of 1992. Most of these 25 studies reported changes in hospital utilization only in the aggregate, and did not distinguish care for women from care for their children. Only 12 of the 25 studies were strong enough to distinguish the impact of managed care. Of these 12 studies, 4 showed a decrease in hospitalizations, one showed an increase, 5 showed no change, and the results are unknown for the remainder. A more recent study by Sisk et al. (1996) found that Medicaid managed care enrollees in New York City reported better access to care and higher levels of satisfaction compared with Medicaid beneficiaries in the fee-for-service program.

A summary of the literature through 1994 indicates that there is little evidence that immunization rates or preventive visit rates are higher in Medicaid managed care than in Medicaid fee-for-service (Rowland et al., 1995). One study provided limited evidence that children received more well-child visits under the Arizona Medicaid program, which uses HMOs to serve the population, than under New Mexico's fee-for-service Medicaid program (Balaban et al., 1994). However, in another study (Mauldon et al., 1994) children in Arizona's Medicaid HMOs received similar numbers of preventive visits and fewer acute care visits than children in New Mexico's fee-for-service Medicaid program.

Studies of Medicaid managed care programs report mixed results in terms of improved access to primary and preventive health services. "Studies show that use of routine preventive services—child health supervision services and immunizations—stays the same or slightly increases under Medicaid managed care arrangements" (Freund and Lewit, 1993; Heinen et al., 1990; Hughes et al., 1995; Hurley et al., 1991). Immunization rates do not meet the standards set forth in Medicaid's Early and Periodic Screening, Diagnosis and Treatment (EPSDT) program in either Medicaid managed care or in Medicaid fee-for-service (see later discussion of EPSDT). This could be because definitions of "necessary services" are sometimes ambiguous, EPSDT requirements are often not explicit in managed care plans, and the separate responsibilities of the state, the plan, and participating providers are frequently not clearly delineated (NIHCM, 1995, p. 13). Wood, Halfon, Sherbourne, and Grabowsky (1994) found that low-income children who sought care in public clinics were more likely to be adequately immunized than those who obtained care through private physicians' offices or HMOs.

In addition to the research literature, an important assessment of how well Medicaid managed care works comes from beneficiaries. In 1995, 21 focus groups of Medicaid beneficiaries in five states showed:

1. experiences varied by state, economic status, region within state, and other factors;
2. enrollment and plan/provider selection processes are critical to smooth implementation of managed care;
3. the most frequently noted advantage of managed care was the guarantee of access to a primary care physician, particularly for beneficiaries who had previously experienced substantial problems finding a physician who participated in fee-for-service Medicaid; and
4. the introduction of managed care did not necessarily eliminate all access problems that beneficiaries experienced under fee-for-service medicine.

Across all states, some managed care enrollees expressed problems in getting care, including making appointments, obtaining specialist care, and getting after-hours care (Frederick Schneiders Research, 1996). In sum, beneficiaries say that how well managed care works depends on many factors.

Children with Chronic Conditions

The population of children with chronic health problems is quite small, although the proportion varies from fewer than 3 percent to as much as 31 percent, depending on the definition of chronic condition. In 1992, fewer than 3 percent of children under age 18 were identified as having a chronic condition, and fewer than 2 percent were identified as being in "fair" or "poor" health by their parents (National Health Interview Survey unpublished tables compiled by the Alpha Center). There is virtually no literature on how children with chronic illnesses fare in managed care compared to fee-for-service systems, in large part because the population of these children is so small, especially within one health plan or provider. Literature focuses on the potential problems of mandating managed care for these children, and the possible problems these children may encounter in managed care systems.

Potential problems with managed care for children with special needs include disruptions of established relationships with providers, difficulties obtaining specialist care or special services, and issues of convenience and accessibility. According to one review,

> Generally, children with disabilities have remained within fee-for-service networks that do not limit access to specialists and allow broader choice of providers. Many of these children have built up relationships, often

with several physicians and other health professionals. "Starting over" with a group of new physicians would place new demands on a group of children and their families who may already be overburdened by coping with the demands of their disabilities, securing the kinds of ancillary and support services they require, and meeting their other school and family responsibilities. (Regenstein and Meyer, 1994)

These problems may occur whenever a child previously enrolled in a fee-for-service system is switched into a managed care system, whether it is under a private insurance program or under Medicaid.

Most Medicaid programs do not currently mandate that children with special needs join managed care plans (Fox et al., 1993). As of 1993, most Medicaid families with special-needs children had a choice about whether to join an HMO, or at least which plan to select, although they did not receive much information to help them make this decision. Most states had some type of "protection" for at least some special-needs children, such as exemptions from enrollment, arrangements for obtaining out-of-plan care, and exclusion of services from HMO contracts. While this trend held through 1995, many states subsequently have obtained federal approval to mandate enrollment of groups of previously excluded children into fully capitated plans (Fox and McManus, 1996b).

A recent evaluation of five states that have received federal approval of their plans for mandatory enrollment in Medicaid managed care showed that in all states except Tennessee all of the plans participating in the waiver program had good pediatric primary care and hospital capacity. However, the pediatric subspecialty networks were more variable, especially in Hawaii and Tennessee. Gaps were found in each of the states for ancillary therapists experienced in pediatric interventions and in some states for children's mental health and home health providers. A major factor influencing the adequacy of provider networks for children was determined to be plans' reimbursement rates (Fox and McManus, 1996a).

The experience of disabled children in managed care plans reveals some areas for concern, but few data are available on health outcomes. One study of AFDC recipients in Wisconsin, for example (Ireys et al., 1996), indicated that fewer than 50 percent of respondents who had requested a referral to an out-of-plan specialist were granted one, while another study of pediatric referrals (Cartland and Yridkonsky, 1992) showed that pediatricians made fewer referrals to subspecialists and to inpatient care for patients in managed care. One fifth of those making referrals for children in the managed care program had at least one referral denied. No attempt was made, however, to validate whether a referral was medically warranted. Smyth, Haas, and Friebe (1995) describe preliminary lessons from Michigan's efforts to enroll disabled children in its Medicaid managed care programs. While the program encouraged appropriate referrals to specialists and linkages with public and private resources, the program had problems related to inadequate reimbursement, lack of knowledge about available resources, poor communication between service providers, lack of interested gatekeepers, and time constraints.

In summary, few studies have been done examining how different types of managed care arrangements affect the health care received by children in general, and children with chronic conditions in particular. What evidence there is suggests that the impacts vary by local conditions, including financing, ideology of the plan offering care, population group, and state and local public health interventions and initiatives. As the health care delivery system evolves, even what little we do know may no longer be relevant to the formulation of public policies.

Influence of Market Dynamics on Managed Care Organizations

Promoters of managed competition have long postulated that given the proper incentives, accountable health plans (distinct provider networks accountable for the health of enrolled populations) would compete first on the basis of price and service, and later, on the basis of quality and health outcomes. If this occurred, the ability to demonstrate positive outcomes for children should become the basis for competition among health plans.

The theory of managed competition depends in large part on having knowledgeable purchasers who would pursue value—the combination of highest quality and service for the best price—with vigor. Some believe that this has largely occurred. By 1993, many more employers were enrolling their workers in lower-cost managed care plans. Nearly 50 percent of employees of large and medium-sized companies were enrolled in managed care, up from just 14 percent in 1986 (U.S. Bureau of Labor Statistics, 1994). The National Committee for Quality Assurance (NCQA), founded in part by large businesses' health benefits managers, developed a widely accepted HMO accreditation process and state-of-the-art indicators for comparing health plan performance (called the Health Employer Data Information Set, or HEDIS). And one of the early promoters of managed competition believes larger employers are increasingly comparing "suppliers" on the basis of cost, quality, and service; pushing them for better performance; and developing more sophisticated and standardized comparative information (Etheredge, 1995).

Despite these developments, sophisticated purchasers are still rare. The Community Snapshot study, which examined purchasing initiatives in 15 communities across the country in 1995, found that, "The majority of purchasers are still using traditional means to control costs, and few are aggressively seeking out better value" (Lipson and De Sa, 1996). A few large employers and employer coalitions are receiving media attention for trying to influence employee choice of plans through financial incentives, contracting directly with providers to achieve greater accountability, and using quality data to make health plan selections. But they are in the minority. Few middle- and small-size firms, which constitute the vast majority of employers in this country, are seeking out value or making purchasing decisions based on anything other than price. The switch to managed care plans is largely reflective of their ability to offer lower prices than indemnity plans, not their ability to offer better quality or value.

Another Community Snapshot analysis revealed that, "The good news is that competition is taking place, even if it is primarily on the basis of price. The bad news is the lack of competition based on measured and reported aspects of quality of care, especially health outcomes" (Miller, 1996). Moreover, "risk-adjusted premiums and capitation rates are not being used to reward plans and providers for caring for sicker patients. Quality measurement remains in an early, developmental stage. And, [a]ccountable [h]ealth [p]artnerships of exclusive relationships between health plans and delivery system organizations have not emerged" (Berenson, 1996).

The gap between managed competition theory and market realities may explain why health indicators for children enrolled in managed care are not uniformly positive. A focus on the bottom line does not encourage plans or their providers to place a priority on lowering the rate of infectious diseases among children or delivering state-of-the-art care to children with special needs. Even though NCQA's most recent version of HEDIS (version 3.0) includes many reporting measures related to children's health care (e.g., immunization status, treatment of children's ear infections, access to primary care providers, and well-child visits), there are still no outcome measures that would indicate how children fare as a result of these services. Managed care organizations refuse to release such information on the grounds that without adequate adjustments for the health status of patients, the results would be meaningless. Yet, the health plans use the data for internal quality improvement purposes. Health plans will report such data only "when their customers—employers and government health programs—make it impossible for them to refuse, industry experts say" (Freudenheim, 1996).

In the meantime, the methods for adjusting capitation rates based on children's health status remain deficient. Fowler and Anderson (1996) demonstrate that under any of the methods now being used, plans would still be underpaid for children with chronic health conditions. Until the risk adjustment field develops further, risk selection will continue to be an important aspect of any HMO's marketing strategy. As long as coverage remains voluntary and enrollees have some choice of plans, those HMOs that can attract a healthier population will always win out over their competitors. This does not bode well for children with costly or special health care needs who are required to enroll in managed care plans. Until the plans have a large number of children with special needs, and the capitation rates they receive reflect these children's additional and unique service needs, HMOs will have an incentive not to enroll them, or to undertreat the children with special needs that they are forced to enroll.

Even if more employers used comparative quality information to make plan selections, it would be surprising if they made children's indicators a priority. Children, as dependents of employees, are not a priority now, or else employers would not have dropped dependent coverage as much as they have. Private coverage (employer and individually purchased) for children declined from 73.6 percent of all children in 1987 to 67.4 percent in 1993 (GAO, 1996). Nor would employers have increased premium contributions for dependent coverage as much as they have in recent years; the percentage of HMO premiums for family coverage paid by employees increased from 24 percent in 1991 to 32 percent in 1994 (KPMG, 1994).

The fact that managed care may not actually change how health care gets delivered may be another reason for managed care organizations' less than stellar performance on children's health. While managed care organizations may want to make some changes in care delivery patterns in the name of efficiency and quality, they are neither pushed by purchasers to make substantial changes nor are providers willing to make such changes readily. The Community Snapshot study found that, "Most purchasers have little interest in changing the health care system; they are simply looking for low-cost venders. Even if they had the interest, the resources available are inad-

equate . . . becoming an aggressive purchaser requires a substantial investment over a long period of time. Even the few companies that have made
such investments want to systematize the process so that they can devote
more resources to their primary business activity" (Lipson and De Sa, 1996).
According to one physician who administers a preferred provider organization, "To the extent that physicians are involved in [integrated delivery sys-
tem] activities or are selling their practices, it is for defensive reasons,
primarily to take back some of the control they have ceded to managed care
organizations or to 'cash-out' while they still can. They do not necessarily
have a vision of better health care resulting from these activities" (Berenson,
1996).

This assessment may seem overly critical in light of some very worthy
community health promotion and public health education activities conducted by managed care organizations. A recent study of the emerging role
of private health care providers and managed care plans in the provision of
public health or population-based activities found nearly 75 such organizations involved in delivering "essential public health services," as defined by
the U.S. Public Health Service, and this estimate was likely to have under-
stated the true extent of such activity (Macro International, 1996). For example, some managed care organizations conduct neighborhood-focused
and community-wide assessments of service needs, coalition-building to
address community health or social service needs, targeted health promotion, and early intervention and prevention activities designed to reduce
domestic violence, accidents, and substance abuse.

The theory of managed care would suggest they are undertaking these
activities because of the financial incentives inherent in capitation payments. Yet the study found "a significant *lack* of connection between these
activities and the business strategy of the . . . organizations. Less than a
quarter of the activities were motivated *primarily* by business-related issues. The predominant primary motivations were altruistic ones . . . [based
on] the organization's mission, community benefit" (Macro International,
1996, p. vi). The study found that capitation was not a motivating factor for
public health activities. These findings suggest that managed care organizations do not undertake prevention-oriented or community health promotion activities because it helps their bottom line. They do so because it helps
them meet their marketing or corporate relations objectives and, in some
cases, contributes to meeting the community benefit obligations of nonprofit organizations.

Communities in which managed care organizations have either community benefit obligations to meet or are owned by "home-grown" organizations, however, are declining in number. Currently, 7 out of 10 HMOs are for-profit, and 81 percent of all new HMOs that formed in 1995 were for-profit, compared to 71 percent of the total industry (Interstudy, 1996). Due in part to mergers and consolidations, the seven largest national managed care firms accounted for almost half (48.6 percent) of all HMO enrollment in July 1996, compared to 34.4 percent six months earlier (Interstudy, 1996). The pace at which acquisitions of small companies by large ones and consolidations or mergers among health plans is taking place portends even less control over managed care organizations by local organizations. When owners are further removed from the communities in which they operate, it raises questions "about the ability of even the best-run and best-intentioned of these organizations to make *long-term* investments in the health of communities and their populations" (Hurley, 1997).

There are some markets where it makes more sense for health plans to cooperate and share in the costs of prevention activities. For example, where there are only a few plans competing in a market and the managed care enrollment level is quite high (as in Minneapolis), the likelihood of any one plan enrolling a member of the community is quite high. Or, where the managed care market is more "mature," that is, it has already squeezed out costs of inefficient care, plans must look to utilization management strategies and patient education to reduce costs of caring for their members. But even in such cases, health plans still tend to focus almost exclusively on their enrollees, rather than the community at large.

One might argue that many of these problems and market dynamics are temporary, that we are still in the first stage of developing a competitive market for health care, and that it is quickly evolving into the second and third "waves." In fact, purchasers are becoming more concerned about quality and health outcomes and increasing their use of HEDIS measures to make health plan selections. Local provider-sponsored organizations are taking control from nationally owned companies. Risk adjustment methods, while still crude, are getting better and will be used increasingly by purchasers to ensure that health plans cannot avoid high-risk patients.

But even so, there is still one facet of market dynamics that serves as a disincentive to invest in children's health: the high turnover rates among enrollees. Among Medicaid AFDC enrollees, an estimated 40 percent go on or off Medicaid during the course of a year (Freund and Lewit, 1993), and this figure does not take into account those who switch among health plans. An analysis by NCQA found that, "In general, fewer than 50 percent of Medicaid managed care plan enrollees were enrolled for longer than 12 months" (NCQA, 1995). Among the general population of preschool-age children, Kogan et al. (1995) found that about one-quarter were without any health insurance for at least one month during their first three years of life. Over one half of these children had a health insurance gap of more than six months, indicating the highly dynamic insurance status of many children. "Turnover among individual plan members or among employer groups certainly erodes, if not undermines, the return on investment logic that drives investor-owned plans" (Hurley, 1997, p. 10).

In summary, the effect of purchasers' focus on price and the resulting competition among plans to offer the lowest price make investment in children's health a frill rather than a necessity. In most of the larger markets in this country, there are still too many competitors to make cooperation of larger community and population-wide health promotion efforts possible. And turnover in any given plan's enrollees makes long-term investment in children's health a losing economic proposition, even though economics may give way to quality and public health concerns in some situations.

Public Policy Interventions
Because managed care per se has not resulted in more positive children's health outcomes, and because market forces often serve as disincentives to invest in children's health, it may be appropriate for government to take some steps to assure that managed care organizations do their part to ensure those outcomes deemed socially and politically desirable. The justification for using public policy to ensure that managed care organizations deliver certain child health services and produce certain outcomes relies in large part on the nature of many children's health services as a public good. When more children are immunized, fewer will rely on public resources should they become ill or suffer long-term disability. Early and adequate prenatal care helps reduce the incidence of low birthweight and disabilities among children, which in turn can diminish the public burden of educating and providing medical services to children with special needs. Ensuring that all children receive regular medical attention allows them to attend school and become productive citizens. In addition to the arguments based on public goods and human capital, there may also be public health issues

that warrant governmental intervention into the operations of managed care organizations and other providers of health care.

Governments at the federal, state, and local level all have different roles to play in the regulation of health care, including financing or paying for health care; assuring the public's health; and regulating health professionals, facilities, and insurance arrangements (Lipson, 1997). Governments' relationships to health plans occur through all of these avenues. For example, through the Medicaid program, states have begun to step up their expectations as purchasers of care from health plans, rather than simply paying the bills submitted. In their role as guarantor of the public's health, states and localities are becoming more involved in assuring the quality, accessibility, and accountability of medical care provided by health plans (ASTHO, 1995). And as managed care plans enroll a greater percentage of the population, demands on federal and state governments have mounted to ensure that the plans are monitored and regulated to protect consumers.

The remainder of this chapter explains how governments at all levels have used, or could use, their purchasing, public health protection, and regulatory authority to ensure that children enrolled in managed care plans are adequately served. The major vehicles or policy interventions include:

1. various federal authorities over HMOs;
2. state licensing and insurance regulations affecting HMOs and other managed care plans;
3. state Medicaid purchasing of managed care;
4. state collaboration with voluntary HMO accreditation agencies; and
5. public health oversight and regulatory actions.

Federal-Level Initiatives

An increasing number of federal laws and programs affect the provision of health care to children in managed care settings. Most of the federal laws pertain to the Medicaid program. (The federal Health Maintenance Act of 1973 and related regulations were more influential at one time. However, Congress has repealed many of the original advantages of federal qualification, rendering the act largely moot [Butler, 1996, p. 5]. In addition, the requirements for federally qualified HMOs are so general as to be largely irrelevant for children's health issues.) Federal Medicaid law establishes the conditions under which states can contract with managed care organizations and pay them on a capitated basis. Among the most important requirements for children are those that mandate that all managed care organizations serving Medicaid recipients: 1) have a quality assurance program and grievance procedures in place, which each state Medicaid agency must oversee and enforce; 2) prohibit discrimination on the basis of health status or health care needs; and 3) provide the full range of EPSDT services, if the provision of these services has been stipulated in the contract between the state and plans.

Besides Medicaid, other key federal programs that promote the health of children in managed care organizations include those operated by the Centers for Disease Control and Prevention (CDC) and the Health Resources and Services Administration (HRSA). In its role as the nation's primary disease surveillance and public health promotion agency, CDC has fostered partnerships with many managed care organizations, Medicaid departments, and local public health initiatives that involve both Medicaid and private managed care organizations (see Morbidity and Mortality Weekly Report, November 17, 1995, for a detailed discussion of CDC's strategy for working with managed care organizations [CDC, 1995]). CDC tries to develop disease prevention and health promotion systems within communities through these partnerships. HRSA, which funds a variety of safety net providers that serve vulnerable children, has developed a comprehensive program to provide training, technical assistance, and financial support to community health centers, maternal and child health centers, rural health clinics, migrant health clinics, school-based health centers, and programs funded under the Ryan White Comprehensive AIDS Resource Emergency (CARE) Act to increase their ability to participate in managed care programs.

State Insurance and Other Regulations Affecting Managed Care Organizations

The federal McCarran-Ferguson Act gives states the authority to regulate the business of insurance (i.e., the business of assuming financial risk for certain occurrences in a group of people). As part of their insurance regulations, every state has enacted an HMO statute or regulation, and approximately 30 states have adopted a model HMO law developed by the National Association of Insurance Commissioners (NAIC, 1990). These laws generally stipulate basic benefits that must be offered; the need for facility licenses (if the HMO owns facilities); minimum net worth, working capital, and reserve requirements; filing of proposed premium rates; assurances that the HMO has adequate provider capacity and contracts; quality assurance and utilization review requirements; rules for marketing and advertising; and basic consumer protection provisions, such as grievance and complaints procedures.

While few of these provisions specifically pertain to children, there are instances in which states have used their regulatory authority to ensure that HMOs meet children's health needs. For example, the rapid adoption of laws in 25 states during 1995 and 1996 that require HMOs to cover minimum lengths of hospital stay for childbirth (Families USA, 1996) reflected a concern for children's health. Extended hospital stays (more than 24 hours after delivery) can be helpful in detecting jaundice and in preventing dehydration among newborns. In addition, Texas issued regulations in 1996 that require "HMOs to refer enrollees to out-of-plan specialists if network providers do not have appropriate training and expertise" (Families USA, 1996, p. 8). This option is particularly important for children with chronic or disabling conditions who need to see specialty care providers.

Besides insurance regulations, states have authority over other aspects of HMOs' or other managed care organizations' business that can be of help to children. For example, as a condition of licensure, Minnesota requires HMOs to file annual "action plans" specifying how they intend to promote community health. The contents of the action plan must include, among other things, information on provider credentialing standards, provider capacity, quality improvement plans, and policies and procedures for serving high-risk or special needs populations. This serves as an incentive for plans to work with groups that can help provide care to children with special needs. The state also requires HMOs to file "collaboration plans" that specify how the HMO will work with public health and community agencies in developing community health promotion programs. As a result of these laws, HMOs are now engaged in a variety of efforts, ranging from promotion of the use of bicycle helmets to detection and prevention of domestic violence, both of which will help to improve children's health status.

In Massachusetts, community benefit guidelines were issued by the attorney general in 1994, requiring nonprofit hospitals and health plans to report annually on the benefits provided to the community to justify their tax-exempt status (see chapter 13, "The Changing Role of Consumer Advocates," for a discussion of the development of these requirements). Such guidelines can be used by states to encourage health plans to engage in health promotion activities that will benefit the entire community, not just enrollees.

The Role of Voluntary/Private Accreditation in Public Policies

Despite their statutory authority to do so, states may not have the resources to monitor, or conduct detailed inspections of, managed care organizations. In some cases, states are collaborating with private sector organizations that have taken the initiative to inspect managed care organizations. The primary private organization responsible for the voluntary accreditation of managed care organizations is NCQA. After its founding by large employer groups interested in obtaining quality of care measures of managed care organizations with which they contracted to provide health care for their employees, NCQA has expanded to help develop similar measures for both Medicare and Medicaid managed care organizations.

HEDIS 3.0, which was released in February 1997, contains many measures pertaining specifically to care received by children. The reporting measures, which were contained in earlier versions of HEDIS, include adolescent immunization status, treatment of children's ear infections, low-birthweight babies, checkups after delivery, children's access to primary care providers, well-child visits at various ages, and whether the plan has a pediatric mental health network, as well as others. Testing measures include substance abuse counseling for adolescents and family visits for children undergoing mental health treatment.

According to NCQA documents, the organization

> . . . is currently partnering with a number of states to incorporate private sector accreditation and/or performance measurement activities into the state regulatory and purchasing process, with the goal of reducing duplication, improving the oversight process and easing the administrative burden on health plans, providers, and regulators. In eight states—Pennsylvania, Florida, Oklahoma, Kansas, Nevada, Rhode Island, Vermont, and South Carolina—an NCQA accreditation review will satisfy the state's licensure requirement for an external quality review. In the state of Vermont, HMOs have the option of undergoing a state review or seeking accreditation from an organization such as NCQA. Rather than create duplicative processes for the evaluation of HMO quality, each of these states decided instead to take advantage of work already performed by the private sector. (NCQA, 1996)

State Medicaid Managed Care Programs

The Medicaid managed care market is growing rapidly. Between 1994 and 1996, an additional 5.5 million Medicaid patients were enrolled in managed care plans, a 71 percent increase (HCFA, 1996). By June 1996, 13.3 million were enrolled in some form of managed care, 40 percent of all Medicaid eligible persons and nearly twice the proportion of three years prior. As Medicaid enrolls more of its beneficiaries into managed care, the managed care organizations that contract with state Medicaid agencies become increasingly responsible for caring for the most vulnerable children in our society, since these programs primarily affect women and children who qualify for Medicaid.

In their role as purchasers of care for low-income children from health plans, states have undertaken several initiatives designed to assure the quality of care received by children, to assure certain health outcomes such as childhood immunization levels or EPSDT screening rates, and to guarantee children's right to see specialists if needed. For example, using EPSDT requirements, states such as Pennsylvania and Oregon are holding health plans more accountable for their performance (NIHCM, 1996).

Based on concerns about Medicaid managed care's potential to disrupt existing patient-provider relationships, some states have also adopted policies designed to ensure that plans establish relationships with traditional community-based providers. For example, Oregon mandates that Medicaid managed care plans contract with county health departments and other publicly funded programs to provide immunizations, as well as screening for sexually transmitted diseases and other communicable diseases. When reviewing proposals, Massachusetts and Arizona among other states view favorably plans that include contracts with community providers. Massachusetts specifies in its request for proposals that plans must make efforts to establish linkages, though not necessarily contracts, with school-based clinics and encourages coordination with public health clinics to serve persons with HIV. Orange County, California's OPTIMA program has made the plan organized by Children's Hospital and University of California–Irvine the default for those who do not voluntarily choose a plan, giving them some advantage.

Public Health Initiatives

A more direct method of protecting and improving children's health is through public health laws and regulations that apply to all providers of health care, including managed care organizations. Most states, for example, have public health laws related to the surveillance and detection of diseases that constitute threats to the public health—infectious diseases such as measles and tuberculosis, or diseases that are caused by environmental factors such as lead poisoning. Governments at all levels mandate that certain types of public health education and outreach programs be conducted, either by governmental agencies or by private organizations. Those interventions that can involve managed care organizations fall into five major categories: direct or supplemental provision of services, mandated provision of services (at some site) by government contractors, coordination of services, surveillance and data collection, and education and outreach programs.

Direct Provision of Services.   State, county, and city public health departments across the country provide public health services to residents with no other source of care. Traditionally, public health departments have provided childhood immunizations (and sometimes adult immunizations), prenatal care, and testing and/or screening for infectious diseases such as tuberculosis and HIV/AIDS. Though health departments are currently trying to cut back on the direct provision of care, especially as Medicaid patients find better access to private providers, they might still serve as an important "safety net" for Medicaid-eligible children in managed care plans as well as for uninsured children. (See the discussion in chapter 16 of the measles epidemic in Milwaukee, Wisconsin, an experience that led the Wisconsin Medicaid program to implement a policy allowing public health departments to bill Medicaid HMOs at Medicaid fee-for-service rates for immunizations they provide to HMO enrollees, thus providing a financial incentive for the managed care organizations to immunize children in-plan. See also Schlenker and Fessler, 1990.)

Mandatory Provision/Screening/Testing.   Several states have laws requiring all service providers, including managed care organizations, to screen for specific health problems. For instance, most states require newborns to be tested for phenylketonuria, and some require them to be tested for HIV. In addition, many state public health statutes mandate that all children be screened for lead. Most public health statutes also mandate that silver nitrate be instilled into all newborn babies. In short, states can mandate whatever they decide is in the interest of "public health," but enforcement is often difficult. The best way to enforce these regulations is to deny access to other public programs—for example, entry into school—unless compliance is proved, or to provide appropriate financial incentives, as in the Milwaukee example.

Coordination of Services Across Sites of Care. Public health departments also coordinate public health initiatives across sites of care. This is an especially important activity for children on Medicaid, who typically gain and lose eligibility for Medicaid (Hughes et al., 1995), and uninsured children. CDC, private foundations, and many state and local governments are currently engaged in setting up immunization registries to which all providers and health plans will contribute and have access. For instance, the state health department in Arizona works with managed care plans and other providers to implement CASA, a computer-based information and monitoring system developed by the CDC to help identify missed opportunities for immunizing children. But this can be done on a voluntary basis, independent of government. For example, health plans in Minnesota are setting up a community registry, so that patients immunized at one site can be identified if they switch plans or receive out-of-plan care. (For a description of the program in operation in Rhode Island, see chapter 16.)

Surveillance and Data Collection. Public health departments are also the primary locus of data collection and surveillance of communicable diseases within each state. CDC has identified many "reportable" diseases—including childhood infectious diseases, tuberculosis, and sexually transmitted diseases—on which data must be collected by each state and urban area. Often these statistics can be used to identify epidemics and areas where public health interventions are warranted. This information can be used as a starting point to examine provider-specific rates of these diseases, as in the Milwaukee measles epidemic example (Schlenker and Fessler, 1990). Ideally, all providers in an area would report these statistics to one central location, with patient identifiers, so that efforts could be coordinated within an area.

Education and Outreach Programs. States and localities often initiate public health education programs for children. California, for example, initiated a community dental disease prevention program for children through the sixth grade. Many states have targeted HIV and other sexually transmitted disease prevention programs, and violence and accident prevention programs, to children and adolescents. Arizona has established a Prenatal Care Education Fund for statewide outreach efforts. Ideally, these efforts include managed care organizations as cooperating partners.

Conclusion

As the dominant form of health care delivery, managed care organizations have a key role to play in helping to improve the health status of children. But it would be risky to rely on managed care organizations to "do the right thing" for children in all cases. Managed care plans are too diverse in their style of practice, methods of containing costs, and use of revenues that exceed medical costs (Clancy and Brody, 1995). In addition, the market forces that determine the form and intensity of competition are too variable across markets and too volatile over time to foster altruistic behavior by all managed care plans. And unfortunately, activities designed to improve children's health are mostly altruistic given the high degree of turnover among plan enrollees, the length of time needed for preventive investments to pay off, and the inadequacy of risk adjustment methodologies to pay plans that provide high-quality care to children with special health care needs.

To realize the potential benefits of managed care, public policymakers must take leadership on many fronts and through a number of policy vehicles to ensure that children's health care needs are not forgotten in the competitive frenzy. Given the rapid evolution of managed care, one can only hope that the policy examples and strategies reviewed in this chapter evolve as well.

References

[ASTHO] Association of State and Territorial Health Officials. 1995 Nov. Ensuring and improving the quality of care in a managed care environment. Draft pending final publication. Washington: ASTHO.

Balaban D, McCall N, Jones Bauer E. 1994 January. Quality of Medicaid managed care: An evaluation of the Arizona Health Care Cost Containment System (AHCCCS). Discussion Paper 94–2. San Francisco: Laguna Research Associates.

Berenson RA. 1996 Sept. New market relationships and their effects on patient care. Paper commissioned by The Robert Wood Johnson Foundation's Program on Changes in Health Care Financing and Organization and delivered at the meeting, A market in turmoil: Evolving relationships. Washington: The Robert Wood Johnson Foundation.

Butler P. 1996. Public oversight of managed care entities: Issues for state policymakers. Washington: National Governors' Association.

Cartland DC, Yridkonsky BK. 1992. Barriers to pediatric referral in managed care. Pediatrics 89:183–92.

[CDC] Centers for Disease Control and Prevention. 1995 Nov. 17. Prevention and managed care: Opportunities for managed care organizations, purchasers of health care, and public health agencies. Morbidity and Mortality Weekly Report 44 (RR-14).

Clancy CM, Brody H. 1995 Jan. 25. Managed care: Jekyll or Hyde? Journal of the American Medical Association 273(4):338–9.

Etheredge L. 1995 Nov. The evolution of a new paradigm: Competitive purchasing of health care. Paper commissioned by The Robert Wood Johnson Foundation's Program on Changes in Health Care Financing and Organization and delivered at the meeting, The new competition: Dynamics shaping the health care market. Washington: The Robert Wood Johnson Foundation.

Evans A, Friedland RB. 1994 May. Financing and delivery of health care for children. Background paper for the Advisory Committee on Reforming American Health Care Financing: Policy and Administrative Choices. Washington: National Academy of Social Insurance.

Families USA. 1996 July. HMO consumers at risk: States to the rescue. Washington: Families USA Foundation.

Fowler EJ, Anderson GF. 1996. Capitation adjustment for pediatric populations. Pediatrics 98(1):10–7.

Fox HB, McManus MA. 1996a March. Impacts of state Medicaid demonstration waiver programs on children: Results from Hawaii, Oregon, Rhode Island, and Tennessee. Washington: Maternal and Child Health Policy Research Center.

Fox HB, McManus MA. 1996b July. Medicaid managed care for children with chronic or disabling conditions: Improved strategies for states and plans. Washington: Maternal and Child Health Policy Research Center.

Fox HB, Wicks LB, Newacheck PW. 1993 Fall. State Medicaid health maintenance organization policies and special-needs children. Health Care Financing Review 15(1):25–37.

Frederick Schneiders Research. 1996 May. Medicaid and managed care: Focus group studies of low-income Medicaid beneficiaries in five states. Paper prepared for the Henry J. Kaiser Family Foundation. Menlo Park, CA.

Freudenheim M. 1996 July 16. The grading becomes stricter on HMOs. New York Times, D1.

Freund DA, Lewit EM. 1993. Managed care for children and pregnant women: Promises and pitfalls. The Future of Children 3(2):92–122.

[GAO] U.S. General Accounting Office. 1996 June. Health insurance for children: Private insurance coverage continues to deteriorate. GAO-HEHS-96-129. Washington: GAO.

[HCFA] Health Care Financing Administration. 1996 June 30. Medicaid managed care enrollment report. Baltimore: Office of Managed Care, HCFA.

Heinen L, Fox P, Anderson M. 1990. Findings from the Medicaid competition demonstrations: A guide for states. Health Care Financing Review 11(4):55–67.

Hughes DC, Newacheck PW, Stoddard JJ, Halfon N. 1995 April. Commentary: Medicaid managed care: Can it work for children? Pediatrics 95(4):591–4.

Hurley RE. 1997 Jan. Managed care research: Moving beyond incremental thinking. Background paper for Agency for Health Care Policy and Research Expert Meeting. Washington, DC.

Hurley RE, Freund DA, Gage BJ. 1991. Gatekeeper effects on patterns of physician use. Journal of Family Practice 32:167–73.

Hurley RE, Freund DA, Paul JE. 1993. Managed care in Medicaid: Lessons for policy and program design. Ann Arbor, MI: Health Administration Press.

Interstudy. 1996 Sept. The Interstudy competitive edge 6.2, part II: Industry report. St. Paul, MN: Decision Resources, Inc.

Ireys HT, Grason HA, Guyer B. 1996. Assuring quality of care for children with special needs in managed care organizations: Roles for pediatricians. Pediatrics 98(2):178–85.

KPMG. 1994. Health Benefits in 1994.

Kogan MD, et al. 1995 Nov. 8. The effects of gaps in health insurance on continuity of a regular source of care among preschool-aged children in the United States. Journal of the American Medical Association 274(18): 1429–35.

Lipson DJ. 1997. State roles in health care policy. In: Litman TJ, Robins LS, editors. Health politics and policy, 3rd ed. Albany, NY: Delmar.

Lipson DJ, De Sa JM. 1996 Summer. Impact of purchasing strategies on local health care systems. Health Affairs 15(2):62–76.

Macro International. 1996 March. Private sector health care organizations and public health: Potential effects on the practice of local public health, final report. Prepared for the Centers for Disease Control and Prevention, Atlanta, GA.

Mashaw JL, Perrin JM, Reno VP. 1996. Restructuring the SSI disability program for children and adolescents. Report of the Committee on Childhood Disability of the Disability Policy Panel. Washington: National Academy of Social Insurance.

Mauldon J, Leibowitz A, Buchanan JL, Damberg C, McGuigan A. 1994. Rationing or rationalizing children's medical care: Comparison of a Medicaid HMO with fee-for-service. American Journal of Public Health 84(6):899–904.

Miller RH. 1996 Summer. Competition in the health system: Good news and bad news. Health Affairs 15(2):107–20.

Miller RH, Luft HS. 1994. Managed care plan performance since 1980. Journal of the American Medical Association 271(19):1512–19.

[NAIC] National Association of Insurance Commissioners. 1990. Health maintenance organization model act. Washington: NAIC.

[NAIC] National Association of Insurance Commissioners. 1996 Dec. The regulation of health risk-bearing entities. Draft White Paper of the Risk-Bearing Entities Working Group. Washington: NAIC.

[NCQA] National Committee for Quality Assurance. 1995. Medicaid HEDIS, Draft Report Washington: NCQA.

[NCQA] National Committee for Quality Assurance. 1996. World Wide Web site.

Neff JM, Anderson G. 1995 Dec. 20. Protecting children with chronic illness in a competitive marketplace. Journal of the American Medical Association 274(23):1866–9.

[NIHCM] National Institute for Health Care Management. 1996 April. Assuring quality of care for children in Medicaid managed care—EPSDT in a time of changing policy. NIHCM White Paper. Washington: NIHCM.

Regenstein M, Meyer JA. 1994 Aug. Low-income children with disabilities: How will they fare under health care reform? Washington: The Economic and Social Research Institute.

Rowland D, Rosenbaum S, Simon L, Chait E. 1995. Medicaid and managed care: Lessons from the literature. Washington: The Kaiser Commission on the Future of Medicaid.

Schlenker T, Fessler K. 1990 July. Measles in Milwaukee. Wisconsin Medical Journal 89(7):403–7.

Sisk JE, Gorman SA, Reisinger AL, Glied SA, DuMouchel WH, Hynes MM. 1996 July 3. Evaluation of Medicaid managed care. Journal of the American Medical Association 276(1):50–5.

Smyth M, Haas D, Friebe M. 1995. The ups and downs for children with chronic illnesses. Managed Care Quarterly 3(4):91–5.

U.S. Bureau of Labor Statistics. 1994. Employee benefits in medium and large establishments, 1993 (and yearly edition for 1986). U.S. Department of Labor. Washington: U.S. Government Printing Office.

Wood D, Halfon N, Sherbourne C, Grabowsky M. 1994. Access to infant immunizations for poor, inner-city families: What is the impact of managed care? Journal of Health Care for the Poor and Underserved 5(2): 112–23.

IV

A SYSTEM FOR THE FUTURE

In light of the great room for improvement in child health status, the widespread dissatisfaction with the current organization of child health services, and the much described risks and opportunities that managed care presents for children, what are we to do next, and how do we avoid some of the pitfalls of previous efforts to improve health services for children?

One reason past efforts may have failed, according to the chapter that follows, is the lack of a clearly articulated statement of children's right to health care. Quite apart from the arguments on behalf of a universal right to health care, it may plausibly be argued that children have a special right to care, because of their complete dependency on adults and because care given or care withheld may well determine the future course of a child's life. A compelling articulation of this moral imperative may help mobilize public opinion.

But clearly articulated principles are not enough. Action is required, and broad-based community-driven action at that. One of the lessons to emerge quite plainly from the last decade in health policy is that it is very difficult to impose change from the top down. Across the country, the models that are working best are those that draw on the strengths of communities, of individual parents and health care consumers. Traditional advocates are discovering new ways of engaging and working with these groups, and with the media, an important partner in any effort to generate public awareness and mobilize collective action. During this process, some new partnerships and coalitions may emerge, in which participants are linked only—but crucially—by their fundamental commitment to children's health and welfare. This commitment needs to be nurtured and developed at all levels of society.

Given that commitment, there is no lack of models, one of the most intrigu-

ing of which is the three-dimensionally integrated system of care described in chapter 14, which would address the concerns raised repeatedly throughout the volume by delivering care that is coordinated across health care and other systems, as well as over time. Better coordination of individual health care services with public health services is also key, predicated on a thoughtful definition and defense of the public health role and mission.

Finally, what begins to emerge is a clear agenda on behalf of children, one that is built on five simple principles: a child-specific standard of care, the appropriate alignment of incentives for providers of care, universal coverage, strengthened community health functions, and investments in appropriate research, education, and data systems.

Simple as these ideas are in principle, putting them into practice requires above all a committed citizenry that is prepared to act and to hold political, business, and community leaders accountable for progress and for the impact of all public decisions on the nation's children. It is a task in which we all have a role to play.

12

A More Equitable Health Care System for Children: The Moral Argument

Jeffrey Blustein

A National Ambivalence About Children

PROTECTING AND IMPROVING children's health, we are often reminded, is a wise investment in the future. It is not just today's children who will benefit: we will all benefit in the long run from a healthier society. Yet despite these frequent reminders and a professed societal commitment to caring for children, many commentators have noted with increasing alarm that the health of our nation's children is in jeopardy and that, if current trends continue, children face an uncertain future at best.

The problem is not that society merely pays lip service to the notion of a societal responsibility for children's health. This criticism neglects the very real advances in children's health that have been achieved through various social programs and policies. The problem is rather that we waver in our commitment to children, perhaps because of a failure to articulate a clear and compelling rationale for society's obligations to children, perhaps because of a failure of political will, or perhaps both. "How will it affect children?" is often the last, rather than the first, question that is asked of proposals to reform the nation's health care system.

This problem is not limited to the area of health care. The body of our social policies, legislation, and case law affecting families and children is riddled with contradictions and inconsistencies. Sometimes children are treated as persons who are entitled to benefits and protections and who have independent interests, and sometimes they are treated as little more than appendages of their parents with no voice or standing of their own.

Sometimes the care and control of children are regarded as private matters, the right and responsibility of individual parents, and sometimes as matters of serious public concern and a responsibility of the entire community.

A brief look at some laws and judicial opinions relating to children bears these tensions out. The first Family Court Act was enacted in Illinois in 1899 and established a paradigm that was followed by all other like state systems. Specialized family courts were to have jurisdiction over three categories of children:

1. The delinquent child, one who had committed an act that if done by an adult would be a crime; because the offender was a child, however, the crime was reduced to the charge of juvenile delinquency and adjudicated in a special court that was private and protected, and that left the child without a criminal record;
2. The status offender, a child who behaved in a way that was not a crime (e.g., staying out late against a parent's wishes); and
3. The neglected child, one whose parents did not provide food, shelter, education, and medical care.

Once established, these judicial interventions to support and protect children soon led to their own abuses. Disregard for the rights of children led the U.S. Supreme Court in 1967 (*in re Gault*, 387 US 1 [1967]) to hold—in a case in which a minor was sentenced to seven years in prison without ever knowing the charges against him, ever confronting the witnesses who testified against him, ever having his parents informed of the danger he faced, or ever having benefit of legal counsel—that children are entitled to basic due process rights in any judicial proceeding, criminal or civil, that may result in their loss of liberty.

A number of other decisions granting rights to children have recently been reached by the Supreme Court. In 1969, in the First Amendment case of *Tinker v. Des Moines Independent Community School District* (393 US 503 [1969]), the Supreme Court held that the right to free speech applied to children and hence protected their right to engage in peaceful political activity and symbolic speech within public schools. In the 1976 right to privacy case of *Planned Parenthood of Central Missouri v. Danforth* (428 US 52 [1976]), the Court declared unconstitutional part of a Missouri abortion statute requiring an unmarried minor female to acquire the consent of her parent or guardian in order to have an abortion performed (unless a physician certified that the abortion was necessary to preserve the mother's life). And in 1977, in *Carey v. Population Services International* (431 US 678 [1977]), the Court overturned a New York law prohibiting the distribution of nonprescription contraceptives to minors under the age of 16 years.

But these cases and others establishing the rights of children to Constitutional protection have been offset by other legislative and Constitutional developments. As children were gaining protection for their rights within the juvenile justice system, that system was being dismantled by many states. The age at which a child could be tried in the criminal justice system was lowered, especially for cases of violent crime. Today, increasing numbers of juvenile offenders are being convicted in adult courts and sent to adult prisons, where they are less likely to receive education and therapy and more likely to be abused by older inmates. In the rush to try juvenile offenders in adult courts, states have paid little attention to the special needs of youthful offenders and the detrimental impact of punishment on their lives.

The Supreme Court has also upon occasion shown a disregard for the rights of children. In the 1977 case of *Ingraham v. Wright* (45 USLW 434 [1977]), the Court ruled that corporal punishment in the schools was not unconstitutional. In 1979, the Court decided (*Parham v. J.L. and J.R.*, 47 USLW 4740 [1979]) that parents could seek state-administered institutional mental health care for their children without an advisory board hearing prior to commitment. This broad parental authority deprived children of the protections afforded all others facing involuntary confinement and left them totally under the power of their parents. The most dramatic recent example of the Court's failure to take the interests of children seriously is the case of *DeShaney v. Winnebago County Department of Social Services* (489 US 189 [1989]). In this case a child was severely and permanently damaged by repeated beatings at the hands of his father. The county department of social services was aware of the danger to the child and failed to act to protect him, although repeatedly requested to do so by hospital authorities identifying signs of abuse. The Supreme Court held that the language of the due process clause that requires the state to protect the life, liberty, and property of citizens established no "special relationship" that required the state to protect this child.

The same ambivalence is reflected in the complex world of foster care and child welfare authorities. Sometimes public policy favors removing children from their mothers when there are signs of prenatal drug use, and sometimes clearly abused children are left in the home because of some notion of the importance of "family preservation." Children are left in foster care for years and not freed for adoption because of the hope that they might one day return to their mothers, but rarely is this hope supported by the social services and family-building efforts that might make it a reality. Once again, there is considerable tension between the notion of the child as part of the parent, as the appendage if not the property of the parent, and the notion of the child as a small constitutionally protected person.

As these examples show, our society is deeply conflicted about whether and to what extent children have independent interests that warrant protection by rights; this conflict in turn is linked to a deeply rooted ambivalence about the respective roles and responsibilities of parents and society in the care and control of children.

Our policy decisions and choices about children's health and care also reflect this ambivalence. In order to understand what is at stake for children, families, and society in the ongoing debates about health care in this country, we must address fundamental issues about the nature and scope of children's and parents' rights, the requirements of social justice with respect to children's health, and our collective responsibilities for the welfare of our children. These principles and values enable us to identify and assess the moral dimensions of the U.S. health care system insofar as it affects the health of children.

Justice and the Rights of Children

As a statement of principle, few would deny that health care ought to occupy a central place in any normative account of our obligations to children. It is not difficult to formulate a rationale for this principle. There are certain basic goods on which the quality of any human life depends, and parental and social authority over children should be exercised in a way that enables them to realize these goods in the course of their development. The details of these goods and their relative weights may vary from one society to another and even within a single society, but generally speaking, they include affectionate care by adults during childhood, knowledge and skills that fit the individual for participation in the life of adult society, intelligence and imagination, a sense of self-worth, and physical and mental health. These and others are what John Rawls calls "primary goods," that is, goods that are necessary for the successful pursuit of virtually any plan of life or, more broadly, the realization of any particular conception of the good, whether or not this can be construed as a plan (Rawls, 1971, p. 62;

Blustein, 1982, pp. 120–30). In this way, health is different from, say, excellence in athletic competition; unlike the former, the latter depends for its value on the details of individuals' specific conceptions of the good and their life goals.

Because as a matter of empirical fact health *care* is necessary for the maintenance and restoration of health, and because those who are responsible for the welfare of children are obligated to respect their need for this good, the provision of health care to children is not morally optional. Moreover, health care is not only a right of children but, according to some theories of social justice, a requirement of justice as well (e.g., Daniels, 1985). Access to health care, like access to education, can determine the range of opportunities available to individuals in society. If equality of opportunity is a demand of justice, then so too is access to health care since it is often a prerequisite for maintaining such equality.

Arguably, the scope of our concern should be expanded beyond access to and availability of traditional services such as medical and surgical care for acute and chronic conditions, routine screening, developmental surveillance, and periodic medical examinations. There are many services designed to deal with nonmedical health-related problems, such as community-based services (e.g., child care and home visiting services) and population-based public health measures (e.g., AIDS or substance-abuse education and prevention programs; injury prevention campaigns; and environmental safety, community safety, and crime prevention programs) (Budetti and Feinson, 1993). Since all of these services have distinct health implications, it can plausibly be argued that the obligations to children that flow from the primary good of health should not be confined to the clinical sphere alone but should encompass provision of these services as well.

It should be noted that the above argument for the obligation to provide health care is specifically related to *children* and that it introduces an additional set of considerations into the usual arguments in the bioethics literature for a general right to health care because it starts with a fundamental fact peculiar to children and those adults who, in relevant respects, remain children: namely, others (parents, teachers, the state) exercise authority over them and intervene to a substantial degree in their lives. This is a descriptive claim. The moral question is how this authority is to be properly exercised. The answer proposed here is that those who exercise authority over children must do so in a way that respects their need for basic human goods, including the good of physical as well as mental health. Children are morally entitled to health care because, unlike most adults, they are dependent on adults who have authority over them and who are therefore *morally obligated* to provide them with the care they need.

Of course it is one thing to argue in this way for health care as a right of each child based on his or her vulnerability. It is quite another to argue that there is a social obligation to provide it and to articulate and defend a certain level of health care to which children generally are entitled. A popularly held view in the philosophical and policy literature on justice in the distribution of health care is that there is a moral right to health care, but that this is a right only to receive an adequate level (or a decent minimum) of health care, not the best health care services available. The arguments for the former narrowly tailored conception of a right to health care are extremely persuasive, but there is not the space to review them here (Buchanan, 1983). The question here is how the idea of a right to an adequate level of care is to be understood in relation to children.

First, children as a group are unique in that they proceed through developmental stages that make their needs for health services different from those of adults (see the discussion of a child-specific definition of medical necessity in chapter 1). The vague notion of adequacy must be spelled out in a way that takes this into account. Second, in defining an adequate level of care for children, the dominant concern should be prevention rather than treatment (Silver, 1994). (This is not an "either-or" claim. Treatment must still be adequate, of course.) One reason for this is the familiar cost-effectiveness rationale: in an economic sense, the largest number of individuals, children as well as adults, can be helped at the lowest cost through public health, health promotion, and other preventive measures. However, there is a moral argument as well for giving priority to prevention in the care of children, based on the moral principle of beneficence, or at least that part of the principle that tells us to prevent harm. A multitude of infectious diseases that in earlier years took a huge toll on children in terms of mortality and morbidity can now be prevented. Another major cause of mortality and morbidity in children is traumatic illness, and here too public health and accident prevention measures have proven effective in reducing the incidence of death and disability (Committee on Pediatric Emergency Services, 1993). Since it is in our power to prevent an enormous amount of pain, suffering, and disability in children, we are morally obligated to do so to the greatest extent compatible with other comparably important moral values. Of course, some children may become ill because of inadequate preventive services, and no set of prospective measures, however well designed and widely available, can completely eradicate disease, illness, and handicapping conditions. Measures should be taken to ensure that sick and disabled children receive the medical services they need, for beneficence requires treatment as well as prevention. But surely it is morally preferable to take proactive steps to prevent harm from occurring in the first place than to ameliorate the harm once it has occurred, and the causes of most mortality and significant morbidity among children can be successfully dealt with preventively.

The larger issue, which so far has only been touched on, is whether there is a moral right at all to health care as a matter of social justice. However widespread the view might be that there is such a right, not all theorists endorse it. Libertarians, for example, argue that there is no pattern of just distribution independent of free-market procedures, no normative ideal for distributing health care independent of the free choices of individuals, that is demanded by justice (Nozick, 1974). Many philosophers believe this approach is fundamentally flawed because it places a premium on the principle of respect for autonomy at the expense of other important moral (specifically, communal) values (President's Commission, 1983). Whatever we think about this, it is clear that specific and special provisions must be made for the care of children, including health care. Infants and young children do not possess autonomy. They must develop it, and its development is contingent on the development of certain psychological capacities, itself contingent on favorable familial and social environments. Indeed, as persons with the potential for autonomy, children have the right to an upbringing that allows and encourages them to exercise their capacities for autonomous action and independent judgment (Blustein, 1982). (What this requires, of course, will depend to some extent on particular features of the society in which children will take their place.) Even among adults, personal autonomy is often limited and tenuous because they lack the material preconditions of leading an autonomous life or because they find themselves in relationships of unequal power, knowledge, or dependence. Among younger children, lack of autonomy is more deep-seated in that it is explained by facts about human psychological development.

Moral rights, in the sense of legitimate claims to treatment as independent, self-conscious agents making choices about their own lives, are of relatively slight concern to children, whose capacities for self-determination are still undeveloped. The rights that are most important for younger children are claim or welfare rights, that is, rights to positive services from others, including health care services. In libertarian theories of social justice in which respect for autonomy is the sole basic moral principle, children are, morally speaking, invisible. They are the recipients of whatever health care (or education, shelter, nutrition) their parents are able and willing to provide for them through free-market procedures. What is missing from this account is an acknowledgment that children have a right to care because they lack the power, knowledge, and skills to secure it on their own, and because parents and others are obligated to ensure their enjoyment of health and other basic goods during the course of their development. Moreover, no matter how well intentioned, individually parents cannot effectively marshal the resources to meet all their children's health needs.

Extreme libertarian opponents of a right to health care argue that health care should be viewed as a service that, like many other services, may be purchased by individuals with the resources to do so and the willingness to spend them in this way, but not as an entitlement. Relatively affluent parents will be able to afford superior health care both for themselves and for their dependents, whereas the poor, if they and their children are to receive even minimally adequate care, must rely on the sympathy and charity of others. This repudiation of a right to health care is blind to the fact that wealth and income in our society are themselves inequitably distributed, and it demeans the poor by putting them in the position of having to rely on the kindness and charity of others for supplying their unmet health care needs.

A more moderate and defensible position—and one that is embraced by justice theorists of various stripes, including utilitarians, Rawlsians, and even some libertarians like Engelhardt (1986)—advocates a two-tiered system of health care in which all members of society are guaranteed a decent minimum of health care and those who are advantaged are permitted to use their own resources to purchase additional and better care. This approach, while allowing inequalities in the distribution of health care resources, avoids the most glaring deficiencies of the extreme libertarian position. As we will see ("The Health Insurance Problem," below), judged from the standpoint of a conception of justice that endorses the use of social resources for the provision of a decent level of health care for all, children's access to health care in the United States depends too heavily on their parents' private resources for purchasing health care services.

Translating Principles into Practice

It has been suggested here that each and every child has a moral right to health care, not only because health is a basic human good, but also because children are dependent on others (principally parents) who control their lives and who must, in turn, exercise authority in a way that respects the child's need for this and other fundamental goods. What distributive justice demands is that all children have equal access to health care that is geared to their developmental level and weighted toward prevention. These are quite abstract principles, and many policy decisions remain about how best to implement them in the context of contemporary social, economic, and political conditions.

An analogy might help. It seems plausible enough to claim that citizens of affluent countries are morally obligated to do more than they presently do to help starving people in other parts of the world. The question remains, however, how to allocate these duties, specifically, what institutions and social arrangements are most effective in fulfilling our duties to aid starving people. It seems uncontroversial that, for this purpose, our resources are not best employed in direct action, but rather should be aimed at maintaining and strengthening private and governmental institutions established to coordinate individual responses to worldwide hunger.

Similarly, if we are to translate moral principles into policies and programs that actually deliver the health care that children need and are entitled to receive, questions must be addressed about the division of responsibility for children's health needs among families, employers, and state and federal governments; financing mechanisms or combinations of mechanisms that best assure children's access to care; and the role that competition and the free market should play. Moral principles should frame and guide our policy deliberations, but which among a number of different policy options ought to be adopted cannot be decided on the basis of these principles alone.

Using these moral principles and the notion of a minimum benefits package for children as a benchmark, let us see how well current health care policies and programs in the United States serve the health care needs of all its children.

The Health Insurance Problem

As suggested in the preceding, no society can guarantee good health for all its children; rather, the proper and obligatory goal is that of ensuring equitable access to an adequate level of health care. But persons can have effective access to health care only if they have health insurance coverage, unless they are either extremely affluent or extremely fortunate. In the United States, the single most important health program for low-income families and children is Medicaid (Newacheck et al., 1995a). However, many poor children do not qualify for Medicaid, a situation that has been exacerbated by the decline over the last two decades in the percentage of children covered as dependents under their parents' employer-based health insurance coverage. Although expansions in Medicaid coverage for children largely offset the decline in private health insurance coverage for children between 1988 and 1992 (Newacheck et al., 1995a), between 1977 and 1987 the percentage of children without any form of insurance grew 40 percent (Newacheck et al., 1995b). Approximately 10 million youngsters in the United States (14 percent of all U.S. children) have neither private nor public health insurance, and contrary to popular perceptions, the majority of these children are non-Hispanic and white (Lazarus et al., 1996, p. 5). In most cases, these children's parents must pay out-of-pocket for care, although most can ill afford to do so.

Medicaid is the single largest payer of health care for children, but it is not the only federal program targeted at pediatric health (Flint et al., 1995). Federally subsidized care for children is provided through multiple and un-coordinated delivery structures, including Title V block grants for prenatal and child health services, public health immunization services, the Special Supplemental Food Program for Women, Infants and Children, and community health centers (Grason and Guyer, 1995; Hughes et al., 1995). (See chapter 6 for a full description of the complex and fragmented service system for children.) A strong argument can be made, if only on economic and efficiency grounds, for replacing this patchwork system of health care financing with a single, comprehensive system of health insurance for children and pregnant women (Hughes et al., 1995).

Moreover, even with some type of health coverage, many underinsured children may be forced to do without common and even relatively inexpensive health care services, and those who gain access to the system do not necessarily have access to the same minimally decent level of care as that available to other children. Poor children with Medicaid coverage have been shown to use preventive care at higher rates than poor children not covered by Medicaid (Newacheck et al., 1995a), but at much lower rates than privately insured children. Compared to privately insured children, poor children on Medicaid are less likely to use a wide range of health services, including preventive care (Lefkowitz and Monheit, 1991) and significantly less likely to have a regular source of care (Wood, 1990). Another study found that poor children with Medicaid were less likely than children living above the poverty line to receive routine care in physicians' offices rather than outpatient clinics and more likely to lack continuity between usual sources of routine and sick care (St. Peter et al., 1992). Together, these sobering statistics raise serious questions about access and equity in the distribution of health care services for more than 30 percent of U.S. children.

The State as Protector of Children

A number of important ethical and policy questions remain. What should be the role of the federal government with respect to securing an adequate level of health care for children? And to what extent should children's health care, prevention as well as treatment, depend on the choices and actions of their parents or guardians, assuming they have adequate insurance coverage to provide their children with the care they need? The discussion so far has not questioned the traditional assumption that parents ought to be in control of their children's health care, but there are some reasons to do so. Finally, when sickness or disability is not or cannot be prevented, how should the burdens of caring for afflicted children be distributed and what are the moral limits of this care obligation? As we will see, questions of justice related to health care for children include, but also extend beyond, those concerned with the adequacy of their health insurance coverage.

Congress recently ended the federal Aid to Families with Dependent Children (AFDC) program, replacing it with a capped block grant program to states, and it continues to explore similar options for the Medicaid program (Flint et al., 1995; Newacheck et al., 1995a; Sidel, 1996, pp. 81–116). Whereas states are now required to make Medicaid payments for specific services to certain groups such as low-income children, block grants would allow states far greater flexibility in setting their own eligibility criteria and benefit levels. Similarly, the Medicaid demonstration projects that have been approved by the Health Care Financing Administration exempt states from the requirement to adhere to federal eligibility and benefit standards (Flint et al., 1995).

It is tempting to discredit the motives of governors who are pressing for the conversion to state block grants and accuse them of being insensitive to the health care needs of disadvantaged children, but this moral insensitivity is only part of the problem. While many states have a history of punitive policies toward the poor (Sidel, 1996), the problem is also one of a lack of political will. States argue that they would be better able to meet the needs of vulnerable populations if they were free to use Medicaid funds in ways that are suited to local conditions, free from burdensome federal regula-- tions, and most observers expect that states would make an effort to continue supporting Medicaid at current levels, at least for the short term. But in the absence of federal regulatory requirements and in the current climate of shrinking federal Medicaid funding, the consequences for children threaten to be dire. As several commentators have noted:

> Block grants would likely become a battleground at the state level as lobbyists and advocates for various groups of beneficiaries, programs, and providers scramble to maintain their share of a shrinking budgetary pie. . . . Children have fared poorly in such circumstances in the past. (Newacheck et al., 1995a, p. 1471)

No less significant is what the dismantling of Medicaid would say about how our society views its responsibilities to its children. Conversion to unrestricted state block grants would render health care coverage for children extremely vulnerable to the vagaries and compromises of the political process. In replacing Medicaid with these grants, our society would be announcing that health care for children was no longer to be regarded as a fundamental right that must be protected; if society took this obligation seriously, its satisfaction would be of the highest importance and it would be largely insulated from politics. Put another way, rather than upholding the *principle* that children are a resource in need of special consideration and protection by the public, we would be declaring that questions about who qualifies for public aid and what benefits they are to receive are henceforth matters of *policy*, to be decided through contentious political processes at the state level. (The distinction between principle and policy is made by Dworkin [1977, ch. 4].) And as suggested earlier, these decisions are not likely to be favorable to children, who lack the political clout possessed by other more effective competitors in the political arena.

Insofar as government fails to assure that children from impoverished families receive the basic health services they need for adequate growth and development, it abdicates certain basic responsibilities. As argued above, the exercise of parental authority should respect children's needs for certain basic human goods, including health, and children have a right to parental care and upbringing that enables them to realize these goods. The needs of children in our society are principally the responsibility of their parents, but for various reasons, some parents may be unable or unwilling to discharge their obligations fully. In these cases the state, in its capacity as protector of those who cannot help themselves (under the doctrine of *parens patriae*), has the legal power and moral responsibility to step in and assume some measure of responsibility for the welfare of these children. The debate about Medicaid and block grants should not be viewed solely in terms of the proper scope of "state's rights," but rather as centering on the question of how government can best protect the rights of children, which it is sworn to do. It is sworn to do so because the obligation to care for children is not only the direct responsibility of their individual parents. There is as well a collective duty that falls on the members of society to ensure that the needs of its young are adequately met, a duty that arises in part from the fact that the common good depends on the health and effective rearing of each new generation.

Parents as Decision Makers and Caretakers

Generally, in our society, where individual freedom and responsibility are regarded as fundamental values, parents are accorded substantial (though not unlimited) discretion to raise their children as they see fit, free from state interference or coercion. Several arguments support this deference shown to parents (Crittendon, 1988, pp. 51–78, 108–120), and they under-lie a fundamental right protected by the Constitution and by case law. (See, e.g., *Parham v J.R.*, 442 US 584 [1979], holding that parents' fundamental right to determine the upbringing of their children extends to the decision to commit them to mental institutions. See also *Wisconsin v Yoder*, 406 US 205 [1972], holding that parents' right to determine their children's up-bringing and education outweighs the state's interest in compulsory school attendance.) First, the raising of children and the special close relationships involved are a source of distinct value in the lives of both parents and children. Public intrusion into the privacy of family life would seriously dam-age the quality of these very personal relationships. Second, freedom from interference in childrearing can be defended on the ground that it protects and promotes diversity in ways of life, a hallmark of liberal democratic and pluralistic society. To be sure, diversity is not an unqualified good; if par-ents' lifestyles include harmful elements, parents have no right to foster such elements in their children. But within broad limits, liberal democratic society will not only permit, but encourage, parents to shape their chil-dren's upbringing in accordance with their particular cultural, religious, and moral beliefs and values as they relate to child care and the division of parental responsibilities, appropriate behavior and methods of discipline, specific values such as the importance of academic achievement, and so forth. Freedom from state intervention creates a zone of privacy in which parents can raise their children in ways that are compatible with these values. Finally, most parents are likely to be sufficiently concerned for their youngsters' well-being to provide what is necessary for their upbringing. There is a strong but rebuttable presumption (consider cases of child abuse and neglect) that parents will be motivated by affection and concern to give their children nurturing that is at least adequate.

Our conventional childrearing arrangements are not without their critics, however. The most radical argue that the rights and interests of children are best secured through some nonfamilial, communal mode of upbringing (following the model of the Israeli kibbutzim, perhaps), or that children should be "liberated" from all forms of adult control much earlier than they are presently (Ladd, 1996). These arguments represent minority positions in academic circles, as well as among the public at large, and in their extreme form, they are unconvincing. They conceive of children as atoms whose interests are entirely separable from the web of relations that constitute the family, or they implausibly assume that the interests and good of children are the only values at stake in the family, or they make unwarranted claims about the decisional capacities of young children. A corollary of this argument that parents have the primary right to make decisions for their children's welfare is that health care reform should preserve and foster significant parental control, including the parents' right to choose their children's health care providers (Hughes et al., 1995, pp. 165–66.).

Of course, there are moral limits to parents' rights, in health care and elsewhere, although it should be acknowledged that these limits are not always well defined and that this has created some ambivalence in our society about the proper scope of parental authority. Whereas the failure to provide health care can be considered parental neglect in some cases, it is not always clear where legitimate parental discretion ends and parental medical neglect begins. To be sure, there are cases in which parents' failure to seek recommended medical treatment subjects their child to obvious, extreme, and irremediable harm, and on these occasions, the state ought to intervene to protect the child. However, parents have rights as well as duties, and, arguably, the child's welfare is only part of what parents should keep in mind when making medical decisions for their youngster (Schoeman, 1985). The child is part of a family in which the interests of some members (even health-related interests) must sometimes and to some extent give way to the interests of others, or to the interests of the family as a whole. This follows from the family's distinctive moral character as a deeply intimate relationship in which individuals share their lives and themselves. The state may be limited to the "best interests" criterion in its dealings with children, but the family would fail to provide its members with many of the goods that make familial life rewarding and valuable if parents were so confined. In addition, as the earlier discussion of cultural and religious differences suggests, we should be careful not to label parents as abusive or neglectful merely because they raise their children in ways that diverge from mainstream values.

Parents' rights to decide about medical care for their children are not only limited by the standard prohibitions against child abuse and neglect. They are restricted as well by the developing maturity of children. It is widely acknowledged that paternalism, which is properly a strong force in the rearing of young children, should begin to relax as children enter puberty and should continue to do so as they advance in adolescence. But here too there are ambiguities, for there are no hard and fast rules about how parents' rights ought to readjust progressively to the growing maturity of children.

Despite an expanding body of professional literature indicating that, with some exceptions, adolescents are capable of making major health decisions and giving informed consent, doubts remain among many parents, physicians, and policymakers regarding the capacity of adolescents to make and accept responsibility for autonomous decisions about their own health care. There are numerous studies in developmental psychology and pediatrics that challenge our traditional notions about the capacities of young people (Brock, 1989; Grisso and Vierling, 1978; Leikin, 1983; Weithornand Campbell, 1982). They converge on a common conclusion: most children over the age of about 14 years have the intellectual capacity and the independence to make at least some health care decisions for themselves. In these cases, parents and other concerned adults may—indeed, should—continue to play a supportive role, but their consent is not morally required.

Financial barriers, however, often stand in the way of young people gaining greater control over their own care. As noted earlier, most children in the United States receive coverage for all or part of their health care needs as dependents under their parents' private health insurance plans. As a result, their parents effectively control their access to health care financing and, in many cases, their access to care. Medicaid coverage is often not a viable option for adolescents, despite its theoretic possibility, because adolescents face serious obstacles created by financial eligibility criteria and stringent requirements related to proving their eligibility for benefits (Ad Hoc Committee on Adolescents and HIV, 1991). A comprehensive approach to ensuring children's access to health care should not only address coverage for children in the broader context of family health care, but should also facilitate coverage for adolescents independent of their parents.

Of course parents are involved in health care for their children not only by way of medical decision making. Our society also looks to parents to assume most of the burdens of caring for sick or disabled children (in fact, as it turns out, most of the work of care is performed by women). Questions about the distribution of care within the family, and about how much we as a society can properly expect parents to do to care for their children, are frequently overlooked in discussions about unfairness in health care. This is partly due to a common, if erroneous, belief that the family, being a private sphere, is beyond the reach of justice, which, it may be thought, regulates dealings among strangers, not among intimates (Okin, 1989, ch. 6). This is also partly due to the way we ordinarily think of children's health care, namely as involving the provision of traditional medical and clinical preventive services, rather than a range of services and programs with impact on the health status of children. However, questions about justice do come up *within* families and not just in the public domain, and a broad discussion of justice and health care for children would address them. Indeed, how care is distributed and managed in the family ought to be a major social concern, since the family is the primary locus of care for children in our society.

Issues of family justice in relation to health care are of two sorts: one concerns the distribution of the tasks of care among family members; the other concerns the degree of onerousness of these tasks for the caretakers. Feminists have drawn attention to the distribution problem, arguing that the division of caring labor in the family is unjust, that it results from the gender discrimination that pervades our society, and that it perpetuates sexism in all areas of social life (Okin, 1989, ch. 6). With respect to justice and the burdens of care, it is clear that family members should and normally do make greater sacrifices for one another than even close friends should or do. What would be supererogatory for those who are not part of our family to do, in other words, what would be morally praiseworthy but not obligatory, is often mandatory for family members. However, there are surely limits even in families to how much we can rightfully require individuals to do for one another. Family members have their own lives to live. They may have important personal goals and interests that would be severely compromised if they had to devote most of their time and energy to the care of other family members. (Of course, when there is no one else to assume the burdens of care, it will often be wrong of family members to refuse to do so, however burdensome the care may be. But this does not make their burdens any more just.) In addition, some caring demands may seriously threaten a family's ability to perform its other valued and valuable functions. One need not be a cynic about families to acknowledge that there are limits to how much we can properly demand of family members on behalf of one another (Nelson and Nelson, 1995, ch. 7).

The implications of these remarks for social policy are significant. First, with respect to the distribution issue, public policy should encourage and facilitate the equitable sharing of responsibility between fathers and mothers for the care of their children. For example, fathers should not be penalized for taking time off from work to care for their sick children. Second, families need support services that help parents raise their children and provide satisfactory care, including health care, whether it be acute or chronic care, comfort care, or rehabilitation. Parents cannot adequately nurture their children if they are forced to choose between caring for their children and caring for themselves, or between caring for their children and tending to the whole range of needs families must serve. To remedy this problem of unjust burdens, parents should have access to a range of supplementary child care services that can relieve them of some of the burdens of care when these become excessive. These include, among others, respite care, homemaker services, alternative care arrangements, and skilled home health assistance. To think of these as aspects of health care policy is to use the term "health care" in a broader sense than that employed in current debates about health care reform. But these services can all have a positive impact on children's health, directly or indirectly, and only such a broad-based approach can effectively protect and promote the health of our nation's children.

Conclusion and Implications

The starting point of ethical analysis about health care for children must be the recognition that children are not the property of their parents, but rather have interests and needs of their own, including health needs, that must be taken into account in decisions affecting them. Children belong to their parents, not as things belong to their owners, but as dependent and vulnerable persons belong to those who are morally responsible for their care and protection. Responsibility for children falls in the first instance on their parents, and any morally acceptable system of health care for children must recognize and respect this. However, the responsibility is not exclusively that of parents. There is also a collective moral responsibility that the members of society have toward children generally, and this is triggered when parents cannot by themselves provide their children with all they need or when parents fail to live up to the standards of minimally decent parenting. Health economists and health policy experts can help us decide whether our society has adequately discharged its collective responsibility to secure health care for children and, if not, whether current trends are moving us closer to or farther away from the realization of that morally mandatory goal. But their academic credentials do not give them any special insight into the moral principles and values that relate to the care of children. We must first articulate these principles and achieve widespread consensus on their central guiding role if we are to have a health care system that is not only fiscally responsible, but morally responsible as well.

In order to convert these principles into policy, we need to recognize that children's health depends not only on hospitals, clinics, nurses, and pediatricians, but also on the income of their parents, their family environment, and their parents' access to a range of nonmedical child care services. We must protect children currently covered by Medicaid and other health safety net programs and work toward expanding health insurance coverage to include all children and pregnant women; health insurance for children should be a comprehensive benefits package and should emphasize primary and preventive care. Financial barriers should not be allowed to prevent pregnant women and children from receiving comprehensive health care. And finally, health policy and law should support and strengthen the capacity of parents and children to make responsible health care choices and to be active participants and decision makers in the care children receive.

References

Ad Hoc Committee on Adolescents and HIV. 1991. Illusions of immortality: The confrontation of adolescents and AIDS. A report to the New York State AIDS Advisory Council.

Blustein J. 1982. Parents and children: The ethics of the family. New York: Oxford University Press.

Brock D. 1989. Children's competence for health care decision-making. In: Kopelman L, Moskop J, editors. Children and health care: Moral and social issues. Boston: Kluwer Academic Publishers.

Buchanan A. 1983. The right to a decent minimum of health care. In: President's Commission for the Study of Ethical Problems in Medicine and Biomedical and Behavioral Research. Securing access to health care, vol. 2. Washington: U.S. Government Printing Office.

Budetti P, Feinson C. 1993 Summer–Fall. Ensuring adequate health care benefits for children and adolescents. The Future of Children 3(2): 37–59.

Committee on Pediatric Emergency Medical Services. 1993. Emergency medical services for children. Washington: National Academy Press.

Crittendon B. 1988. Parents, the state, and the right to educate. Australia: Melbourne University Press.

Daniels N. 1985. Just health care. New York: Cambridge University Press.

Dworkin R. 1977. Taking rights seriously. Cambridge, MA: Oxford University Press.

Engelhardt HT. 1986. Foundations of bioethics. New York: Oxford University Press.

Flint S, Yudkowsky B, Tang S. 1995 Nov. Children's Medicaid entitlement: What have we got to lose? Pediatrics 96(5, pt. 1):967–70.

Grason H, Guyer B. 1995. Rethinking the organization of children's programs. Milbank Quarterly 73(4):565–97.

Grisso T, Vierling L. 1978 Aug. Minor's consent to treatment: A developmental perspective. Professional Psychology 9:412–27.

Hughes R, Davis T, Reynolds R. 1995 Summer. Assuring children's health as the basis for health care reform. Health Affairs 14(2):158–67.

Ladd RE, editor. 1996. Children's rights revisited. Belmont, CA: Wadsworth.

Lazarus W, Lipper L, Hughes D, Morrow E. 1996. America's uninsured children and the changing policy environment. Washington: The Children's Partnership.

Lefkowitz DC, Monheit AC. 1991. Health insurance, use of health services, and health care expenditures. AHCPR Pub. No. 92–0017. National Medical Expenditures Survey Research Findings 12. Rockville, MD: AHCPR.

Leikin S. 1983. Minors' assent or dissent to medical treatment. Journal of Pediatrics 102:169–76.

Nelson HL, Nelson J. 1995. The patient in the family. New York: Routledge.

Newacheck P, Hughes D, English A, Fox H, Perrin J, Halfon N. 1995a Nov. 8. The effect on children of curtailing Medicaid spending. Journal of the American Medical Association 274(18):1468–71.

Newacheck P, Hughes D, Cisternas M. 1995b Spring. Children and health insurance: An overview of recent trends. Health Affairs 14(1):244–54.

Nozick R. 1974. Anarchy, state, and utopia. New York: Basic Books.

Okin S. 1989. Justice, gender and the family. New York: Basic Books.

President's Commission for the Study of Ethical Problems in Medicine and Biomedical and Behavioral Research. 1983. Securing access to health care, vol. 2. Washington: U.S. Government Printing Office.

Rawls J. 1971. A theory of justice. Cambridge, MA: Belknap Press.

St. Peter R, Newacheck P, Halfon N. 1992 May 27. Access to care for poor children. Journal of the American Medical Association 267(2):2760–4.

Schoeman F. 1985. Parental discretion and children's rights: Background and implications for medical decision-making. The Journal of Medicine and Philosophy 10:45–61.

Sidel R. 1996. Keeping women and children last. New York: Penguin.

Silver G. 1994 June. Why a rising tide doesn't lift all the boats: Medicaid and medical care for children. American Journal of Public Health 48(6): 893–4.

Weithorn LA, Campbell S. 1982. The competency of children and adolescents to make informed treatment decisions. Child Development 53:1589–98.

Wood DL, et al. 1990. Access to medical care for children and adolescents in the United States. Pediatrics 86(5):666–73.

13

The Changing Role of Consumer Advocates

Susan Sherry, Carol Gentry, and Robert Restuccia

FOR ONCE, Costa Billias, a rambunctious 13-year-old, was not grinning and cracking jokes. An aspiring linebacker in the Pop Warner Football League, he had found out he would not be able to play. Because of his mother's illness, the family had lost access to health insurance.

He protested the injustice in a school essay. That led to this day, when Costa told his story to Massachusetts legislators and an auditorium full of people. "I have to tell you how hard it is, being a kid without health insurance," he said. "Please *do* something."

Costa's speech, which drew a standing ovation, was one of a host of inspirational events in the Children's Health Outreach Project, a multiyear campaign that, in July 1996, prodded Massachusetts to become the first state with a comprehensive insurance program for all children up to age 18—over the opposition of the governor. Some of the players in the drama were even younger than Costa. At one assembly for the legislature, fifth and sixth graders marched in carrying giant paper dolls that represented the state's 160,000 uninsured children.

Some of those present had stood in the same state house auditorium in 1988, when Massachusetts debated and passed a universal health care law, the key piece of which—the mandate that employers cover their workers—was never fully implemented, although several significant access programs were. The 1988 victory was won through the efforts of professional advocates with a strong media-based strategy and a working alliance with the liberal Democratic political leaders then in power. The business community was an enemy, the state medical society was apathetic, the unions were distracted by the effort to protect their own health benefits, and the public at large was uninvolved. By contrast, in 1996 many of the participants had direct experience with the failings of the health care system. The state teachers' union enlisted local teachers in grassroots organizing of uninsured parents, and the state medical society donated a full-time lobbyist. The 1996 victory was won through an intensive, broad, district-based campaign addressed to a relatively conservative Democratic legislature with a Republican governor.

What made the 1996 success possible was a huge shift in thinking and approach on the part of consumer advocates in Massachusetts. Changes in the political and health care environment between 1988 and 1996 helped to create this shift. In this chapter, we describe the ways in which advocacy for children is changing, with examples drawn primarily from our work at Health Care For All, a 10-year-old advocacy group that mobilizes at-risk groups to gain control over health care decision making, and Community Catalyst, a six-year-old project that provides consumer groups around the country with technical assistance in strategy development, leadership training, health policy analysis, and organizing techniques.

A Crossroads

Shifts in the political and health policy environments have brought consumer and child health advocates to a crossroads where they must decide between continuing advocacy as usual or investing resources in new approaches. Many organizations are finding that success depends on choosing a path that requires them to work differently than in the past. Further progress in health reform demands that they put consumer empowerment at the center of their agenda, using their advocacy and policy skills for support. This vision requires an explicit commitment to expanding racial, ethnic, and class diversity at all levels of organizing, advocacy, and policy analysis. Organizations must realize the necessity of carrying out a number of different campaigns and projects based on the needs of people and the changing health care environment. They have to develop new skills and restructure themselves. But the reasons to embark on this route are powerful.

The failure of national health care reform shows why it is so important to institutionalize a strong role for consumers in the health care system. In the debate about national reform, the vested interests gained the upper hand because the voting public had not been drawn into the debate in a meaningful way. Consumers were the audience, not the actors.

Similarly, in Massachusetts, the public's distance from the health reform struggle showed in polls taken after the passage of the state's universal health care law in 1988. Despite a year and a half of well-publicized debate, 28 percent of Massachusetts residents said they had never heard about the issue. More tellingly, 41 percent of the *uninsured* knew nothing about it.

The need for a fresh approach to engaging the public is now more critical than ever. Conservative political shifts at the national and state levels have led to tightened public funding, threatened reductions in health benefit and coverage standards, anti-government public sentiment, and unsympathetic attitudes toward poor people and programs for poor people ("compassion fatigue"). Traditional lobbying approaches, in which liberal activists expect or insist that government do "the right thing," are not likely to be effective in this environment.

With the shift to a market-based health system, government has transferred much of its decision making to private players who are not directly responsive or responsible to the voters. Public hospitals are becoming private nonprofit hospitals and nonprofit institutions are converting to investor-owned for-profit organizations. Responsibility for the care of low-income and at-risk children is being handed over to private health plans that are trying to realign their finances to survive in the new health care marketplace. If child advocates focus only on the traditional arenas—financing and regulation of public programs—they run the risk of being left out of critical decision making. The chaos created by the shifts in the marketplace, however, can offer new opportunities for advocates to find allies.

The challenge that child advocates face is illustrated by a 1995 survey of key members of state legislatures and representatives of children's advocacy groups (SLLF, 1995). The state legislative leaders said:

- They cared about child and family issues, but did not receive much information about them.
- They seldom heard from their constituents on child and family issues.
- Advocates for children had acquired an image as "elitists" who viewed the legislative process and elected officials with disdain. Advocates were perceived as partisan, having no interest in dealing with Republicans, only with Democrats, and even then, just with the liberals.
- Children's advocacy organizations had little political clout.
- Groups that advocated for children had no clear-cut agenda, no sustained strategy for legislative success, and no training on how to work

with legislators effectively. Sometimes they worked at cross-purposes with one another.

The state legislative leaders and the advocacy organizations saw a need for both professional lobbyists for children *and* a higher degree of grass-roots political activity on behalf of legislative initiatives for families. The report calls on state legislators to make a greater effort to learn about children's issues without being prodded. But given the realities of the political process, the report concludes that "if leaders are to become more engaged with child and family issues, those who advocate for children and families will have to change their tactics. There is no escaping the fact that the leaders we interviewed have a broadly unfavorable perception of the advocacy community."

All too frequently, advocates attempt only to speak *for* the community, acting on its behalf, instead of organizing the community to speak for itself. Legislators and policymakers know the difference. If they do not hear on their home turf about the concerns advocates want addressed, they will not act. Like generals without an army, advocates get trampled by opposing forces. Effective advocates must mobilize people who are not yet engaged in the debate to join in a cause that promotes their own interest and that of their children. This requires identifying local community-based opportunities for action or intervention. Advocates must focus as much, or more, attention on the community and community residents as they do on the state house and policymakers.

To accomplish this, advocates must develop new skills and a genuine constituency. The usual intelligence, educational credentials, and research skills are no longer enough to succeed in advocacy work; logic and facts often collide with the raw, gritty essence of political decision making, which is frequently influenced by those interests with ready access to decision makers and resources, as well as by trade-offs among unrelated issues and interests. Eloquence and depth of commitment are not enough either, although those are vital. Effective health care advocacy for children today requires:

- Skills in community organizing to build credibility for the movement, so that it will be grounded in "real people's" needs and experiences.
- A commitment to empowerment of the constituents that advocates claim to represent. Institutionalizing the involvement of people who

have experienced problems with the health system must be an explicit organizational goal. This involvement ensures that advocacy organizations speak effectively to the real needs of people.

- A thorough understanding of the new health system and its pressure points. Policy skills should be directed to identifying new pressure points and to enabling constituents to intervene in these decision-making arenas.
- Coalition-building among groups with divergent views but a common goal.

The following sections describe how these skills have been successfully employed in Massachusetts and other states, to amplify the message, build political muscle, and win meaningful improvements in health services for children. A range of state and local groups have partnered to reach out in new ways to find and support families with a stake in helping themselves—and their children—by working for change.

Leadership Development

The most important task of a children's advocate is to motivate and train parents, other caring adults, and children themselves to become advocates on their own behalf. The benefits of this approach extend beyond the necessity of building a political movement: children benefit in many ways as their parents become knowledgeable and assertive. When people see that they are not alone, that others share their dilemma, they realize that it is the *system*, not *they*, that is flawed. In working to change the system, they lose their fear and gain a sense of personal power that they can pass on to others, forming a chain of hope.

This is how it can work.

Sylvia Pierce and Health Care For All

Jim Pierce, a plumber, was on his way home one night when he was killed by a robber. His wife Sylvia Pierce, a schoolteacher, was pregnant with their fourth child. In one moment of violence she lost her husband, most of the family's income, and their health insurance.

She quit her teaching job because the children needed her at home, and the family lived on modest survivor's benefits. Their income, though low, was just a bit too high for them to qualify for food stamps. Sylvia was able to enroll her two oldest children in a state-run insurance program, and at first Medicaid covered her and the two youngest children. But Medicaid dropped Sylvia following the birth of her child and dropped her two youngest children a year later. She found out the state-run program had a waiting list, so the three of them were left uninsured.

One day, the school sent home an open letter to parents from Health Care For All, asking whether they needed health insurance for their children. Sylvia received the letter because Health Care For All and the local teachers union had launched a joint effort to inform parents about available health services and to develop a grassroots constituency for improved health access. Sylvia wrote back. A few weeks later, she got an invitation through the school counselor to speak at a local meeting of teachers, health care workers, public officials, and others who were concerned about children's need for health care. A shy person, Sylvia was at first leery of speaking to 250 to 300 people. But Cheryl Gresek, a Health Care For All activist who had lost her insurance after having a disabled child, called and shared her own story. Sylvia no longer felt isolated; she realized she could help her own children and others. So she went to the conference and told her story. It was so riveting that she was asked to speak to Boston's business leaders, the director of the state's Medicaid program, and others.

Recently Sylvia became a part-time parent organizer for Health Care For All. She goes where the parents are—school open houses, soccer games, bingo nights—and sets up a booth to inform people about health programs available for their children and also about how to be part of Health Care For All's efforts to improve and expand those programs. She reaches many through the churches.

"I know what it feels like when your child is sick and you're afraid to call the doctor because you don't have health insurance and you don't have the money. I've been there," Sylvia says. She dispels the stereotype of the uninsured as lazy people milking the system and calls herself "the reality factor for the people who sit behind the desks and make the decisions."

Elizabeth Byers and Oregon Health Action Campaign
In the early 1990s, Oregon received a Medicaid waiver that allowed it to curtail some services, expand coverage to 120,000 uninsured people, and move all Medicaid participants into managed care. State officials said this new Medicaid program, called Oregon Health Plan, would vastly improve access to care. But Elizabeth Byers of Salem, a volunteer with the Oregon

Health Action Campaign, was skeptical. A single mother who had been on Medicaid since suffering a stroke at age 36, she had never seen a doctor except in the emergency room in her four years on the program. She had not been able to find a private physician who would take Medicaid patients.

In February 1994, when she received a lengthy list of Salem doctors who supposedly had agreed to participate in Oregon Health Plan, she called a friend who also needed a doctor and suggested they split up the list and start making calls. The friend had a friend who was willing to help, and soon they had a group of five callers. Their impromptu survey of 40 medical offices found only one physician who agreed to take new Oregon Health Plan patients without restrictions, and another who said he would see children.

Working under the name Project Equality, the group presented the report to state officials and the media. Oregon Health Plan officials, who had ignored concerns about provider capacity when they were conveyed by professional advocates, suddenly paid attention because legislators were listening and asking questions. The resulting pressure on the health plans produced an immediate response, the establishment of a new nurse-practitioner clinic site by one of the major health plans contracting with Medicaid, and a long-term commitment to ensuring access.

Next, Project Equality took on a more sophisticated project: a questionnaire for Oregon Health Plan patients that attempted to find out how well they were being served by their managed care plans. When a state official questioned whether the group knew how to conduct such a survey, the group persuaded him to attend monthly meetings to help develop the questionnaire. The group recruited 20 people who had served as previous volunteers for the Oregon Health Action Campaign, and fanned out to find survey subjects in clinics, unemployment offices, and other likely places. The data they collected in 350 interviews indicated that 25 percent of patients had no access to primary care, even though the state was paying up to $125 a month in premiums to private health plans for them. Some people could get to their assigned physician only by hitchhiking. Because of language barriers at some medical offices, small children were having to translate serious medical information for their parents.

By asking those surveyed if they would like to become involved in Project Equality, the group kept expanding. Today, it has a place at the table whenever the state makes decisions about Oregon Health Plan, including decisions about the new Medicaid contract provisions that will apply to the health plans. Bill Baugher, manager of the Oregon Health Plan delivery system, said that as far as he is aware, Project Equality is the first group of welfare families to organize on their own behalf.

Having the group looking over his shoulder is "good for me," he says. "We have not developed a perfect system. When things go wrong, we need to know. The only way the Oregon Health Plan is going to be successful is to have their input."

Carolyn Landry-Billias and Health Care For All

Three years ago, Carolyn Landry-Billias and her husband were going through tough times in the family business. They had to decide whether to make the mortgage payment or keep up the premiums on the health insurance plan that covered them and their twins. They let the health insurance lapse, thinking they could pick it back up when times got better. But a few weeks later, Carolyn was diagnosed with chronic active hepatitis C, a viral disease that will eventually kill her unless she can get a liver transplant. Now the family no longer qualified for insurance; one salesman told Carolyn it "would be like insuring a burning house." Distraught, Carolyn was to receive one more blow, this time from an unexpected source: Even though she had always paid cash for office visits, her doctor refused to keep treating her because she was uninsured.

"I was really lost," Carolyn recalls. "Scared, confused. I literally went to bed for a month." One day she saw an article in the newspaper about the possibility that a local hospital would be closed. It mentioned Health Care For All, so she called.

When she was put through to Mark Rukavina, then director of community organizing, she cried and unloaded all her hurt and frustration and anger on him. When she collected herself and apologized for going on and on, he told her, "The problem is, Carolyn, you haven't said enough." He encouraged her to share her story with a number of groups—eventually including a televised health reform rally with President Bill Clinton before 15,000 people.

A physician who heard Carolyn offered to accept her into an experimental treatment program, which is still going on. Although her spine is deteriorating and her strength sometimes flags, Carolyn has become a key organizer in the North Shore suburbs of Boston, urging expansion of health care coverage and caution in the restructuring of local hospitals and health plans. She writes op-ed pieces for the local newspaper and speaks at area churches. Several times, she has been interviewed on television about health issues. She remembers how quiet she used to be, and says she has never been a leader—then realizes that a leader is, in fact, what she has become. She says, "I still can't believe I do the things I do."

Leslie Mansfield and Maine People's Alliance

Like many Americans, Leslie Mansfield suffered the inequities of the health insurance system in silent despair until someone showed her a specific way to fight back. Her awakening as an activist came in the early 1990s with a knock on the door from an organizer for the Maine People's Alliance. When he started talking about the need for health care reform, Leslie let him know he was preaching to the converted.

Her husband, a builder, had insured them and their two children under a small group plan through his business. But when their son Jamie was diagnosed with diabetes at age 3, the premiums began to go up. Within two years, they had jumped from $190 to $650 a month. In addition, the family had to buy Jamie's medical supplies and pay off their 20 percent share of his hospital bills, at $10 or $15 a month. Leslie took a job as a waitress to keep the family afloat.

So when the canvasser from Maine People's Alliance asked Leslie to help, she readily agreed. Leslie became a leader in Maine People's Alliance's successful effort to ban the insurance company practice of refusing coverage to individuals with preexisting conditions and to establish community rating for Maine's small group and individual health insurance markets. The next thing she knew, she was being asked to go to Washington to talk to the National Press Club. She was terrified, but thoughts of her son propelled her. Soon after her successful presentation in Washington, she was interviewed on CBS News. Another news program invited her to respond to President Clinton's State of the Union Address.

Today, she is a board member of the Maine People's Alliance and writes op-ed columns for the local newspaper about health insurance. She is now working to win consumer representation on the board of the Maine Medical Center because she is concerned that its clinics are not being placed where they are most needed. She has become a "squeaky wheel," she says with a laugh.

"Some people think no one is going to listen to what we have to say, but I think we should try," she says. "I'm a big believer that communication can make a difference."

Identifying potential leaders like Leslie and the others and developing their skills require a serious long-term investment in constituency building. Just finding such people in the first place requires creativity and effort, whether it is recruiting them from among help line callers or conducting door-to-door outreach. Then, these potential leaders must be brought together so they see that they are not alone and given training so that they can collectively address their concerns. Providing clear, understandable information in a variety of educational formats is a critical component of this organizing process.

While these efforts do not equal a mass movement, personal stories carry the power to make a significant impact on health policy. The legislators who complain that children's advocates are elitist change their view when they hear from people like Sylvia Pierce, Carolyn Landry-Billias, Elizabeth Byers, and Leslie Mansfield. Their involvement helps to ground advocacy organizations in the concerns of real people.

New Alliances and Strategies
In addition to involving new activists, many successful advocacy groups are going well beyond a traditional focus on public benefit programs.

Identifying New Sources of Funding for Programs
In Massachusetts, Health Care For All had built a grassroots political base of parents through local school outreach, organizing projects around local hospital controversies, and its toll-free Health Help line. Thousands of Massachusetts families called in; some who got help enrolling their children in existing programs were grateful and became volunteers. Others found there was no program for their children, and were encouraged to join the movement. The political base and number of parent-activists kept growing.

Initially, many of these activists threw themselves into the Clinton effort to achieve national health reform. But when that effort died, Health Care For All decided it was time to reframe the health access debate around children. Health Care For All filed and successfully promoted legislation that would add 25 cents to the price of a pack of cigarettes. Seventy percent of the estimated $100 million in new revenues will provide new coverage for uninsured children and the rest will buy prescriptions for the low-income elderly.

While parent-activists formed the core of the campaign, to be successful, Health Care For All had to form an unconventional alliance that included providers, insurers, and the business community. This alliance was made possible by Health Care For All agreeing not to oppose repeal of the universal health law's employer mandate in exchange for support of the cigarette tax. Realistically, Health Care For All knew that the mandate could not be implemented over the objections of a Republican governor and more conservative legislature.

Among the groups that pushed for passage of the final legislation were Associated Industries of Massachusetts, the Massachusetts Business Roundtable (the chief executives of the largest firms in the state), and United Way's "Success by 6" Leadership Council, which backs programs that benefit young children. The chairman of one of the largest banks in New England and the former chief executive of the telephone company found themselves in the unaccustomed position of lobbying in concert with union leaders, advocates of a single-payer health plan, and other progressive groups.

The importance of the business community's contribution to the passage of the bill cannot be overstated. Building relationships with people who had not previously been thought of as allies, people who could not possibly be demonized as "tax-and-spend liberals," Health Care For All created an unbeatable coalition.

The children's health campaign became a vehicle for Massachusetts physicians to demonstrate their concern for their patients as well. The emergence of managed care in Massachusetts, as elsewhere, had changed the balance of power among health insurers, hospitals, and doctors. In the face of this, the state medical society was seeking a stronger alliance with consumer groups. Its commitment went beyond lip service to the commitment of meaningful lobbying resources.

Insurance Market Reforms

Another unconventional alliance emerged in Maine, after consumer organizations were blocked from expanding public health access programs by constrained state spending and a hostile governor. The Maine People's Alliance not only sought to build a stronger grassroots base through a variety of outreach approaches, it attempted to address access issues by pursuing insurance market reforms. Through local forums, Maine People's Alliance identified many young families who had trouble obtaining or affording individual health coverage; it also identified many small businesses that had trouble obtaining small group coverage. Maine People's Alliance broadened its constituency by reaching out to businesspeople. Before, small business lobbyists' opposition to increased state spending had led consumer advocates to assume that small business was the "enemy." Maine People's Alliance's willingness to develop a new constituency paid off. Many of the new consumer activists identified through this campaign continue to play a leadership role in campaigns to expand access and implement Medicaid managed care in the state.

Another new approach for Maine People's Alliance was its decision to form an alliance with Blue Cross/Blue Shield. Historically, Maine People's Alliance had opposed the Blues' policy agenda of rate deregulation and rate increases, an agenda driven by the Blues' status as insurer of last resort, required to take high-risk applicants while its competitors could avoid them. Together, Maine People's Alliance and the Blues waged a successful multi-year campaign to restrict severely other companies' ability to turn down customers with preexisting conditions and hike rates to unaffordable levels to get rid of families like Leslie Mansfield's. Maine People's Alliance's link with the Blues on market reforms continues despite its opposition to other elements of the company's policy agenda, including its attempt to convert to for-profit corporate status.

Managed Care Monitoring

The Oregon Health Action Campaign's investment in organizing families on Medicaid has positioned it as a major player in implementation of the state's Medicaid waiver. While historically involved in advocacy around Medicaid program decisions and regulations, Oregon Health Action Campaign's investment of resources in community organizing has greatly strengthened its role. The direct involvement of people in the program ensures that Oregon Health Action Campaign is able to identify problems right away and articulate them effectively. Oregon Health Action Campaign's broad constituency covers the full political spectrum, from conservative rural areas to more liberal urban areas. The physician shortage issue identified by Project Equality found a highly sympathetic ear among rural legislators. Project members now participate in Medicaid contracting and state regulation of managed care, through regular meetings with state officials, public hearings, and written comment.

A survey that turned up the need for Spanish translation and cultural competence at medical clinics led to a community outreach and health leadership development project in the Hispanic community. These new leaders are now helping rewrite the state's Medicaid managed care regulations and pressing local hospitals for more responsive services. The Oregon Health Action Campaign is also providing health policy staff to the state's Hispanic Human Service roundtable.

Like Oregon Health Action Campaign, the Illinois Campaign for Better Health Care has found that its ability to influence Medicaid managed care policy has been enhanced by its commitment to work with low-income constituencies and local community organizations. Illinois's efforts to implement Medicaid managed care have been plagued by significant implementation and oversight problems going back to the late 1980s (GAO, 1990; Krol, 1994). Child and legal service advocates had consistently communicated with the media, state policymakers, and federal officials about the abusive marketing techniques of some HMOs and access problems, but with few results.

With a federal waiver for mandatory Medicaid managed care pending, an unresponsive state bureaucracy, and a growing number of state residents moving into managed care, Campaign for Better Health Care judged that the time was right to interest the media in covering continued problems. Stymied by a lack of adequate state data, Campaign for Better Health Care worked closely with its grassroots member organizations to identify cases of marketing abuses by HMOs. These case examples were incorporated into a policy report prepared by the Center for Community Health Action (CCHA, 1996b). Prior to the release of the report, Campaign for Better Health Care helped to link journalists with community organizations and additional Medicaid clients so they could see firsthand the human dimension of the marketing abuse problems.

The extensive media coverage that resulted provided support for the federal Health Care Financing Administration's later decision to condition approval of the state's waiver on the use of independent counselors to assist clients in selecting managed care plans. As importantly, Campaign for Better Health Care's effort significantly heightened coverage of more general health policy and Medicaid issues both in the mainstream press and in the ethnic and neighborhood media that reach large segments of low-income people in Chicago.

Scrutinizing Mergers

In New Hampshire, consumer advocates seized an opportunity to address access issues when an out-of-state health plan applied to take over a local

HMO. Advocates knew that rural areas already had too few doctors and poor health indicators, especially for children and adolescents. In this sparsely populated state, parents whose children had special needs found themselves relying upon a limited number of pediatric specialists. Meanwhile, health plans were competing to tie up physicians in exclusive provider contracts, which preclude providers from participating in other health plans, effectively preventing them from seeing patients enrolled in those plans. From its work with community and parents' groups, New Hampshire Citizen Action understood that this move threatened to create significant access problems for families not able to enroll in whatever health plan had locked in their specialist or primary care provider.

Fortunately, the application to take over the local HMO required a review by the state insurance department. New Hampshire Citizen Action sought formal intervener status in the review hearings and used it to raise access issues, request that exclusive provider contracts be forbidden, and insist that the merged entity be required to dedicate several million dollars to address rural health needs. Following this unexpected intervention, the health plans initiated a series of meetings to negotiate with the community groups.

The negotiation and hearing process produced a ruling that banned exclusive provider arrangements for specialists and underserved areas. In addition, the merged health plans were required to dedicate $5 million to rural health delivery improvements and an additional $17 million to a state trust fund for other community benefits. While in the end the HMO merger fell through for unrelated business reasons, state regulatory precedent was established. Public attention to the issue from the insurance hearings also led to a new state law banning exclusive provider arrangements.

Combining Research with Community Outreach

In Boston, Health Care For All and the Center for Community Health Action used a high-profile research project to show that nonprofit teaching hospitals had accumulated millions of dollars in cash reserves while allowing community needs to go unmet. The research report was a catalyst for an organizing effort that gave neighborhood residents more say in how hospitals allocate their resources.

Despite the fact that Boston had 12 nonprofit teaching hospitals—some of the wealthiest in the country—many of the city's neighborhoods had poor health status, with infant mortality rates that rivaled those in developing countries. As competitive pressures increased, many of these nonprofit institutions invested heavily in expansion to prosperous suburbs, disregarding pressing needs in their immediate communities. Some defined their market not just regionally, but globally, attracting international celebrities who wanted world-class hospital care. Advocates questioned the priorities of these tax-subsidized institutions.

The project undertook a two-pronged effort to address these inequities. First, discussion with community leaders was initiated to determine what they saw as the greatest needs for health care resources. The Boston At Risk project was one element of this community outreach effort. The project developed a participatory adult education curriculum about community health and the health care system. (The model has served as a useful starting point for other local community action projects in both urban and rural settings.) Simultaneously, support and publicity were mobilized for a Harvard University School of Public Health research project on the financial status of teaching institutions. Conducted by Nancy Kane, the research identified $2 billion in discretionary cash available to the city's hospitals (Kane, 1993). After conducting training sessions for community leaders on the research results, the report was released to the press.

Health Care For All subsequently organized community leaders in public campaigns questioning hospital priorities. As part of that campaign community leaders worked with the Attorney General, who regulates all charitable entities. The result was the formulation of standards by the Attorney General's office on nonprofit hospitals' responsibility to the community. Hospitals throughout Massachusetts are now expected to consult with communities and allocate substantial resources to "community benefits." Improvements won to date include translation services, capital investment in neighborhood health centers, funding for neighborhood outreach workers, and expansion of free care to cover prescription drugs and physician services. Many of these services benefit children.

Helping to Structure the Disposition of Charitable Assets as Nonprofit Health Institutions Convert to For-profit Status

As hospitals and health plans attempt to survive in a competitive environment where bigger is better, nonprofit health care institutions are converting to for-profit status. This unprecedented phenomenon can jeopardize critical community health services and millions of dollars of charitable assets intended for public benefit (CCHA, 1995, 1996a; Hamberger et al.,

1995). In central Massachusetts, a broad community coalition of senior citizens, Latino groups, and social service agencies formed to represent public interests in two local conversions. With training and legal policy support from Health Care For All, the coalition has engaged in direct negotiations with the converting institutions and the Attorney General. As a result of this community involvement, final approval of a local hospital conversion was conditioned on maintenance of free care, interpreter services, and access for disabled community members. The coalition also negotiated strong community participation in the mission development and governance structure of the fund that will receive charitable proceeds from the sale.

In North Carolina, the pending sale of a county hospital that is the primary service provider for the community has been the object of a local organizing campaign by North Carolina Fair Share. With policy support from the Center for Community Health Action, North Carolina Fair Share initiated a local outreach campaign that included public forums to identify community concerns about the sale's impact on health services. Religious leaders and social service agencies not previously involved with health advocacy became engaged in the campaign. Following the forums and meetings with the hospital administrators, North Carolina Fair Share crafted service delivery criteria, including criteria for charity care access, that the county should incorporate into any sale agreement. County officials acknowledged the need for increased attention to such health delivery issues and, in response, formed a task force with community participants to address these concerns.

Conclusions

The above examples illustrate how legal and policy expertise can be used to promote health care organizing. Analytic efforts do not stop at monitoring changes in the system, but must help find new policy-related opportunities for organizing consumers around the priorities they—not state policymakers—have set. It is important to note that many of the organizing campaigns and activities described did not begin as legislative fights. Challenging a hospital to become more responsive to the community or conducting a local school drive to enroll children in existing health programs are ways in which policy expertise can be applied outside the walls of government. While ultimately government intervention was a critical element in these successful campaigns, the organizing activity was not initially focused on government. Many of the key campaign elements were directed at the local and institutional level rather than at the state house or Medicaid office.

It is also of note that several of these successful advocacy efforts intervened in policy arenas other than the public benefits programs that traditionally have been the primary focus of child advocates. Private insurance underwriting practices in Maine, market-driven corporate mergers in New Hampshire, and the competitive behavior of private nonprofit institutions in Boston all provided opportunities for successful policy intervention and leadership development. Advocates became successful players in the new government and regulatory arenas that are increasingly important in a health care system that is more private and market-driven.

By sharing their expertise, professional advocates turn volunteers into sophisticated activists. Medicaid beneficiary Elizabeth Byers now helps state officials design surveys, and waitress Leslie Mansfield collects and analyzes hospital documents. It is no coincidence that both of these women decided to go back to school once they were trained as volunteer advocates. The skills that people develop in their own communities enable them to assume broader leadership roles.

The advocacy approach described here is far from a final product. Much remains untested, and new learning continues as more advocates create new organizing projects to build and sustain a consumer movement for health. Components of the approach, however, can be articulated.

Assessment of the Environment
Given the increasingly complex nature of the U.S. health care system, understanding what is happening to consumers is a difficult task requiring constant monitoring. Analysis must be focused on:

1. health industry restructuring and financial analysis of the system;
2. community needs;
3. political forces; and
4. regulatory agencies.

The rapid changes brought about by a market-oriented health system mean that advocates must constantly be on the lookout for new opportunities and pressure points, because as the system evolves, consumers can play a major role in shaping how government and health care institutions respond to these new developments. This type of broad, systemic monitoring allowed the advocates described above to identify new means of organizing consumers to represent their interests. Five years ago, few advocates would have identified a health plan merger as a tool for directing new resources to rural health system infrastructure development, yet it became that in New Hampshire. Similarly, advocates in Maine were able to take advantage of competitive shifts within the health insurance industry to tackle the previously esoteric world of insurance underwriting, allying with Blue Cross and Blue Shield against other elements in the insurance industry.

Technical Supports

By monitoring systems changes, children's health advocates can help to identify areas for further research and develop possible policy avenues for organizing consumers to represent their interests. The capacity to engage in new areas of legal and policy research can play a critical role in enabling consumers to have significant impact on policy for vulnerable constituencies, as has been the case with the wave of conversions of nonprofit health care institutions to for-profit status. Armed with in-depth legal research, consumer advocates around the country are playing a key role in shaping new regulatory intervention that is creating new charitable foundations devoted to meeting the needs of at-risk populations as well as preserving community health services.

When the ability to analyze emerging policy issues is coupled with the capacity to emphasize the human dimension of the issue, a media strategy can be especially effective. The story of Leslie Mansfield's experience with insurance underwriting practices helped to make the issue of experience rating understandable to the media and the public. The Central Massachusetts Community Health Coalition's articulation of the community health services that could be put at risk by a nonprofit hospital's conversion moved media coverage of the issue from the business pages to the front page of local newspapers.

In all of the campaigns described above, technical information was translated into lay language and a variety of educational formats were used to make it accessible to community people who are not policy experts.

Organizing

The process of organizing and leadership development has a number of steps:

1. Identification of potential activists and leaders through carefully targeted outreach and organizing campaigns or support services such as school-based outreach, help lines, door-to-door outreach, or community surveys.
2. Engagement of individuals who learn what they can do to promote change through appeals, hearings, and self-advocacy.
3. Organizing campaigns, bringing together diverse individuals and organizations around single issues, system reform, or multi-issue community-based action.
4. Development of volunteers' skills through constant support, information, and training.
5. Activation of volunteers to participate in negotiations with local hospitals and health plans, offer legislative or regulatory testimony, conduct outreach to others in similar circumstances, and talk to the media. Taking action is a means of informing both policymakers and the general public.

It is a constant challenge to place organizing and empowerment at the center of advocacy work, given the pressure to respond to day-to-day legislative and policy crises. As the political environment and health care delivery system continue to change dramatically, this approach will need to be adapted. However, to make government respond to the needs of children, power must be generated at its richest source—the homes and schools and churches and businesses of our communities. This cannot be accomplished if advocates spend their time in their offices talking to people like themselves. It cannot be accomplished by remaining above the nitty-gritty of politics. Yes, public officials *should* act in the interests of children and families. But they need their constituents to tell them what those interests are. Mobilizing that constituency must be advocates' top priority.*

References

[CCHA] Center for Community Health Action. 1995 Nov. Converting to for-profit health care: What advocates should know. State of Health 9(8).
[CCHA] Center for Community Health Action/Consumers Union. 1996a Oct. The conversion of nonprofit health care organizations into for-

---

*Those who would like to explore ways to strengthen constituency involvement or to develop skills in community organizing should contact Community Catalyst, 30 Winter Street, 10th Floor, Boston, MA 02108. Telephone: (617)338-6035.

profit corporations: The community health assets training manual. Boston: CCHA.

[CCHA] Center for Community Health Action and Illinois Campaign for Better Health Care. 1996b May. Illinois managed care marketing abuses: Dangerous precedent, dangerous future. Boston: CCHA.

[GAO] General Accounting Office. 1990 Aug. Oversight of health maintenance organizations in the Chicago area. Washington: U.S. Government Printing Office.

Hamberger E, Finberg J, Alcantar L. 1995 Aug.–Sept. Pot of gold: Monitoring health care conversions can yield billions of dollars for health care. Clearinghouse Review 29(5).

Kane NM. 1993 May. Report on the financial resources of major hospitals in Boston. Boston: Department of Health and Hospitals.

Krol E. 1994 June 24. State health plan for poor comes up short. Chicago Tribune, Section 1, p. 1.

[SSLF] State Legislative Leaders Foundation. 1995. State legislative leaders: Keys to effective legislation for children and families; a report. Centerville, MA: Children and Families Program, State Legislative Leaders Foundation.

14

Developing a System of Care for All: What the Needs of Vulnerable Children Tell Us

Neal Halfon and Miles Hochstein

Introduction: Market and Organizational Trends Affecting Children

IN THE LAST TWO DECADES, two major policy questions have confronted those interested in improving the delivery of health services to children: how to ensure access to appropriate health care services (the insurance question) and how to assure that health services are organized to meet children's needs (the systems question). Those addressing the first question have focused on the important role of health insurance in providing access, as well as on the role of nonfinancial barriers such as lack of transportation, outreach, and translation services. Those addressing the systems question have focused on the kinds of services that should be provided for children and on how different health and related services can be coordinated into family-centered, community-based systems of care; increasingly, they have focused on issues of quality as well. More recently, the recognition that much of the inability to coordinate the vast array of programs potentially available to children (a systems issue) is a function of how services are financed and administered (an insurance issue) also has fueled new efforts to integrate services through decategorization of separate funding streams (Hughes et al., in press).

While issues of access and appropriately designed systems of care are important for all children, they are especially important for those children who are most vulnerable, such as children with chronic and debilitating medical problems, those suffering from serious emotional problems, children who have been abused and neglected, and children born to teenage parents. The effort to provide better and more accessible care for highly vulnerable children promises to improve the capacity of the health care system to respond adequately to the needs of all children, improving health development and minimizing severe disability and dysfunction.

These issues have taken on a new urgency in recent years due to several related trends that are fundamentally changing the organization, financing, and delivery of health care. These trends include:

• *The erosion of private employer-based health insurance.* The number of children with employer-sponsored health insurance has been steadily declining over the past eight years, with approximately 600,000 children losing coverage each year. For those who have not lost insurance eligibility, coverage has been restricted, a circumstance that particularly affects children with multiple or special health needs (GAO, 1996; Newacheck et al., 1995a). As we rapidly approach a time when less than 50 percent of children will be covered by private employer-based health insurance, the rationale for using an employer-based system to cover children may be called into question.

• *Politically imposed limits on Medicaid expansion.* The absolute number of uninsured children has remained reasonably constant at about 14 percent in spite of the deterioration in employer-based coverage, because the Medicaid program has rapidly expanded since 1989. The Medicaid program has played a particularly important role for vulnerable children, who are disproportionately covered by Medicaid and whose systems of care have often been constructed with flexible Medicaid dollars (Newacheck, 1995c). However, cost control concerns, entitlement downsizing, and the transition to managed care make it unlikely that Medicaid will be able to continue to fill in new gaps, nor is it likely to be as available to pay for special services. Other recent policy changes such as the tightening of eligibility requirements for Social Security Income and the elimination of Medicaid benefits for immigrants will further constrict the pool of children eligible for Medicaid.

• *The growth of managed care.* Marketplace restructuring has been led by the growth of managed care and the rapid rise of vertically integrated health care corporations that have the ability to integrate the delivery and financing of services and spread financial risk across the system (Halfon et al., 1996; Miller, 1996b). The increasing use of managed care for Medicaid beneficiaries may improve access and availability of services for some children, but it is likely to disrupt many established provider relationships for children with special needs (Ireys et al., 1996).

• *The growth of managed competition.* The macro-marketplace is being redefined by aggressive competition among large corporate managed care organizations on the basis of price and, purportedly, quality (Miller, 1996a). The dearth of accepted child-specific quality measures justifies skepticism about whether competition on the basis of quality can take place at this time for children, particularly for those children who are most vulnerable (McGlynn et al., 1995).

• *The transformation of the social role of medicine.* The metamorphosis of the health care system from an amalgamation of not-for-profit entities and private practices into a for-profit market involving large corporate units has made economic issues increasingly central to all health care encounters. A health care system emphasizing the social allocation of resources is in the process of being replaced with a market-based, commodity-oriented system.

For those concerned with addressing either the access or the systems question for America's most highly vulnerable children, these trends present formidable challenges as well as potential opportunities. Past correctives such as the expansion of Medicaid, the use of Title V monies for expanded services, and the development of new categorical service programs may not be an option, nor are they necessarily viable strategies in the emerging health care market. The real policy challenge lies in using these marketplace changes and long-term financing trends to maximize access and to fashion a system of services that meets the needs of the most vulnerable children.

Vulnerable children are found at one end of a continuum of vulnerability that includes all children, and because children may move from a condition of relative well-being to one of relative vulnerability in a relatively short time, reforms that enable the health system to respond to highly vulnerable children have the potential to benefit all children.

In this chapter we first discuss childhood vulnerability in conceptual terms and then consider how certain groups of children are particularly vulnerable. We then consider four different kinds of barriers to addressing the needs of highly vulnerable children and suggest a set of policies that can move the United States toward a system of health care that responds effectively to the needs of children at all levels of vulnerability.

Conceptualizing Inherent Vulnerability and Enhanced Vulnerability
What is vulnerability? In its most basic sense, vulnerability means that an individual is at risk of poor health outcomes (Aday, 1993). When speaking of childhood vulnerability, it is important to consider two dimensions: risk factors associated with the condition of childhood itself (the inherent vulnerability of childhood), and the particular patterns of risk factors that make some children more vulnerable than others (enhanced vulnerability). Standard models of vulnerability typically use socioeconomic status variables like income, race, sex, and age to define vulnerable populations (Aday, 1993). These models may also include measures of the density of social relationships, reflecting the capacity of a rich network of supportive friends and community-oriented professionals to buffer an individual's risk. Such models may also include a measure of an individual's human capital (years of education and skills acquired), factors that can also buffer risk.

If adult models of vulnerability are applied to children, it quickly becomes apparent that, by adult standards, all children are inherently vulnerable and many are disproportionately vulnerable. In terms of social status, children are young and have no independent income, and they are disproportionately members of racial and ethnic groups that are discriminated against. Their social network is relatively limited, and, in terms of human capital, they have little education and no marketable skills, and the development of their innate capabilities is entirely dependent upon an appropriate nurturing environment. By adult standards children are all, by their very nature, crowded into the vulnerable end of the spectrum of human vulnerability, notwithstanding the innate resilience of some children (Werner, 1990) and the social buffering provided by many families and communities (Bronfenbrenner, 1986; Garbarino, 1990).

The policy issue for vulnerable children is therefore one of addressing not only the inherent vulnerability of childhood, but conditions of enhanced vulnerability as well. Any young, defenseless, growing, developmentally malleable, financially and emotionally dependent individual will face serious *inherent* risks. The plasticity of a child's mental and physical development, the dependency of children on caregivers, the patterns of illness associated with childhood, and children's need to integrate their growing functional capacities all constitute unique characteristics of children's health, and define the dimensions of children's inherent vulnerability (Perry et al., 1995).

These issues pertain to all children. However, when we identify vulnerable children we are identifying children whose additional vulnerabilities, or risk factors, intersect and interact in negative ways with the inherent vulnerabilities associated with the condition of childhood itself. Enhanced vulnerability can have biological origins, in a genetic deficit or chronic medical condition, or can be a function of social variables like low parental competence, chaotic family circumstances, and the absence of buffering community resources (Bronfenbrenner, 1986; Garbarino, 1990). Enhanced vulnerability can also be a consequence of social policies that deny care or create barriers to care, or can result from failures of service coordination. Whether of biological, social, or policy-related origin, the factors that place children at risk of poor health outcomes are risk factors precisely because of the ways in which they interact with the inherent vulnerabilities associated with the biologically and socially determined condition of childhood itself.

Examples of Vulnerable Children

Vulnerable children often have multiple needs that are serious and in many cases life threatening, and require a comprehensive set of medical and non-medical services. The number of vulnerable children is increasing, as are the demands they place on the service system (Aday, 1993). Because of their complex and multifaceted needs, these children can be difficult to care for, and are often not adequately cared for under the existing patchwork of children's programs (Halfon and Berkowitz, 1993). Needless to say, without legally defined protection they are not likely to be better off in a competitive managed care marketplace.

There are many classes of children who suffer from chronic disorders and from adverse social situations who fit the definition of "highly vulnerable," including babies born to teenage mothers, and many teen mothers themselves, children who are severely emotionally disturbed, children living in homeless families, substance-abusing teens, and others. Some have argued that children with multiple needs are becoming more the rule than the exception, and it is suggested that nearly half the child population now has some special needs.

We have chosen four classes of vulnerable children as exemplars to illustrate the extent and nature of unmet needs and the problems faced in developing service systems and potential reform strategies: children with chronic illnesses, children in foster care, young adolescents (aged 10–14 years), and immigrant children. These groups do not represent an exhaustive list, but help to illustrate the kinds of issues that must be addressed when formulating political and systemic responses to different kinds of vulnerability in child populations. While each group is defined by a distinct set of circum-stances and etiologies, the kinds of reforms needed to serve these groups of children better involve some common themes that apply to all children.

Children with Chronic Medical Conditions

There is no one universally accepted definition of chronic illness (Perrin and MacLean, 1988; Perrin et al., 1993b; Stein et al., 1993). In general a chronic illness or health condition is one that lasts a substantial period of time. Many chronic illnesses are lifelong even when symptoms are episodic. For practical purposes the National Center for Health Statistics opera-tionally defines a chronic condition as one that has lasted or that ordinarily would last more than three months. Chronic health conditions can be caused by genetic abnormalities or other insults; by infections, accidents, injuries, and environmental exposures; or by combinations of one or more of these etiologies.

There is a basic difference in the profile and distribution of chronic con-ditions affecting children and those affecting adults. Adults are typically af-fected by a small number of relatively common diseases that represent the final common pathways of a lifetime of insults or traumas (e.g., heart dis-ease, emphysema, chronic obstructive pulmonary disease, cirrhosis, chronic hepatitis, nephritis, and various neoplasms). By contrast, children are af-fected by a large number of rare diseases with genetic or prenatal origins in addition to common insults and the residua of prematurity. Only asthma and common and milder forms of congenital heart disease occur with suffi-cient frequency to affect more than 1 or 2 percent of the child population. Be-tween 10 percent and 30 percent of all children in the United States have some sort of chronic health problem (Newacheck and Taylor, 1992), and the number appears to be on the rise (Newacheck and Halfon, 1997). Data from the National Health Interview Surveys indicate that between 1960 and 1994 the prevalence of the most severe disabling conditions increased more than threefold, from approximately 2 percent in 1960 to 6.7 percent in 1994.

Children with disabling chronic conditions are more than three times as likely to be hospitalized as are nonaffected children and, when hospitalized, they have twice the average length of stay for each hospitalization (Newacheck and Halfon, 1997). In 1993 the approximately 6.2 percent of children who were disabled accounted for 31 percent of hospital days. Chil-dren with disabilities also have six times greater use of allied health profes-sionals (occupational therapists, physical therapists, social workers, etc.)

than those without disabilities (Newacheck and McManus, 1988). It has been estimated that children with disabling chronic conditions in general use at least twice as many health services resources as other children and that the 2 percent that are most severely affected consume 25 percent of the child health dollar (Newacheck et al., 1993).

Because of these unique needs, children with chronic conditions often receive their care through special university-affiliated programs and regionalized specialty centers that provide multiple services under one roof. Because of the scope and intensity of their service needs, children and families with special health care needs require a unique relationship with a health care provider and benefit when multiple services are configured into a system that is family centered, community based, and child focused (Brewer et al., 1989). The special role of health care providers for the family with a chronically ill child cannot be overestimated. The continuation of that relationship as a source of support, guidance, and advocacy based on mutual participation and respect depends on a health care system that is organized to foster such relationships (Perrin and McLean, 1988).

The health care needs of children and youth with chronic illnesses and disabilities demand intensive, comprehensive, and coordinated health services (Perrin et al., 1993a). These children often have a great need for medical services, including primary care; specialty treatment services from allied health professionals including occupational and physical therapists; rehabilitation services; mental health services; prescription drugs; durable medical products; nutritional services; specialized respite and day care services; and case management.

In order to develop systems of care for children with special health care needs, it is important to develop or foster community-based case management services and better coordination among various levels of care providers (including families, primary care providers, specialists and ancillary providers) and financing services. While many children with complex medical problems are dependent on medical technologies and intensive nursing procedures, there is a growing trend spurred on by improved portable technologies and efforts to contain costs to provide more of this kind of care at home (Perrin et al., 1993a).

Children's chronic illnesses can also place a severe financial burden on families, contributing to a child's overall vulnerability. On average, families with children with special health care needs have three times the level of expenditure per child. Approximately 62 percent of disabled children were covered by private health insurance in 1993, with 15 percent, or approximately 495,000 children, without health insurance (unpublished tabulations by Paul Newacheck, 1996). The major reason that children are uninsured is the inability of their families to pay for insurance. Even for those children who are covered by private health insurance, coverage is increasingly incomplete. Many private health insurance plans impose limits on covered expenses and increase deductible and coinsurance rates (McManus et al., 1992). Because families provide most of the care for children with special health care needs, the resulting caregiving demands can place substantial economic and emotional burdens on a family, resulting in income lost due to a diminished likelihood of maternal employment outside of the home, family disruption, and divorce (Breslau and Mortimer, 1981).

Managed care is rapidly becoming the dominant delivery modality for vulnerable children including those with chronic illnesses (Fox et al., 1993; Perrin and McLean, 1988). As of 1996, 13 states had enrolled children with chronic conditions into capitated Medicaid programs by using special waiver authority. Data from a limited number of studies suggest that managed care offers the opportunity to increase access to appropriate care for children with chronic illnesses by increasing the use of primary care services and decreasing emergency room utilization (Manning et al., 1984; Mauldon et al., 1994; Perkoff et al., 1976). Notwithstanding the potential benefits of managed care, there is little evidence to support the contention that managed care plans are providing a full continuum of comprehensive services to children with chronic conditions (Newacheck et al., 1994). Moreover, the transition to managed care threatens to exclude relatively high-risk children from some of the potential benefits of managed care as health plans maneuver to avoid enrolling higher-risk and higher-cost children (Ireys et al., 1996). Appropriate utilization may also be restricted for children with chronic illnesses through limitations on referrals to pediatric subspecialists (Cartland and Yudkowsky, 1992; Horwitz and Stein, 1990). An initial evaluation of four mandatory Medicaid managed care programs in Hawaii, Oregon, Rhode Island, and Tennessee indicated several problematic areas including disruption of provider relationships and limited availability of subspecialists and ancillary providers (Fox and McManus, 1996; Fox et al., 1993). Because of the absence of well-developed risk-adjusters and clinically predictive evaluation instruments, the inclusion of children with complex chronic medical conditions can pose problems for a managed care organization and for the communities responsible for the financing and monitoring of the care for such children (Fowler and Andersen, 1996). Partly in response to these concerns, it has been proposed that chronic illnesses be handled in "carved out" risk pools (Fowler and Andersen, 1996; Neff and Andersen, 1995). However, this is only a temporary solution, given marketplace forces and state Medicaid programs' desire to discharge their responsibility for this population through capitated contracts.

Several organizational innovations have been attempted to improve the comprehensiveness and integration of services for elderly individuals with chronic conditions that may have applicability to children. Social health maintenance organizations (SHMOs) and the related Programs of All-Inclusive Health Care for the Elderly (PACE) are a modification of the basic health maintenance organization (HMO) model, providing additional social and support services as well as long-term care options to the frail elderly. Both of these models have pediatric applications. At present the Health Care Financing Administration is sponsoring a small demonstration project in Washington, DC, aimed at creating a limited SHMO-like program for children with chronic disabling conditions cared for in the District's Special Health Care Need Program. Several children's hospitals around the country are forming multispecialty pediatric practices designed to better compete in a managed care market, and the children's hospital in Houston has announced plans to set up its own HMO.

Children in Foster Care

Children in foster care face enhanced vulnerability because of the disruption of their primary familial dependency relationships and their consequent dependence upon a system of care that is often incapable of serving their complex health and related needs. Children are placed into foster care when the state determines that the child's family can no longer provide a minimally safe environment for that child, most commonly because of abuse or neglect. Since both state and federal laws view removal of children from their biological family as an extreme intervention, children are usually placed in foster care only in cases of serious danger and family dysfunction. In 1992, 442,000 children (7.5 per 1,000) were in foster care, up from 262,000 (4.2 per 1,000) in 1982 (U.S. Dept. of Health and Human Services, 1996). Some children enter foster care for a matter of months, and others will spend years of their lives moving from home to home, facing additional challenges and potential traumas with each transition experience.

Children in foster care experience higher rates of chronic medical, mental health, and developmental problems (Dubowitz et al., 1992; Halfon et al., 1995b; Hochstadt et al., 1987; Schor, 1982, 1989; Swire and Kavaler, 1977).

Studies indicate that from 20 to 40 percent of children in foster care suffer from chronic medical conditions, and 40 to 80 percent suffer from mental health problems. Like other vulnerable children, children in foster care often suffer from multiple conditions. In one study of young children in foster care, more than 28 percent had three or more conditions (Halfon et al., 1995b).

Like other children with multiple needs, children in foster care require a comprehensive continuum of services and standards of service delivery, similar to those developed by the Child Welfare League of America and the American Academy of Pediatrics (AAP, 1994; Child Welfare League of America, 1988). These standards include a comprehensive needs assessment to determine the full scope of their health and developmental needs when they enter the system and access to a range of specialty medical and mental health care, rehabilitation services, and other developmental supports.

However, because of the rising number of reported and documented cases of abuse and neglect, child welfare agencies have increasingly transformed themselves into "child protection" agencies, with less orientation toward the overall welfare of children. Health services have never been a priority for the child protection system, except when medical exams are necessary for court or legal reasons, and increasing social worker caseloads often make health concerns a low priority (Halfon and Klee, 1987, 1991). This tendency is exacerbated by the fact that most children in the foster care system are currently covered by Medicaid. In many states Medicaid programs impose strict limits on the availability of mental health and developmental services, two sets of services that are essential for this population. Many states are electing to exclude or carve out children in the child welfare system from Medicaid managed care and maintain some, if not all, of their care in the fee-for-service Medicaid program. However, this is not universally the case, and when children in foster care are placed into managed care, many of the same concerns arise regarding comprehensiveness, coordination, and availability of appropriate providers that apply to children with chronic conditions. And again, a carve-out strategy is only a temporary solution, buying time until more enduring solutions emerge.

Managed care poses some real challenges for this population. Their unique pattern of morbidity, their high level of mobility, their changing eligibility status, and their need for special court and legal procedural-based services all demand special attention from the individual or team entrusted with their care (Halfon et al., 1994). A lack of standardized assessment protocols, risk assessment instruments, and quality measures means that there are few procedural supports to guarantee the provision of high-quality care.

Several model programs have developed around the country to improve the availability of comprehensive services for this group of children (Simms and Halfon, 1994). Special vulnerable child clinics have sought to use multidisciplinary teams to provide comprehensive assessment, care coordination, and case planning, in addition to routine diagnostic and treatment services (Figure 14.1). Los Angeles County has launched what eventually

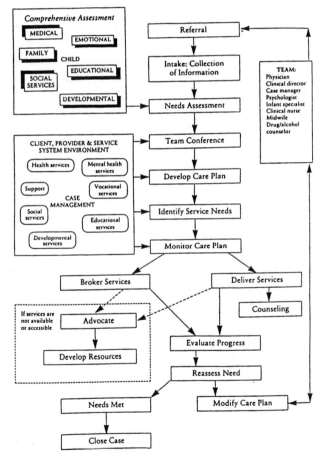

Figure 14.1
A case management system for vulnerable children. (From Halfon et al., 1991; copyright © 1991 by the Center for the Vulnerable Child; reprinted by permission.)

could become a SHMO for 73,000 children in its child welfare system. The Protective Services Child Health System is creating regionalized comprehensive assessment centers, each surrounded by a geographically dispersed primary, specialty, and ancillary service provider network. Public health nurses serve as care coordinators, linking the assessment centers with both the child welfare system and the provider networks. At present Los Angeles has one center running, with two more scheduled to open in 1997, and more than 30 public health nurses serving as care coordinators.

Young Adolescents

Early adolescence has been identified as a time of enhanced vulnerability. The inherent vulnerability of young adolescent children (aged 10-14 years) is a function of profound biologically determined developmental changes, their changing relationships with parents and peers, and related age-specific biological, psychological, and social issues. One problem is that many parents appear to withdraw from involvement with their children's lives beginning in the middle-school years, confusing early strivings for independence with a readiness and a desire to be free of parental supervision. The increased requirements of parental employment in recent years mean that many young adolescents are alone from the time they leave school until a parent returns from work, and it is during unsupervised hours that young adolescents are most likely to be involved in risk-taking behaviors (U.S. Congress, 1991).

While 10- and 11-year-olds have the lowest expected death rate of any group in the population (Ellickson et al., 1993), numerous morbidities begin to manifest themselves during these critical years, as lifelong patterns of health-related behavior begin to take root (Kelder et al., 1994). Young adolescents face a high risk from injuries (Bell and Bell, 1993). Motor vehicle accidents are the leading cause of death, and firearm deaths are increasing rapidly, particularly for black males (Carnegie Council on Adolescent Development, 1995). Unintentional injury and motor vehicle accidents account for about 10 percent of early adolescent mortality and are the leading causes of death in this age group (Ellickson et al., 1993; National Center for Health Statistics, 1995). Young adolescents are frequently victims of assault, with 12- to 15-year-olds particularly vulnerable (Bureau of Justice Statistics, 1994). The use of alcohol and cigarettes is widespread, with more than 14 percent of eighth graders reporting binge drinking in the previous two weeks (University of Michigan Institute for Social Research, 1994). Sexual activity now begins at an earlier age than in previous years, for both boys and girls. For girls, sex in the early adolescent years is often forced, with 60 percent of sexually experienced girls 13 years and under reporting involuntary intercourse (Alan Guttmacher Institute, 1994). Births among young adolescents are rising, with 12,000 births to girls under 15 in 1992 (National Center for Health Statistics, 1995). For girls depression is a major issue, and suicide for young adolescents of both sexes is on the rise (Carnegie Council on Adolescent Development, 1995).

Service systems must address a range of health needs, including integration of personal medical services with community-based health and support functions. Assuring better health for young adolescents requires that health services reach into the community and encourage parents to remain actively involved in their children's lives. When parents cannot or will not do this, adult mentoring and other social support strategies are particularly important for this age group (Lowry et al., 1996). Peer-mediated programs to promote health and education have also been found to be particularly effective in reaching young adolescents (Carnegie Council on Adolescent Development, 1995). Programs that seek to develop basic life skills may be appropriate for some young adolescents.

Young adolescents often lack adequate insurance coverage, with one in seven adolescents having no insurance (Carnegie Council on Adolescent Development, 1995). Children between the ages of 10 and 18 are among the least likely persons in the U.S. population to be insured. Furthermore, when young adolescents do have insurance, many important preventive and treatment services like psychological and abuse counseling are often not covered (Carnegie Council on Adolescent Development, 1995). Other needs, like contraceptive services, are made more difficult to meet because of bans on the provision of contraceptives in school health clinics. Many adolescents face additional barriers to the receipt of adequate care because of patterns of care-seeking behavior that are at odds with conventional health services (Lieu et al., 1993). The dearth of minority physicians and the lack of specific training of physicians to deal with adolescent issues pose additional problems.

For young adolescents there is a strong need to broaden the availability of conventional health insurance coverage. When coverage is supplied through a managed care plan, it is particularly important that the managed care plan have links to the school, and if no school health clinic exists, that the managed care plan be supportive of its establishment, particularly in middle schools where such clinics are usually absent. At the same time, it will be important to expand provider training concerning adolescent health issues. Young adolescents require a broad range of services, including appropriate preventive services, and while managed care can excel in the provision of good primary care, the psychosocial services required by young adolescents are less often available (Blum and Bearinger, 1990; U.S. Congress, 1991).

The expansion of health insurance coverage for young adolescents, desirable in itself, needs to be matched by two additional, and more fundamental, changes. The first is the development of strategies to increase the positive involvement of parents in their young adolescents' lives. The second is the development of integrated systems of health care and education, the creation of relationships between health services organizations and the primary institutions (schools) in which children spend their days so that the other adults in their lives, including teachers, community workers, and medical personnel, help supervise children at an intensity level appropriate to guide children away from injurious behaviors and provide the health-related services they may need.

Immigrant Children and the Children of Immigrants

Children who are immigrants or who are U.S. citizens by virtue of their birth in the United States but whose parents are immigrants represent a large and rapidly growing population in certain states. The percentage of children and youth who are foreign born has been steadily increasing, from 1.2 percent in 1970 to 3.4 percent in 1990. The percentage of children who are foreign born increases with age: 1.2 percent of children less than 5 years old and 6.5 percent of children 15 to 19 years of age are foreign born. These proportions vary by race and ethnicity, with 32 percent of Asian children being foreign born and 15.8 percent of Hispanic children and youth being foreign born. In some states, like California, New York, Florida, and Texas, these percentages are even higher (U.S. Dept. of Health and Human Services, 1996).

The health risks of immigrant children are a function of higher rates of health problems and risk exposures. By virtue of their immigration status or that of their parents, these children experience greater residential mobility, have fewer family supports, and have less access to health care than non-immigrants of similar economic status. In California, where a large number of children are born to immigrant parents or families in which one parent is an immigrant (Brown et al., 1996; Hayes-Bautista et al., 1994; National Health Foundation, 1995), a recent population-based survey of two relatively impoverished areas of Los Angeles found that 80 percent of parents of two-year-old children interviewed were not U.S. citizens (Halfon et al., 1997). Immigrant families in this study were found to have at least one member working, yet also had fewer economic resources and were less likely to be insured or have continuous Medicaid coverage than citizens in the same neighborhoods. They reported numerous barriers to the receipt of routine care for their children. Immigrant children also experience a high rate of illness due to exposures in their native lands or during their travel to the United States (Mendoza et al., 1991).

The health risks of immigrant children are also a function of new policies that threaten to deny them access to basic health services (Mendoza et al., 1991). For a variety of reasons anti-immigrant sentiment has melded with anti-welfare sentiment, to pass powerful state and federal legislation that potentially restricts access for all immigrants, whether authorized or not, to a range of important social welfare services including Medicaid, the Special Supplemental Food Program for Women, Infants, and Children (WIC), and food stamps (Ziv and Lo, 1995). The welfare reform measures enacted in 1996, which will severely limit the availability of Medicaid to authorized and unauthorized immigrants in the United States beginning in 1997, will have a dramatic impact on access to care and on health status. A study recently carried out in California suggested that 146,000 noncitizen children will lose Medicaid coverage in California alone as a result of new federal eligibility changes (Brown et al., 1996).

Understanding the Barriers to System Change

David Hamburg, president of the Carnegie Corporation, has suggested that all children need individual attention, attachment, protection, encouragement, stimulation, and guidance (Hamburg, 1992). A health care system that was more appropriately financed and organized could play an important role in helping families provide these essential functions, addressing both inherent vulnerability and enhanced vulnerability. For children the mismatch between needs and services is particularly acute because the conceptual framework of insurance is inappropriate for a population whose basic needs involve a predictable range of preventive and health-related support services. In reengineering the health system for highly vulnerable children, four sets of barriers to change need to be addressed: financial, organizational, procedural, and conceptual.

Financial Barriers. The mechanism for financing health care for most U.S. children does not guarantee them security of coverage (Halfon et al., 1995a; Starr, 1992). Health care costs have continued to rise and the interests of children have been easy to sacrifice, as the imperative to control costs drives both government and private corporate payers to reduce expenditures by any means necessary. Finding new money for service or insurance expansions will be difficult, and it will even be difficult to maintain many child health and related services at current funding levels in the present political environment. Moreover, many vulnerable children require a comprehensive continuum of care that includes preventive, treatment, and rehabilitative services delivered not only by medical providers but by schools and social welfare, mental health, and child development organizations. This requirement raises fundamental questions regarding fiscal responsibility and methods for sharing or transferring financial risks across agencies and sectors.

Organizational Barriers. The organizational mismatch between the needs of children and the dominant adult-oriented health care system has its historic origins in several interrelated trends (Halfon et al., 1996). These range from how the social role of children has changed over the past century to how children's programs have been conceived by policymakers as welfare or second-chance programs for the exceptional child in a family that is often assumed to be unable to meet the child's needs directly. While there really has not been a child-centered focus in U.S. policy since the Progressive era (Skocpol, 1992), beginning in the 1930s with the passage of Title V, an opportunistic set of child health policies has been created in successive waves when the attention of policymakers could be secured. In the 1960s and early 1970s, EPSDT, Head Start, Medicaid, WIC, child abuse programs, and community mental health programs were all created, each with its own funding stream and eligibility and administrative requirements. The 1980s and early 1990s brought federal child care supports, early intervention programs, school-based health services, and child abuse prevention and family protection programs. Except for broad funding capacity provided by Medicaid, most of these other programs support community-based prevention, intervention, and health-related support services that are neither funded at levels that allow them to serve all who are eligible, nor easily integrated with the personal medical services of the old fee-for-service system, nor likely to be better integrated into the new world of managed care and competitive markets.

Procedural Barriers.   Procedural barriers are those barriers that stem from the absence of the techniques, tools, and other processes that are necessary either to reengineer the new managed care environment for children or to protect children from the excesses of a profit-motivated system expanding without significant restraint. Necessary tools include well-developed quality measurement techniques and quality improvement systems that can be used to guarantee that the care received by a child with diabetes, cystic fibrosis, or a severe emotional disorder is of high technical and interpersonal quality. Needed tools also include risk adjustment mechanisms that allow for the development of capitation and other reimbursement mechanisms capable of accounting for the differences in needed resources, based not only on the diagnosis and presumed severity of the child's ailment, but also on family and social circumstances that may indicate a need for additional services and resources. Additionally, clear medical necessity criteria are needed, based on a clearly articulated child standard that can be used by health plans to determine exactly what covered benefits are permissible for a given child with a specific disease.

Conceptual Barriers.   Perhaps the most important barrier in fashioning a system that makes sense for children is the inadequate conceptualization of the difference between adults and children, and what those differences mean for financing and organization of the health care system and for the tools that are necessary to make it work. The powerful marketplace forces that are reshaping the health care system into large managed corporate entities often tend to view all consumers equally, creating generic one-size-fits-all health plans. This compounds the longstanding tendency of health insurance plans to ignore important differences between children and adults and to instead treat children as little adults. For the unique health care needs of children, and especially of vulnerable children, to be not only acknowledged, but a driving force in reengineering the system, the conceptual framework for financing and organizing health services for children must change in a way to promote more attention to their unique needs.

Overcoming the Barriers to System Change

Financial Barriers: Coordinating Services for Vulnerable Children

Children face growing access problems due to a lack of health insurance, unstable health insurance coverage, or being underinsured. The continued erosion of employer-based coverage and the potential of politically imposed limits to Medicaid expansion are exacerbating the impact of these trends. A significant portion of children with disabling chronic conditions, adolescents, and immigrant children are now uninsured. Many children with disabilities are insufficiently covered to receive necessary habilitative services, and many children in foster care with significant mental health problems are restricted to a few visits per month for psychological services under Medicaid service caps. While only limited data are available, it seems that the growth of for-profit managed care is not likely to solve these problems, and in fact may make the situation worse. Creating financial access in an era of fiscal austerity, deficit reduction, and balanced budgets is a real challenge.

The Desirability of Insurance for All.   It clearly would be desirable to provide all children in the United States with appropriate health insurance or health services coverage. Such coverage would guarantee children access to a full range of acute, chronic, and rehabilitative health services, as well as appropriate preventive and health-promoting services. At the present time, this full range of services (personal, community-based, and other) is financed through employer-based private health insurance, Medicaid, out-of-pocket expenditures by families, and a wide range of federal, state, and local community health and health-related support programs. In planning for the future, one of the key questions is how best to use whatever the total potential allocation of resources is for children to maximize the production of health in the child population. Strategic integration of funding mechanisms and decategorization of existing funding streams will play a key role in maximizing child health.

Traditional Insurance May Be an Inappropriate Financing Mechanism. In conceptual terms, however, health insurance may not be the appropriate conceptual and operative framework for financing health care for children, because it is based on a model of insurance against unexpected costs (Starr, 1992). Most children's health care costs, for low-risk as well as for high-risk children, can be anticipated. If a health insurance–based system is to be relied upon, its expansion must be accompanied by a restructuring of the risk-based payment system to create new incentives that are more appropriate to the predictable needs of different groups of children for different kinds of comprehensive services. One political strategy that might enable a formal recognition of the different nature of children's health risks would be to separate children's health insurance enrollment from adults'. For example, when an employer offers a plan to its employees, a distinct· children's package with different services could be offered. If this strategy were to be pursued, it would be possible to cover a broader and yet less expensive set of services for a larger number of children, and to build in provisions for school-based health services or other options designed to meet children's unique needs (Starr, 1992).

Expanding the Existing Employer-Based System.   While it is an interesting intellectual exercise to consider removing children entirely from an employer-based system of coverage, such a radical change, at least at the present time, would be destabilizing to the health care market and might not guarantee children any greater security in funding or services. Instead, short-term strategies should involve consideration of options to help diminish or reverse the erosion of employer-based coverage. Rosenbaum and colleagues have outlined and analyzed the range of strategies to expand health insurance for all children (Rosenbaum and Borzi, 1996). These include mandatory options such as employer mandates and a Medicare-like program for children ("Kidicare") as well as a much broader range of incremental voluntary options. Newacheck et al. (1996a) and Rosenbaum and Borzi (1996) have suggested that one of the most politically feasible strategies to bolster the current employer-based insurance system for children would use an incremental approach involving premium subsidies at either a state or national level.

Wraparound Services Can Build on Basic Insurance Coverage.   While having a basic insurance plan will continue to be necessary for basic access to care, such insurance will not be sufficient to provide the breadth and depth of services that many vulnerable children and their families need. Financial access and the provision of what have come to be known as wraparound services are important considerations for all vulnerable children. At present these services are provided through a fragmented array of different programs that vary from state to state and between local jurisdictions within a state. For example, many children with chronic medical conditions receive wraparound services through Title V programs for children with special health care needs. Fox and colleagues (Newacheck et al., 1996b) have suggested that several different funding streams be consolidated at the state level to create a more uniform wraparound insurance program for children with special health care needs. Such a pool might be constructed with funds from Medicaid, EPSDT, Title V, and a variety of other programs.

Decategorization of Public Funding Can Improve System.   An important noninsurance strategy that has emerged to alter financing, intended not to expand but to improve coordination and integration of services, calls for the decategorization of many of the currently categorically funded programs (Newacheck et al., 1995b). Decategorization promises to create flexible funding pools that could be used by local communities to develop their own set of customized service packages. Decategorization could make it easier for children and parents to gain one-stop access to a range of health and health-related services in newly rationalized community-organized delivery systems. However, decategorization also promises to make it more difficult for advocates and legislators to know how allocated monies are being spent and requires increasingly sophisticated accountability procedures. Will funding for vulnerable children be politically sustainable under decategorization, or will decategorization become a mechanism for unreasoned cost cutting by localities freed from administrative oversight? It is clear that increased reporting and quality assessment of health plans and other providers are essential concomitants of programmatic decategorization of funding streams. To date, attempts to create flexible funding pools from categorical funding streams have met with only limited success (Hughes et al.).

Financing Is Inextricably Entwined with Delivery System.   Discussing financial access without acknowledging the important role that managed care is playing, and the fiscal rules that govern managed care plans, ignores an important set of financial realities. Since private managed care organizations are becoming the fundamental unit of service delivery within the health system, fiscal alternatives to expand services must reconcile the financial demands of managed care organizations' short-term profit-maximizing mission with society's interest in long-term investment in child health development. In order for private managed care organizations to embrace initiatives to broaden the scope of services or to develop linkages across sectors, these initiatives will have to demonstrate both improved health outcomes and cost savings potential.

Determining whether funds are saved and who accrues those savings is a fundamental policy conundrum. For example, home visiting programs and other early intervention programs targeted at high-risk children have proven cost effective in improving health status, cognitive functioning, and academic performance while decreasing dependence on public assistance (Olds et al., 1993). However, few of these successful demonstration programs have been implemented on a larger scale, in part because the cost savings and other benefits accrued to public sector programs and not to the private sector institutions providing the services. Currently, a managed care organization that makes a significant health investment in a potentially learning disabled child and saves a school district thousands of dollars in special education services can anticipate no economic reward for its prevention activities. Lacking formal financial and organizational relationships with other sectors that may benefit from its prevention activities, the managed care organization has no economic incentive to generate savings that will accrue only to those other sectors. Innovative financing schemes will be required to tie socially desirable and economically beneficial outcomes in other sectors to the financial incentives that are offered to managed care organizations. Developing a prevention credit and other forms of crediting for desirable health inputs may serve to break the policy logjam.

Organizational Issues: Overcoming Barriers to Integrating Services for Vulnerable Children

Examination of the specific needs of highly vulnerable children suggests that integration of different kinds and intensities of service and the provision of those integrated services across an extended time frame are particularly important to improve the quality of care. We believe that there are three types of integration that are fundamental to the achievement of an ideal health care system for children: vertical, horizontal, and longitudinal. A "three dimensionally" integrated system should be the goal of any coherent set of reforms.

Vertical Integration. Market forces are already driving managed care organizations to link primary, secondary, and tertiary care as a means to increase production efficiency and to achieve an efficient allocation of generalists and specialists. Such vertically integrated systems can be good for children, if they are specifically adapted to cope with the unique challenges posed by the nature of the developmental process. But tightly organized, medically focused, vertically integrated managed care organizations also pose threats to children. For example, many managed care organizations do not have the capacity or the willingness to provide the specialized nonmedical services that many children require. In a more extreme case, a cost-conscious managed care organization may insist that access to pediatric subspecialists is not "necessary," and rely on adult specialists alone (Cartland and Yudkowsky, 1992). With the appropriate standards and quality measurement tools, vertically integrated managed care could be fashioned to deliver reasonable quality medical care, but without them it will be difficult for families or public agencies charged with ensuring accountability to know the quality of care that is being delivered (McGlynn et al., 1995).

Horizontal Integration.   Because the health needs of high-risk children affect multiple domains of function, it is important that their health coverage and the health system in which they receive services have the capacity to provide multidisciplinary care. Horizontal integration (between health and health-related services, and including education and other social service organizations as well) will require the active cooperation between private sector managed care organizations and various public institutions. SHMOs have demonstrated the feasibility of providing horizontally integrated social services for the elderly (on a limited basis), but horizontally integrated care for children remains a prisoner of a long history of policy and service fragmentation. The potential benefits of horizontally linked services are clear, but traditional conceptual, organizational, and financial boundaries between health services and other social services continue to create barriers to their realization.

Longitudinal Integration.   Longitudinally integrated services address children's developmental vulnerability and assure that children receive time-critical care when needed, that coverage is continuous, and that children accumulate a single, complete developmental health record that accounts for all health inputs, evaluations, and adverse events. Longitudinal integration further implies that over the child's developmental trajectory, each new contact with the health services system coherently reflects the child's previous contacts with the system and advances the child's development and well-being. Longitudinal integration means that care is provided within the time framework of the full two decades of childhood and adolescence, and that medical necessity is understood in terms of a procedure's impact not only upon present functional level, but upon functional level two and three decades in the future.

Longitudinal integration for children will be difficult to achieve. In the public sector, planning horizons of more than a few years are rare, and no single organization is empowered to track and guard a child's health over a two-decade span. In the private sector, managed care organizations generally operate under market-defined time frames that shape their business strategy and that reflect their necessary concern with cost control and economic survival. Preventive services that may reduce utilization of services at some distant future date, when a given child may no longer be enrolled in the managed care organization, would not appear to represent sound business practices in this context, notwithstanding their apparent ethical and public policy value. The time frames that publicly traded corporations must consider, reflected by quarterly financial statements and stock market value, may be discordant with the public interest in the long-term health and well-being of child populations. For these reasons, it is important to foster incentives that can reward a longer-term focus than may be sustainable by companies that must rely on private financial markets. If incentives are inadequate to encourage long-term investments in the health of children, then mandating a wider range of preventive services should be considered.

It is possible to envision a single organization for children that functions something like an HMO, but is horizontally integrated with other health-related services, like a SHMO for the frail elderly, and also offers a measure of long-term longitudinal integration. Such an organization we have called elsewhere a health development organization. In contrast with HMOs, which receive capitated funding streams designed to maintain the health of an adult population at a given level, the health development organization would be mandated to actively develop the health of children in its full longitudinal context. Incentives for the health development organizations would be designed to encourage the long-term creation of healthy populations, based on best estimates of the long-term value of preventive services, and as research proceeds, by providing health development organizations with some of the economic rewards associated with reducing the burden of childhood illness on other sectors of the economy.

Children's developmental vulnerability and unique health characteristics suggest their need for three-dimensional integration, so that as they pass through crucial developmental stages, their contact with the health system is not disrupted, and they continue to receive a complete and comprehensive array of essential health and health-related services. SHMOs for the frail elderly have pointed the way with their integrated provision of social and health services. SHMOs for children like those being created in Washington, DC, for children with disabling chronic conditions and in Los Angeles for children in foster care represent promising innovations. The three-dimensional integrated health development organization represents the next logical step in system design for vulnerable children.

Procedural Barriers: Creating the Tools for Integrated Systems of Care

New Tools Are Needed.   Building three-dimensional integrated systems of care for children with multiple needs will be facilitated by tools that allow managed care organizations and other public agencies to improve coordination and integration of services, provide adequate financing for a range of interrelated services, and improve outcomes management and quality measurement and improvement processes. Without such tools, it will be difficult to leverage the current system, difficult to help customize and reengineer existing managed care organizations, and difficult to make the important connections between managed care and other health-related service providers.

Quality Measurement Tools Are Needed.   One of the premises of managed competition is that competition between health care plans will be based on both price and quality of care. While there has been extensive work done in the development of quality measures for adults, current methodologies for measuring quality of care for individual children and families are quite limited (McGlynn et al., 1995). Moreover, because children's health services include personal medical care services delivered in managed care organizations, as well as health-related social and other support services provided through early intervention programs and developmental disabilities programs, tools are needed to measure the quality of services provided not only at the health plan level but at the community level (Ireys et al., 1996). The development of multilevel quality measurement tools will allow for greater accountability of health care plans and communities to produce desired health outcomes.

The development of appropriate quality measurement tools for children in managed care plans is quite challenging, for the same reasons that children are vulnerable: their developmental plasticity, their dependency on adults and others, and the pattern of their disease profile and its expression. For adults, a specific health outcome tool (e.g., SF 36) can be used for a range of diseases in order to determine functional outcomes, but for children, changing developmental expectations demand that measures of functional status reflect the changing developmental capacity of the child (Jameson and Wehr, 1994). Moreover, for external quality-monitoring purposes, the low prevalence of many chronic conditions in childhood such as diabetes or different types of heart disease suggests that there will never be enough children in a given plan with one of these diseases to produce a sufficient sample size to judge differences in technical quality and outcomes between plans. Development of appropriate quality measurement tools will require a significant research and development effort by those federal agencies that have undertaken efforts aimed at improving the quality of health services (Agency for Health Care Policy and Research and Maternal and Child Health Board), as well as by the agencies within the National Institutes of Health that are concerned with specific disease entities. The 1997 national conference, *Improving Quality of Care for Children: An Agenda for Research*, convened by the Association for Health Services Research and funded by the Maternal and Child Health Bureau, Health Care Financing Administration, Centers for Disease Control and Prevention, Agency for Health Care Policy and Research, and the National Institutes of Health, is a step in this direction.

Measurement of Health Status and of Risk Status Also Requires New Tools. A related set of tools is needed to assess health and risk status. The customization of managed care for children requires child-specific instruments that can measure the multiple domains and determinants of health status, including the child's own inherent capacity and the influence of the child's environment, family, and other factors. Again, there has been a burgeoning effort in the adult health area to develop health risk appraisal instruments in order to determine functional status of an individual and to assign the appropriate level of service to the individual within a managed care organization. Unfortunately, similar efforts have not been as widespread for children. Like quality measurement tools for children, health risk appraisal tools must account for a child's changing developmental capacity and for the role of a variety of external factors that have a profound influence on the child's functional status, including parents, neighborhood, and community issues. Determining the role and contribution of these social factors is important not only in determining level and breadth of needs, but in monitoring longitudinal outcomes and determining for what the health plan can reasonably be held accountable. Such health risk appraisal instruments are particularly needed for vulnerable subgroups such as children in foster care, immigrant children, and homeless children. In recent years, attempts have been made to develop functional status measures for children with chronic illnesses, as well as for adolescents (Starfield et al., 1995a; Starfield et al., 1995b; Stein and Jessop, 1982). These have been useful but have had limited application. In this area too, a major research and development effort is necessary to improve the quality and performance of such measures and to integrate such measures into the intake and referral processes of managed care plans.

Risk Adjustment.   Assuring that children receive the scope and intensity of services necessary requires financial arrangements that adequately reimburse health plans based on children's needs. Evidence from the early years of managed care suggest that HMOs selectively enrolled healthier populations. Many of the most vulnerable populations have not been traditionally served within commercial managed care settings, yet are destined to be enrolled in these plans in the next few years. The development of appropriate risk adjustment mechanisms that allow for appropriate financial rate adjustments is a necessary prerequisite for allocating resources in an efficient way for this population. While there has been a great flurry of activity in the development of risk adjusters in the last several years, recent reviews suggest that the current methodologies for adult populations are not translatable to children with chronic medical conditions (Fowler and Andersen, 1996). Risk adjustment methodologies that use prior utilization as a core basis for determining risk may not work well for children whose health status may vary significantly from year to year (Fowler and Andersen, 1996; Manton et al., 1994; Neff and Andersen, 1995). Several projects are currently under way to develop risk-adjusted capitation rates for chronically ill or disabled populations (Fowler and Andersen, 1996; Kronic et al., 1995; Starfield et al., 1995a).

Monitoring and Surveillance.   In addition to the tools necessary for reengineering services at the health plan level, community-wide monitoring and evaluation systems are necessary. Such community-wide systems would monitor the health and developmental function of children, monitor the provision of services by different managed care organizations, and evaluate the linkage mechanisms and coordination functions that are used to create comprehensive continuums of care. Answers to questions such as "Does a particular managed care organization provide bridges to social service providers when such providers are determined to be a medically appropriate component of a child's treatment plan?" can then be answered and used in considering future contracting with a plan. The results of such community-wide surveillance and monitoring activities can be shared with providers, policymakers, and the public through periodic report cards and other reports. Such monitoring efforts can serve as the basis of community-wide quality improvement efforts targeted at holding managed care organizations accountable, as well as creating guidelines for the development of better systems of care. A good example of such a monitoring and quality improvement effort is the activities of New England SERVE. This multistate project has surveyed managed care organizations and other providers, established guidelines for service system development, and participated in a number of systems quality improvement efforts based on its monitoring activities.

Conceptual Barriers: Moving Toward a National Child Standard

Wehr and Jameson (1994), in an influential analysis of children's health insurance design options, suggest that in order to provide children with the legal safeguards for the new world of managed care, a child standard of coverage is required. Such a child standard would be based upon the important physiological and clinical differences between children and adults and would be used to leverage appropriate definitions of medical necessity and secure appropriate levels of coverage. We believe that a child standard is necessary as a fundamental way of reconceptualizing what children need, and beyond its potential legal uses, would have other uses as well. A child standard could provide practical policy guidance for the coverage of vulnerable children, and suggest the kinds of institutional and systemic contexts in which vulnerable children can most benefit.

Practically, a child standard would be based on the unique health characteristics of children, such as their developmental vulnerability, their dependency on adults, and their unique patterns of morbidity, and would define the difference between adult and child health care needs. It could be used by health planners, insurance benefits managers, and others to establish and judge the adequacy of benefit levels; it could also be used as a practical yardstick in evaluating quality measures to assure that they were developmentally sensitive and captured important variation that typifies certain childhood conditions. It would also become the practical guide in evaluating how well new organizational forms like child SHMOs and health development organizations are working.

Legally a child standard serves as a backstop for arbitrating conflicts between a family and a health care plan. One important legal role might be in defining the scope of medical necessity. Medical necessity definitions and requirements could specify that medically necessary care includes care that will maintain or improve the child's medical, emotional, and developmental status. As a legal standard, it would also provide a powerful leverage point for advocates monitoring how well a specific health plan was performing for children in their community. At the policy level a child standard could be promulgated through a national commission on standards and quality of care. While such a commission does not currently exist, the recently formed Presidential Commission on Quality of Health Care is a step in this direction.

In a symbolic role, a child standard represents a constructive way to spark the political process to support a greater focus on the health needs of children through public and private programs. While such a standard is based on rational arguments concerning how children differ from adults and on the overwhelming scientific evidence about the lifelong consequences of not attending to health and developmental problems early in life, in the political process it is more than rationality that carries the day. A child standard can play the role of igniting the political imagination of the country on the side of civic responsibility and the need to pay proper attention to the unique needs of children.

Conclusion

Some of the financial, organizational, procedural, and conceptual barriers that we have noted suggest divergent kinds of policy approaches to assuring that the health interests of vulnerable children are protected. The financial barriers point to the need to expand and reinforce the existing employer-based insurance system, supplemented as it is through Medicaid and Title V and other federal and state programs. Although imperfect, this system still provides most children with insurance, and in the near term it will need to continue to do so. Administrators, child advocates, and politicians understand how it works. The kinds of modest policy actions that are needed to enable it to hobble along for another few years are also fairly easy to grasp: an expansion of the use of premium subsidies or an eligibility extension for benefits may enable the system to make it through to the next year, with only the additional children who have no insurance paying the price. In another sense, however, the foundation upon which this familiar system has been built—fee-for-service payments, physicians in private practice, employer-based insurance, and governmental willingness to fund stop-gap coverage—is rapidly changing under the pressure of sweeping health systems change, perceived federal budgetary limitations, and the growth of large-scale corporate medicine, which is by its very nature particularly sensitive to the demands of shareholders to maximize profits. Patching together the old system can work only for so long, and so more fundamental reforms must also be considered.

Fortunately, some of the same forces that are undermining the current system, including in particular the desire of employers to control costs and the consequent growth of large integrated managed care organizations, suggest the potential shape of solutions to some of the problems now faced by children. The emergence of vertically integrated managed care organizations may make it possible to develop even more comprehensive three-dimensional integrated systems of care for children. If the appropriate financing mechanisms can be developed (a big "if"), managed care offers the possibility for a population-based approach to health care delivery that has only been dreamed of in this country until now. Yet to save managed care organizations from the pressures of market-driven cost controls, it will be vitally important for policymakers to pursue two interconnected policy tracks, seeking to overcome both the procedural barriers and conceptual barriers discussed above. The first track requires developing the tools and measurement capacities to understand exactly what is happening to children in large managed care organizations, and the ability to fairly reimburse managed care organizations relative to their actual risk. The second essential issue is the deployment of better standards of care for children, standards that are supported by the force of law. Children do not complain, they do not write to elected representatives, and they are, by their very nature, inherently vulnerable. Legal standards of care have the potential to assure the protection of children, and properly framed, no ambitious politician will want to be on the wrong side of that issue. As a package, tools and standards can work, transforming the managed care organization from a potential threat to child health to its best guarantor. Carefully developed assessment tools make it possible for both policymakers and providers to monitor what managed care organizations do, and a child standard makes it possible to define what they are legally required to do. Together these elements can humanize, moderate, and customize managed care to meet all children's needs better.

With new sophistication in measurement of health and of risk, and with new legal standards that would assure not only minimum levels of care, but minimum breadth and duration of care, it is possible to envision the emergence of an entirely new kind of health care organization, one that goes far beyond the narrow medical focus of the managed care organization as we know it today, an organization that forms effective long-lasting links between service providers and families and their children. This health development organization would offer three-dimensional integrated care to its enrolled population, and begin to address some of the serious flaws in the way the U.S. health care system cares for vulnerable children. It is vulnerable children who most need integrated systems of care. It is often the families of vulnerable children who are least capable of playing the integrating role, whether that integration is needed between the levels of care offered by a managed care organization, or between service organizations, or over time. Health development organizations could represent a major advance for all children, but none will benefit more directly from the promise of the health development organization than those who are most vulnerable.

References

Aday LA. 1993. At risk in America: The health and health care needs of vulnerable populations in the United States. San Francisco: Jossey-Bass.

Alan Guttmacher Institute. 1994. Unpublished data. In: Carnegie Council on Adolescent Development. 1995 Oct. Great transitions: Preparing adolescents for a new century. New York: Carnegie Corporation of New York.

[AAP] American Academy of Pediatrics, Committee on Early Childhood, Adoption and Dependent Care. 1994. Health care of children in foster care. Pediatrics 93:355–8.

Bell NJ, Bell RW. 1993. Adolescent risk taking. Newbury Park, CA: Sage Publications.

Blum RW, Bearinger LH. 1990. Knowledge and attitudes of health professionals toward adolescent health care. Journal of Adolescent Health Care 11:289–94.

Breslau N, Mortimer EA. 1981. Seeing the same doctor: Determinants of satisfaction with specialty care for disabled children. Medical Care 19:741–58.

Brewer EJ, McPherson M, Magrab PR, Hutchins, V. 1989. Family centered, community based, coordinated care for children with special health care needs. Pediatrics 83(6):1055–61.

Bronfenbrenner U. 1986. Ecology of the family as a context for human development research perspectives. Developmental Psychology 22: 723–42.

Brown ER, Wyn R, Fong K, Valenzuela A, Morales L, Cumberland WG, Ong P, Becerra R. 1996 June. 830,000 California immigrants may lose MediCal and become uninsured. Policy brief. Los Angeles: Center for Health Policy Research, University of California, Los Angeles.

Bureau of Justice Statistics. 1994. Criminal victimization in the United States, 1992. NCJ-145-125. Washington: U.S. Government Printing Office.

Carnegie Council on Adolescent Development. 1995 Oct. Great transactions: Preparing adolescents for a new century. New York: Carnegie Corporation of New York.

Cartland JDC, Yudkowsky BK. 1992 Feb. Barriers to pediatric referral in managed care systems. Pediatrics 89(2):183–8.

Child Welfare League of America. 1988. Standards for health care services for children in out-of-home care. Washington: CWLA.

Dubowitz H, Geigelman S, Zuravin S, Tepper V, Davidson N, Lichenstein R. 1992. The physical health of children in kinship care. American Journal of Diseases of Children 146:603–10.

Ellickson PL, Lara ME, Sherbourne CD, Zima B. 1993. Forgotten ages, forgotten problems: Adolescents' health. RAND.

Fowler L, Andersen G. 1996. Capitation adjustment for pediatric populations. Pediatrics 98(1):10–17.

Fox H, McManus M. 1996 March. Impacts of state Medicaid waiver programs on children: results from Hawaii, Oregon, Rhode Island and Tennessee. Policy Center.

Fox HB, Wicks LB, Newacheck PW. 1993. State Medicaid health maintenance organization policies and special-needs children. Health Care Financial Review 15:25–37.

[GAO] General Accounting Office. 1996 July 9. Medicaid and uninsured children. GAO/HEHS-96, 174e. Washington: U.S. Government Printing Office.

Garbarino J. 1990. The human ecology of early risk. In: Meisels SJ, Shomkoff JP, editors. Handbook of early childhood intervention, pp. 78–96. New York: Cambridge University Press.

Halfon N, Berkowitz G. 1993. Health care entitlements for children. In: Jensen MA, Goffin SG, editors. Visions of entitlement: The care and education of America's children, pp. 175–212. New York: State University of New York Press.

Halfon N, Klee L. 1987. Health services for California's foster children: Current practices and policy recommendations. Pediatrics 80(2):183–91.

Halfon N, Klee L. 1991. Health and development services for children with multiple needs: The children in foster care. Yale Law and Policy Review 9:71–96.

Halfon N, Berkowitz, G, Klee L. 1991. Developing an integrated case management program for vulnerable children. Child Welfare.

Halfon N, English A, Allen ML, Dewoody M. 1994. National health care reform, Medicaid and children in foster care. Child Welfare 73:99–115.

Halfon N, Inkelas M, Woods D. 1995a. Nonfinancial barriers to care for children and youth. Annual Review of Public Health 16:447–72.

Halfon N, Mendonca A, Berkowitz G. 1995b April. Health status of children in foster care: The experience of the Center for the Vulnerable Child. Archives of Pediatric and Adolescent Medicine 149:386–92.

Halfon N, Inkelas M, Wood D. Schuster M. 1996. Health care reform for children in families: The financing and restructuring of the U.S. child health system. In: Andersen R, Rice TH, Kominsky G, editors. Changing the U.S. health care system, pp. 229–54. San Francisco: Jossey-Bass.

Halfon N, Wood D, Valdez RB, Pereya M, Duan, N. 1997. Medicaid enrollment and health services access by Latino children in inner-city Los Angeles. Journal of the American Medical Association 277(8):636–41.

Hamburg DA. 1992. Children's security and the nation's future. In: Van De Water PN, Schorr LB, editors. Security for America's children: Proceedings of the fourth conference of the National Academy of Social Insurance, pp. 13–17. Dubuque, IA: Kendall/Hunt Publishing.

Hayes-Bautista DE, Schink WO, Rodriguez G. 1994. Latino immigrants in Los Angeles: A portrait from the 1990 census. Los Angeles: ALTA California Policy Research Center, Community Partners.

Hochstadt JN, Jaudes PK, Zimo DA, Schachter J. 1987. The medical psychosocial needs of children entering foster care. Child Abuse and Neglect 2:53–62.

Horwitz SM, Stein REK. 1990 May. Health maintenance organizations vs. indemnity insurance for children with chronic illness: Trading gaps in coverage. American Journal of Diseases of Children 144:581–6.

Hughes DC, Halfon N, Brindis CD, Newacheck PW. In press. Improving children's access to health care: The role of decategorization. Bulletin of the New York Academy of Sciences.

Ireys HT, Grason HA, Guyer B. 1996 Aug. Assuring quality of care for children with special needs in managed care organizations: Roles for pediatricians. Pediatrics 98(2):178–85.

Jameson EJ, Wehr E. 1994. Drafting national health care reform legislation to protect the health interests of children. Stanford Law and Policy Review 5(1):152–76.

Kelder SH, Perry CL, Klepp KI, Lytle LL. 1994. Longitudinal tracking of adolescent smoking, physical activity and food choice behaviors. American Journal of Public Health 84:1121–6.

Kronic R, Dreyfus T, Zhou A, Lee L. 1995. Risk adjusted reimbursement for people with disabilities: A diagnostic approach for the states of Missouri Medicaid Working Group.

Lieu TA, Newacheck PW, McManus MA. 1993. Race, ethnicity, and access to ambulatory care among U.S. adolescents. American Journal of Public Health 84(10):1621–25.

Lowry R, Kann L, Collins JL, Kolbe LJ. 1996. The effect of socioeconomic status on chronic disease risk behaviors among US adolescents. Journal of the American Medical Association 276:792–7.

Manning WG, Leibowitz A, Goldberg GA, Rogers WH, Newhouse JP. 1984. A controlled trial of the effect of a prepaid group practice on use of services. New England Journal of Medicine 310:1505–10.

Manton KG, Newcomer R, Ventelless JC, Lowizimore GR, Harrington C. 1994. A method for adjusting capitation payment to managed care plans using multivariate patterns of health and functioning. The Experience of Social Health Maintenance Organizations 32(2):277–97.

Mauldon J, Leibowitz A, Buchanan JL, Damberg C, McGuigan KA. 1994. Rationing or rationalizing children's medical care: Comparison of a Medicaid HMO with fee-for-service care. American Journal of Public Health 84:899–904.

McGlynn E, Halfon N, Leibowitz A. 1995. Assessing the quality of care for children: Prospects under health care reform. Archives of Pediatric and Adolescent Medicine.

McManus M, Newacheck P, Kelly R, Mackiln M. 1992 May. High cost of children: The unknown liability. Business and Health.

Mendoza F, Ventura S, Valdez RB, Costello RO, Saldivar L, Balsden K, Matorell R. 1991. Selected measures of health status for Mexican American, mainland Puerto Rican, and Cuban American children. Journal of the American Medical Association 265(2):227–32.

Miller RH. 1996a. Competition in the health system: good news and bad news. Health Affairs 15(2):107–20.

Miller, RH. 1996b. Health system integration: A means to an end. Health Affairs 15(2):92–106.

National Center for Health Statistics. 1994, 1995. Unpublished data reported in Carnegie Council on Adolescent Development. 1995 Oct. Great transitions: Preparing adolescents for a new century. New York: Carnegie Corporation of New York.

National Health Foundation and The Center for the Study of Latino Health at UCLA. 1995 Nov. Barriers to health care for US citizen children of undocumented parents. Los Angeles: UCLA.

Neff JM, Andersen G. 1995. Protecting children with chronic illness in a competitive marketplace. Journal of the American Medical Association 274(23):1866–9.

Newacheck PW, Halfon N. 1997 submitted. Prevalence and impact of disabling childhood chronic conditions. American Journal of Public Health.

Newacheck PW, McManus M. 1988. Financing health care for disabled children. Pediatrics 81:385–94.

Newacheck PW, Taylor WP. 1992. Childhood chronic illness: Prevalence, severity and impact. American Journal of Public Health 82:364–71.

Newacheck P, McManus M, St. Peter R. 1993 June. Children's use of preventive care services. San Francisco: Institute for Health Studies, University of California.

Newacheck PW, Hughes DC, Stoddard JJ, Halfon N. 1994. Children with chronic illness and Medicaid managed care. Pediatrics 93:497–500.

Newacheck PW, Hughes DC, Cisternas M. 1995a. Children and health insurance: An overview of recent trends. Health Affairs 14(1):244–54.

Newacheck PW, Hughes DC, Brindis C, Halfon N. 1995b. Decategorizing health services: Interim findings from the Robert Wood Johnson Foundation's Child Health Initiative. Health Affairs 14(3):232–42.

Newacheck PW, Hughes DC, English A, Fox HB, Perrin J, Halfon N. 1995c. The effect on children of curtailing Medicaid spending. Journal of the American Medical Association 274:1468–71.

Newacheck PW, McManus M, Fox HB. 1996a May. An incremental and voluntary proposal for expanding children's health insurance. Institute for Health Policy Studies.

Newacheck PW, McManus M, Fox HB. 1996b. Three options for providing universal health coverage to children. Maternal and Child Health Policy Research Center.

Olds D, Henderson C, Phelps C, Kitzman H, Hanks C. 1993. Effect of prenatal and infancy nurse home visitation on government spending. Medical Care 31(2):155–74.

Perkoff GT, Kahn L, Haas PJ. 1976. The effects of an experimental prepaid group practice of medical care utilization and cost. Medical Care 14: 432–49.

Perrin JM, MacLean WE. 1988 Dec. Children with chronic illness: The prevention of dysfunction. The Pediatric Clinics of North America 35(6): 1325–37.

Perrin JM, Shayne MW, Bloom SE. 1993a. Home and community care for chronically ill children. New York: Oxford University Press.

Perrin E, Newacheck P, Pless I, et al. 1993b. Issues involved in the definition and classification of chronic illness. Pediatrics 91(4):787–93.

Perry BD, Pollard RA, Blakley TL, Baker WL, Vigilante D. 1995 Winter. Childhood trauma, the neurobiology of adaptation, and "use-dependent" development of the brain: How "states" become "traits." Infant Mental Health Journal 16(4):271–91.

Rosenbaum S, Borzi PC. 1996 March. Health insurance coverage for children: Background and options in reform. Washington: Center for Health Policy Research, George Washington University Medical Center.

Schor EL. 1982. The foster care system and health status of foster children. Pediatrics 69:521–8.

Simms NM, Halfon N. 1994. The health care needs of children in foster care: A research agenda. Child Welfare 73:505–24.

Skocpol T. 1992. Comment on Paul Starr "A new deal for the young." In: Van De Water PN, Schorr LB, editors. Security for America's children: Proceedings of the fourth conference of the National Academy of Social Insurance, pp. 29–31. Dubuque, IA: Kendall/Hunt Publishing.

Starfield B, Weiner J, Mumford L, Steinwachs D. 1995a. Ambulatory care groups: A categorization of diagnosis for research and management. Health Services Research 26(1):53–74.

Starfield B, Riley AW, Green BF, et al. 1995b. The adolescent CHIP: A population-based measure of health. Medical Care 33:553–6.

Starr P. 1992. A new deal for the young. In: Van De Water PN, Schorr LB, editors. Security for America's children: Proceedings of the fourth conference of the National Academy of Social Insurance, pp. 17–24. Dubuque, IA: Kendall/Hunt Publishing.

Stein REK, Jessop D. 1990. Functional status II(R). A measure of child health status. Medical Care 28:1041–55.

Stein REK, Bauman LJ, Westbrook LE, Coupey SM, Ireys HT. 1993. Framework for identifying children who have chronic conditions: The case for a new definition. Journal of Pediatrics 122:342–7.

Swire MR, Kavaler F. 1977. The health status of foster children. Child Welfare 56:635–53.

U.S. Congress, Office of Technology Assessment. 1991 April. Adolescent health, Vol. 1: Summary and policy options. OTA-H-468. Washington: U.S. Government Printing Office.

U.S. Department of Health and Human Services. 1996. Trends in the well being of America's children. Washington: U.S. Government Printing Office.

University of Michigan Institute for Social Research. 1994 Dec. Monitoring the future study. Unpublished data. In: Carnegie Council on Adolescent Development. 1995 Oct. Great transitions: Preparing adolescents for a new century. New York: Carnegie Corporation of New York.

Wehr E, Jameson EJ. 1994 Winter. Beyond benefits: The importance of a pediatric standard in private insurance contracts to ensuring health care access for children. The Future of Children 4:115–33.

Werner E. 1990. Protective factors and individual resilience. In: Meisels SJ, Shomkoff JP, editors. Handbook of early childhood intervention, pp. 97–116. New York: Cambridge University Press.

Ziv TA, Lo B. 1995. Denial of care to illegal immigrants: Proposition 187 in California. New England Journal of Medicine 332:1095–8.

15

The Role of Public Health in Assuring a System of Health Care for Children

Maxine Hayes and Deborah Klein Walker

PUBLIC HEALTH DEPARTMENTS perform many different functions. They are responsible for the health of populations or communities, but they have defined and executed this broad mission in different ways in different parts of the country and at different times. This has led to some confusion, even among public health professionals, about the proper role of public health in today's health care environment, in which public health departments are being challenged to articulate and defend their role and as public health budgets across the nation are being cut.

In fact, the swift changes that are occurring in the U.S. health care system argue for the need for a strong and continuing public health function, to assess how changes are impacting population health, to enforce standards of care, and to assure availability of care. In particular, public health can provide a strong unifying voice for mothers, children, and their families.

This chapter provides an overview of the current shifts in the general public health system as well as a description of the current maternal and child health system supported by the Title V Maternal and Child Health (MCH) block grant. Examples of MCH activities in two states are described. In the concluding section, recommendations are presented for assuring that public health continues to function as the ultimate point of accountability at all levels of government in the design and implementation of a system of health care for children.

The Changing Role of Public Health

In order to articulate the role of public health in building a health care system for children and adolescents, it is important to understand the history of public health in the United States, as well as the changes currently occurring.

Since the first state public health department was established in Massachusetts in the mid-nineteenth century, state and local health departments in the United States have shared the mission of improving population health status. Originally, they focused on combating infectious diseases and improving sanitary conditions. Although infectious diseases pose somewhat less of a challenge today, as disease outbreaks and epidemics have been eliminated or significantly reduced through the introduction of vaccines and antibiotics, the emergence of HIV/AIDS and the reemergence of tuberculosis indicate that public health still has a role to play in the battle against communicable diseases.

In addition, public health agencies today focus on social and community issues such as social and behavioral problems, for example, violence in its various forms, including domestic violence and child and elder abuse. They also collect and disseminate the information necessary to do needs assessments and community planning.

Finally, public health agencies focus on prevention and on assuring a system of care for all citizens. They seek to achieve these goals by educating and informing the public, enforcing laws and regulations, developing and implementing standards of care, training and educating health care workers, and in some situations providing direct clinical services to those who have no other options.

Public Health Departments as Direct Service Providers

It is this last role—the provision of direct health care services—that has predominated as the most visible public health function in recent times and that is most in question today. There are many areas of the country where public health departments have become a provider of health care services to populations that might otherwise lack access to health care: poor and uninsured individuals, the vast majority of them pregnant women and children. This pattern is especially evident in the South and West, where city and county health departments play a major role in the delivery of direct medical services. In the northern and New England states, public health departments have been organized differently, and medical services for the poor and uninsured are delivered in community health centers and in local medical facilities using public health dollars but not by public health agencies themselves. Nonetheless, over time, many people, including many health care professionals and advocates, have come to see public health departments as one set of service providers and the private sector as another, and have lost sight of the other key public health functions that public health departments perform. In fact, many health departments have themselves become so consumed in providing direct clinical care that they have not had time to hone the community systems development and health planning skills necessary to perform all the other population-based public health functions effectively.

It was to clarify the myriad roles of public health departments that the Institute of Medicine, in the late 1980s, articulated the three core functions of public health: assessment, policy development, and quality assurance (Institute of Medicine, 1988). These core functions have been further developed into a set of ten essential public health services (Grayson and Guyer, 1995):

- Monitoring health status to identify community health problems.
- Diagnosing and investigating health problems and health hazards in the community.
- Informing, educating, and empowering people about health issues.
- Mobilizing community partnerships to identify and solve health problems.
- Developing policies and plans that support individual and community health efforts.
- Enforcing laws and regulations that protect health and ensure safety.
- Linking people to needed personal health services and assuring the provision of health care when otherwise unavailable.
- Assuring a competent public health and personal health care workforce.
- Evaluating effectiveness, accessibility, and quality of personal and population-based health services.
- Conducting research for new insights and innovative solutions to health problems.

The Impact of Managed Care

As managed care has grown and coverage for the uninsured has expanded, those public health agencies that have been providing direct services have had to choose between becoming competitors in the marketplace for Medicaid patients (by becoming community health centers, for example) and abandoning the delivery of clinical care altogether. Beginning in the late 1980s, some public health departments had already begun to relinquish their role as direct providers of clinical services to focus more on assessment, policy development, and the other health assurance strategies. To effect this transition, clinical staff at local health departments need to develop new nonclinical public health skills, and public health practitioners need to be assured that the patients they were previously serving will be served by others in more integrated settings (Baker et al., 1994; Roper et al., 1992; Turnock et al., 1994).

Indeed, much more clarification is needed of the role of public health departments in assuring the provision of medical care, regardless of the setting or payor. Although many recognize the key contributions of public health entities in the assessment and policy development functions, there is much less understanding and consensus about the ways public health agencies perform the assurance function. The mandate to assure a system of care for the population is present in federal law relating to the maternal and child health population (see discussion of Title V below), but there is no comparable federal statute for adults. Hence, there is a great deal of confusion about public health's broader authority over the entire system of care.

Just as many public health agencies are moving away from the delivery of medical care, many traditional providers of medical care (e.g., hospitals and health maintenance organizations [HMOs]) are becoming more interested in the traditional population-based public health functions. Part of this interest is related to outreach activities and public relations opportunities in the community, and part is due to pressures from accrediting bodies and state regulatory authorities. For example, hospitals are now required to prepare a community needs assessment for accreditation. In some states (e.g., Massachusetts), the Attorney General requires all not-for-profit hospitals to provide community benefits in exchange for their tax-exempt status. In addition, some managed care organizations, understanding that prevention activities save dollars, have sponsored community-based education and screening programs, especially in areas where they have gained enough market share to have a long-term interest in the community's health.

As these various roles are sorted out and the responsibilities of public health departments defined or redefined, it is instructive to examine public health departments' role with respect to maternal and child health. This is an area in which, more than any other, public health departments have retained their focus on populations (Association of Maternal and Child Health Programs, 1994) by providing children's services and playing a role in assuring access to care and coordinated services. State MCH agencies are involved in a variety of systems development activities for mothers and children whose aim is the integration of a wide variety of players and structures.

As the examples below illustrate, they are working within a new paradigm that emphasizes a community-based, consumer-driven focus that integrates public and private systems across diseases and health outcomes.

Title V of the Social Security Act

The role of public health in building a system of health care for children is best demonstrated through the work of the Title V program. Operating in all 50 states and jurisdictions as a federal/state partnership since its authorization in 1935 as part of the Social Security Act, Title V mandates state maternal and child health programs "to improve the health of all mothers and children" (Guyer, 1990; Lesser, 1985).

Significant amendments were made to the program in 1981 and 1989. In 1981, seven categorical programs, the largest of which were the Maternal and Child Health Services and Crippled Children's Programs, were consolidated into a single Maternal and Child Health block grant, allowing states a significant degree of flexibility and discretion in setting their own priorities to reflect their own needs. In 1989, amid concern that greater accountability was needed, the block grant was amended to require state programs to

- develop a population-based needs assessment;
- implement a program responsive to the state's needs assessment and related to Year 2000 objectives;
- develop community-based networks of preventive and primary care for pregnant women, infants, children, and adolescents; and
- develop family-centered, community-based, coordinated care systems for children with special health care needs.

Each state MCH program is also required to plan, develop, and evaluate systems of preventive and primary care, and must develop standards that allow effective and fair monitoring and assurance of quality.

While state MCH programs do provide direct services to special populations or to fill gaps in services, this is not the primary purpose of Title V. Because the needs of the MCH population are so complex, and because meeting these needs and improving the health of mothers and children requires more than simple financing of care, there has been a focus on developing adequate and appropriate infrastructure at all levels of government to ensure access and eliminate fragmentation among health and related services for all women and children. In 1991, the MCH Bureau estimated that 75 percent of the MCH block grant dollars to states were spent on services to improve health care systems, to prevent health problems, and to maximize resources at the state and local level. Examples of state efforts in these categories include

- infrastructure and capacity building (e.g., needs assessment, planning, legislation, coordination, quality assurance, standards development, monitoring, and training);
- population-based services (e.g., newborn screening, lead poisoning prevention, immunization, Sudden Infant Death Syndrome (SIDS) counseling, injury prevention outreach, and public education);
- enabling services (e.g., case management, health education, transportation, translation, home visiting, and nutrition); and
- services for children with special health care needs (e.g., assurance of the availability, accessibility, and quality of services to these special children and their families at the community level).

Examples of MCH Programs at Work

Within states, MCH Title V agencies work to design and implement systems of care to improve the health and well-being of children and their families in local communities. The following examples are drawn from the National Governors Association's Issue Brief, "Protecting the Health of All Women and Children through Title V" (June 30, 1995).

Infant Mortality

In Washington State, the First Steps Program, created by the Maternity Access Act, has been improving maternal and infant care for low-income families since 1989. The program is a collaborative effort of the state Department of Social and Health Services, the Department of Health, the federal Title V program, and community agencies. The program is administered jointly by the state Medicaid agency and the state Title V program. The two departments developed a public advisory steering committee, which provides guidance and oversight in the effort to improve access to prenatal care and to integrate prenatal care services.

First Steps has increased access to medical care for pregnant women and infants by modifying income guidelines and increasing reimbursement rates for Medicaid maternity and pediatric care providers. The client application process was streamlined, allowing eligibility to be determined within 15 days, and staff from the Department of Social and Health Services were stationed in community settings to assist with the application process. Two key components of the First Steps program are Maternity Support Services, managed by the Title V program, and Maternity Case Management. These nonmedical services include community health nursing, nutrition and social work visits, childbirth education classes, and child care reimbursement for bed rest and visiting hospitalized newborns. These nonmedical services were added to the state Medicaid program, making federal Medicaid matching dollars available to the state. First Steps has also provided needed health services across the state through a wide range of providers, such as county health departments, community clinics, Indian health agencies, social services agencies, and local government programs.

Recent evaluation data indicate that women receiving Maternity Support Services are 20 percent more likely to receive adequate prenatal care than women who do not receive such services. Moreover, since First Steps began six years ago, Washington has seen a 25 percent decline in the low-birthweight rate among infants born to Medicaid-eligible women. Today it has the lowest infant mortality rate among all 50 states.

The state MCH program was instrumental in establishing a foundation for, and facilitating the development of, the First Steps Program. Title V administrators pressed state legislators and kept them well informed on the importance of a comprehensive approach to maternity care access, using outcome data that had been collected and analyzed for many years prior to the First Steps legislation. Without these data, the design of the program would not have been as comprehensive. Title V resources were also key to developing the interdisciplinary approach reflected in the Maternity Support Services component of First Steps. In 1990, the state enacted Second Steps. This program has expanded children's eligibility for health services and provided "bridge" grants to support local communities' efforts to improve children's access to care. Today, Washington State provides health care coverage for all children through age 18, up to 200 percent of the federal poverty level, by combining Medicaid expansions with coverage for low-income families through the state-sponsored Basic Health Plan.

School Health

In Massachusetts, the Title V agency has taken the lead in developing comprehensive school health programs in communities across the state. Title V resources have been used to support the development and implementation of a system of school-linked and school-based services for school-aged children and adolescents.

The Title V agency collects and provides data regularly on a wide variety of indicators related to the socioeconomic condition, health status, and general well-being of children, youth, and families. These data are available at the city, town, and census tract levels to enhance community needs assessments, monitor overall child health status, and evaluate school and community health activities. Title V funds were used to conduct youth health surveys in the schools where school-based health centers were being developed.

The Title V agency has been the leader in a number of policy development activities crucial to building safe school environments that assure access for all children across the state. For example, Title V staff took the lead in the development and adoption of absentee and inclusion policies for children and youth with HIV/AIDS, curriculum guidelines for the incorporation of HIV/AIDS prevention activities, a major revision in the regulations regarding the administration of medications in school settings, and guidelines for the maintenance of safe schools, including violence prevention activities and guidelines for safe playgrounds. A recently developed school health manual by Title V staff will facilitate the further development of all components of a comprehensive school health program.

In order to assure that comprehensive school health programs are in place, Title V resources have been used to provide regular training opportunities for school nurses and other school personnel, provide ongoing technical assistance to all school systems for health and related issues, develop standards and guidelines for practice, facilitate the licensing process for school-based health centers, and facilitate links to a variety of other health and social services (e.g., dental health, nutrition, mental health, genetic counseling). In addition, Title V funds were used to establish the first school-based health center in 1986. Today there are more than 30 centers supported by Title V block grant funds and resources from a state excise tax on cigarettes passed in November 1992. Title V staff are actively working with the state Medicaid agency to assure that school health services are well integrated into the managed care system for children and adolescents.

Finally, Title V resources are being used to develop and maintain active partnerships and collaborative working coalitions at the local and state levels with education and other agencies, private organizations, youth, and families. In sum, Title V MCH staff and resources have been used to support school-linked and school-based programs in order to enhance the health status and well-being of children and youth in communities across the state.

Summary, Implications, and Recommendations

As we enter the twenty-first century and look back on the contributions of the Title V program to public health, it is imperative to understand the importance of sustaining and bolstering a locus of accountability for the health of women and children, regardless of what service delivery and financing systems emerge.

Historically in this country, as well as in most other nations, women and children have been singled out for special public interest and responsibility. The reasons include

- the vulnerability of pregnant women and of children and youth during critical formative periods of growth and development;
- the efficacy of prevention and early intervention with women of childbearing age, and with children and youth, which yield long-term benefits in adult productivity and life expectancy as well as cost savings for remedial services;
- the special needs of children with chronic conditions and of adolescents, which warrant careful attention in policy and program development;
- the need for services to be tailored to the specific needs of women and youth, in light of their different physiological and developmental characteristics, which influence risk for and progression of disease and disability, as well as utilization of services;
- the lack of political power of children and still limited political power of women;
- the dependence of youth on families as well as on community and social institutions;
- the interrelatedness of children's health status, educational achievement, and social development, and the importance and influence of family and community on these factors; and

• the disproportionate representation of the underserved, including the poor and people of color, among women of childbearing age, children and youth, and their families (Association of Maternal and Child Health Programs, 1994).

Although the Title V program is the locus of accountability for the health of women and children in this country, it currently lacks the clout, visibility, resources, and strong statutory base and structure to carry out not only the very broad mandate given to it by Congress in 1935, but the leadership role in developing systems of care for children given to it by Congress in 1989.

Additionally, over the past decades, much has happened to change the health care environment, including the emergence of health care reform; managed care; and reforms in Medicaid, education, mental health, and most recently welfare. In the future the human service system will change in many other ways as the federal government transfers many of its current functions to the states. With these changes, it is imperative that our nation does not lose sight of the need for a strong locus of accountability for children. This locus of accountability is needed at *all* levels of government in order to assure assessment (exchange and analysis of the health information upon which systems are built), planning, design, coordination, development, and implementation of systems of care. Without a strong locus of accountability and leadership, a well-functioning system of care will never evolve.

It is important to reexamine key issues related to maternal and child health policy and systems. What should the locus of accountability for maternal and child health look like? Where within governmental bodies and communities should it be located? What is it accountable to? How should it be structured? What vertical powers should it have? What unique roles and responsibilities should it have? What core capacities, competencies, and skills should it have?

The current Title V statute is a good starting point for answering these questions, but it should be significantly enhanced and strengthened.

• *A strong federal/state partnership should continue to exist to accomplish the core functions of public health with respect to the maternal and child health population.* This partnership should have as its mission the creation of systems of care at the community level to enhance the health and well-being of all mothers, children, youth, and their families. Efforts should focus on maintaining capacity at the state and local level to assure that systems of care that address the total environment of the child (i.e., physical, emotional, social) are in place and maintained.

• *The primary locus of accountability for the MCH population should remain at the state level.* Within states this accountability has been housed within the state health agency. We think this arrangement should continue, even though, in light of the devolution of more and more responsibilities for human services to the state, a concern emerges about the source of oversight needed to galvanize a national agenda for children. Every state needs a designated MCH entity that is well known and accountable to the public to assure that services and policies are in place to protect and promote children and their families.

• *A strong federal locus of accountability should exist.* Most recently, this locus has been the MCH Bureau within the Health Resources and Services Administration, but it is questionable whether the Bureau's current capacity, structure, or placement provides it with the visibility, clout, and capability to be effective. An entity is needed that would be directly accountable to the secretary of the Department of Health and Human Services, the administration, and the Congress. It would need a strong statutory base with regulatory power to monitor the health status as well as the health systems in place that affect the health and well-being of children. This would require a strong policy development function drawn from a very strong health information and data capacity with the ability to analyze national trends, a strong surveillance capability that links relevant databases from multiple sources, and strong links to the National Center for Health Statistics, Centers for Disease Control and Prevention, National Institute of Child Health and Development, and the agencies responsible for child welfare, mental health, and education.

• *Title V of the Social Security Act should be reviewed and strengthened with respect to other key legislation affecting the MCH population.* First, the Title V statute should be reexamined and strengthened to give authority to all levels of government to serve as the point of accountability for all children and families. Perhaps the statute should be revised to resemble the Older Americans Act, which delineates structures and processes at every level of government. Second, history has taught us the need for statutory language in all other relevant statutes linking back to Title V or its replacement in order to build systems of care for children. For example, Title V in 1989 had language in its statute requiring links to Medicaid, but no link to the Title V statute exists in the Medicaid statute. Reciprocal statutory links are needed in legislation concerning child welfare, education, mental health, and other child-related areas to promote a coordinated system of care for children. These statutory linkages at the federal level would also pave the way for parallel behavior at the state level.

In sum, the locus of accountability at all levels must be responsible for agenda setting, for providing information to decision makers at all levels of government, and for convening periodic summits on the status of children's health. At a time when market forces and evolving public policy decisions are bringing about dramatic changes in the health care system, a focal point with responsibility for setting a national and state agenda for children's health and well-being is desperately needed. Without this focal point, policymakers and communities may lose sight of children. The agenda should take into consideration the developmental needs of children at different ages as well as their dependency on the families and environments in which they live for optimal growth and development. This requires adequate capacity in the core functions of public health and the ability to convene regular summits to report on how children are faring. National standards must be developed and the capacity created to assist states in operationalizing these standards.

The linking of the state MCH block grant requirements for Year 2000 health objectives with the needs assessments of states is the history we now have to build upon. Adequate technical assistance and consultation for states and local communities are needed to provide oversight and accountability. Systems performance measures need to be developed, but there must be capacity to assist states in operationalizing systems measures as well.

References

Association of Maternal and Child Health Programs. 1994. Beyond security: The need for a maternal and child health focus and roles for Title V in health care reform. Washington: Association of Maternal and Child Health Programs.

Baker RL, Melton RJ, Stange PV, Fields ML, Koplan JP, Guerra FA, Satcher D. 1994. Health reform and the health of the public. Journal of the American Medical Association 276(16):1276–82.

Grayson HA, Guyer B. 1995. Public MCH program functions: Essential public health services to promote maternal and child health in America. Baltimore, MD: Child and Adolescent Health Policy Center, Johns Hopkins University School of Hygiene and Public Health.

Guyer B. 1990. The evolution and future role of Title V. In: Schlesinger MJ, Eisenberg L, editors. Changing in a changing health system: Assessments and proposals for reform, pages 297–324. Baltimore, MD: Johns Hopkins University Press.

Institute of Medicine. 1988. The future of public health. Washington: National Academy Press.

Lesser AJ. 1985. The origin and development of maternal and child health programs in the United States. American Journal of Public Health 75: 590–8.

Roper WL, Baker EL, Dyal WW, Nicola RM. 1992. Strengthening the public health system. Public Health Reports 197(6):609–15.

Turnock BJ, Handler A, Dyal WW, Christenson G, Vaughn EH, Rowitz L, Munson JW, Balierson T, Richards TB. 1994. Implementing and assessing organizational practices in local health departments. Public Health Reports 109(4):478–84.

16

Models of Collaboration: Strategies for Improving Children's Health in a Managed Care Environment

Phyllis Brooks

CHILD HEALTH PROFESSIONALS in the United States are at varying stages of coming to terms with managed care. Troubled by the existing patchwork of services for children, they welcome managed care's promise of accessible and integrated services and its emphasis on prevention, while remaining wary about the potential abuses inherent in a capitated system of payment, among them the incentives to provide fewer services and to enroll only the healthiest children.

Nonetheless, at this moment when the organization of the entire U.S. health care system is in question, it seems critical to identify the unique needs of children and get at the root of some of the disturbing trends outlined in the first section of this book. To shape a more equitable, accessible, and cohesive system of care, child health professionals and advocates need to collaborate in new ways and to rethink how services are structured

This chapter is based on presentations made at the United Hospital Fund's 1996 conference "Child Health in a Managed Care Environment: Balancing Personal and Community Health Needs" by Thomas Barela, M.D., a Phoenix-based pediatrician; Robert M. Bilenker, M.D., acting chairperson of the department of pediatrics and head of the Comprehensive Care Program at the Metro Health Medical Center in Cleveland, Ohio; William H. Hollinshead, M.D., Medical Director of the Division of Family Health of the Rhode Island Department of Health; Paul Nannis, Milwaukee Commissioner of Health; Deborah Klein Walker, Assistant Commissioner of the Bureau of Family and Community Health, and the Massachusetts Department of Health; and Donna Zimmerman, former executive director of Health Start in St. Paul, Minnesota.

and how responsibility for services is assigned. This kind of restructuring requires considerable thought and energy, at a time when much attention is necessarily diverted to defending those public programs that have, for the last three decades, provided a measure of relief and support to children and their families. At such a juncture, the temptation is to focus on protecting those services that exist rather than seeking to expand services or develop more ambitious collaborations. However, some enterprising child health professionals, public health officials, and managed care administrators across the country have begun to collaborate in the design of programs that may serve as models for their colleagues elsewhere.

This chapter describes six such collaborative approaches: the partnership between the Massachusetts Division of Medical Assistance and Department of Health in the development of managed care contracting standards; collaboration among the Milwaukee Department of Health and various managed care plans in the wake of a measles epidemic; links between the school-based clinics of Health Start in St. Paul, Minnesota, and various managed care plans; how two initiatives for children with chronic conditions in Cleveland and Phoenix have adapted to managed care; and how Rhode Island has developed a system for collecting, analyzing, and disseminating the types of health status information necessary to track children's health status.

New Partnerships
New care schemes demand improved communication among various entities that historically may not have had the smoothest working relationships, or any working relationship at all. Different state agencies, small provider groups, and managed care plans are now finding that their individual success depends on the degree of cooperation with each other.

Between State Agencies
Collaborations work best when there is some congruence of mission and when each partner has something to offer. This was the case in Massachusetts, where the Division of Medical Assistance, the state agency responsible for administering the Medicaid program, partnered with the Department of Health, the agency responsible for all public health initiatives, including maternal and child health programs.

Like Medicaid agencies around the country, the Massachusetts Division of Medical Assistance found itself called on to assume new responsibilities with the transition to managed care. With managed care comes responsi-

bility for contracting for services, conducting extensive outreach and beneficiary education, and monitoring the success of managed care plans in
meeting contract specifications as well as long-term population health
goals. Although Massachusetts has a relatively mature managed care market
and a long history of paying for public health services (e.g., primary care,
school health) on a contractual basis, these significant new responsibilities
required new kinds of expertise and working relationships (Walker, 1996).

The Department of Health, on the other hand, had considerable experience in traditional public health functions, including outreach to vulnerable populations and designing programs to meet the needs of women and
children, who constitute so large a proportion of the Medicaid population.
Despite this experience, and despite the mandate, embodied in federal regulation, that public health departments serve as the ultimate point of accountability for population health, the department had relatively little clout
and no clear authority over the managed care plans that would be treating
the state's most vulnerable children.

Together, however, the two offices undertook a highly successful collaboration with respect to managed care implementation beginning in 1993.
As the state's largest buyer of medical services, the Division of Medical Assistance had significant bargaining power, and was prepared to benefit from
the Department of Health's expertise in maternal and child health issues in
determining the range of services needed to serve the low-income state residents enrolled in the program. For their part, the health department staff
got a crash course in health care contracting and reimbursement.

The success of the collaboration depended on effective communication.
To facilitate the sharing of information, the two agencies created an internal working group, which includes staff from both offices, to develop joint
work plans, with shared responsibility for achieving the work plan objectives. In addition, an external advisory committee was formed, comprising
advocates and representatives from the state chapter of the American Academy of Pediatrics. A health maintenance organization (HMO) work group
was also formed, which includes representatives from all the HMOs under
contract to the Medicaid agency; the work group meets monthly with Medicaid office staff and public health staff (Walker, 1996).

The collaboration among the two offices has been most effective in establishing standards and quality improvement projects for managed care
contracts. The Medicaid agency is now incorporating in its contracting
specifications a quality improvement system that is implemented with the
assistance of the Maternal and Child Health (MCH) Title V staff in public

health. A baseline for each HMO is established by an independent agency using information contained in plans' medical records regarding their achievement of Early and Periodic Screening, Diagnosis and Treatment (EPSDT) standards. Medicaid and health department staff use this baseline in working with plan physicians to develop a strategy for improving the plan's performance. The plan's success in meeting the goals is evaluated at contract renewal time; some managed care plans in the state have lost their approval as Medicaid providers because of their failure to meet the goals.

In a related effort to establish the best way to incorporate children with special needs, the health department obtained a grant to study the best options for this population. Together, the health department and Medicaid agency have surveyed every parent of a child receiving Supplemental Security Income or in the state's Part H early intervention program as well as every primary care provider serving Medicaid beneficiaries; it is using the findings to design health improvement strategies and will document the results. Finally, the MCH Title V staff in public health are overseeing the Massachusetts Bright Futures project, which establishes a set of outcomes— including the provision of immunizations, well-child visits, and anticipatory guidance for adolescents—as target quality standards for all purchasers and providers in the state. Medicaid was the first purchaser in the state to pay fully for the needed care and require reporting on performance indicators related to the Bright Futures goals. Ultimately, the state hopes that other purchasers will fully implement these goals also.

The Division of Medical Assistance and the Department of Health have also worked together to develop standards for school-based health centers (see chapter 15 for a full discussion). Because the Medicaid agency recognizes school-based health centers as important primary care providers, it requires all managed care plans to have linkages with school-based health centers. In turn the health department establishes the standards and certifies that school-based health centers have met them; MCH staff work with the centers to help in resolving issues of confidentiality, exchange of information, and terms of reimbursement (Walker, 1996). Other areas of collaboration include improving prenatal health care, services for children with special health care needs, and primary care for children.

The health department's special expertise has also been put to use in training benefits managers about how best to educate people with disabilities and chronic illnesses, as well as adolescents, about health care services and options. Like other health departments around the country, the Massachusetts health department has also developed considerable expertise around issues of cultural sensitivity and methods of communicating with diverse communities, which it is sharing with the Medicaid office; this kind of expertise will be in increasing demand as states move toward enrolling greater proportions of their Medicaid beneficiaries in managed care plans.

The experience in Massachusetts demonstrates that public health strategies can be used productively to improve managed care services. More broadly, it illustrates the benefits of collaboration. For the health department, its collaboration with the Medicaid agency was a crucial first step toward partnerships with other health care purchasers; its experience in working with the state's largest public purchaser of health care services will, it is hoped, provide an entree to other health care purchasers, bringing the state closer to the goal of establishing and enforcing universal standards for children's health care. This goal is predicated on the recognition that children's health status will not improve unless all providers and purchasers can agree to the same set of goals for child health.

Between Public Health Agencies and Managed Care Plans

Clearly, there is much to be gained by collaboration among state agencies, which may traditionally have had slightly different portfolios, but which share the mission of improving the health of the state's population and can pool their authority and expertise to influence the behavior of managed care plans. Too often, however, the relationship between public agencies and the managed care plans that they oversee is adversarial or, worse, nonexistent.

Such was the case in 1990, when five years into its managed care initiative, Milwaukee experienced a measles epidemic: 1,100 cases of measles and three deaths, mostly among disadvantaged preschool-aged children. Eighty-three percent of the children were enrolled in managed care plans. Subsequent analysis revealed that of all the preschoolers enrolled in the managed care plans, two-thirds were not appropriately immunized. No accountability for delivering immunizations had been built into the system. Of the 233 children hospitalized for measles, 33 percent identified the emergency department as their primary source of care. In the wake of the crisis, the health department immunized 20,000 children in a ten-week period, 55 percent of them enrolled in managed care plans (Nannis, 1996).

This crisis aptly demonstrates what can happen when the transition to managed care takes place quickly and without a developed plan for how public health agencies and managed care plans interact. In the press of state politics, the temptation is to minimize the magnitude of the shift. Experience in Milwaukee, however, powerfully indicates that time is needed in order to pay adequate attention to issues of provider capacity and accessibility, from a logistical as well as a cultural and linguistic point of view; to provide adequate consumer education; to avoid disrupting existing relationships among providers and patients; to develop the data systems for fiscal and clinical tracking across systems; and to make adequate provisions for oversight (Nannis, 1996). Particularly important is the development of formal relationships between managed care organizations and the public health department. In Milwaukee, there was no history of collaboration between the two sectors prior to the measles epidemic.

In the wake of the crisis, however, the health department worked closely with the city's managed care plans to develop specific strategies for averting such disasters in the future and for achieving specified public health goals. The health department is now reimbursed at a rate negotiated in advance with the managed care organizations if it provides lead tests or immunizations at one of its four clinics to a child enrolled in a managed care organization. Managed care organizations now have clear financial incentives to provide these services themselves and to do outreach and education of their members. The health department has worked aggressively to develop relationships with staff, particularly nursing staff, at managed care plans, so it can make referrals back to the plan once it has provided services; referrals are most often made by the city's 104 public health nurses, who are trained in advocacy and case management and who have direct access to providers in each of the managed care plans. Although the public health clinics welcome the uninsured, the goal is to make the public health clinics the last resort for children enrolled in managed care plans (Nannis, 1996).

In addition, the state has identified immunizations as a priority area, and requires plans to submit timetables with a plan of action and follow-up. The state is using the Our Kids Count Immunization Record System to track which children are immunized and with which vaccines. The health department and the managed care plans are also working together on a variety of public health initiatives, including ones focused on violence, infant mortality, and lead poisoning. In 1995 the number of lead screens performed by all sectors was approximately 30,000, up from 800 in 1993, and for the first time, the number of screens performed by the private sector exceeded the number performed by the public sector. Managed care plans are moreover expected to provide uniform data on enrollees, including prevalence and cause of mortality, morbidity, and disability; timing and frequency of immunizations; and effectiveness of interventions (Nannis, 1996).

The experience in Milwaukee demonstrates how much can be accomplished once health departments and managed care plans decide to collaborate; it also demonstrates that the consequences of lack of collaboration can be tragic.

School-Based Health Clinics and Managed Care Plans

Collaboration may be particularly difficult in cases where managed care plans are perceived as competing for the same patient population as, or threatening the existence of, providers who have a stake in the community or who have been serving populations that have traditionally been ignored or avoided. This is the case in many states with regard to providers serving populations with special needs, for example, people with HIV/AIDS or people with mental illness.

It is also the case with school-based health centers, which have typically grown up in areas with inadequate primary care infrastructures and which are designed for the hard-to-reach adolescent population. There are currently very few school-based health centers countrywide that have agreements with health plans and few health plans with experience in delivering school-based care. Nonetheless, the advent of managed care threatens the existence of most school-based health centers.

One organization that was able to develop fruitful relationships with managed care plans was Health Start, a nonprofit organization in St. Paul, Minnesota, that serves women, children, and teenagers in a variety of public health, community-based, and primary care settings. It is known for its school-based health center program, which started in 1973 and today operates eight school-based health centers for adolescents in St. Paul. These centers offer comprehensive services, including primary and preventive health care, mental health services, basic laboratory services, and referrals to subspecialists (Zimmerman, 1996).

Seventy percent of the students served by Health Start's school-based health clinics are enrolled in some form of managed health care, whether a commercial plan or a Medicaid managed care plan. Health Start's leaders sought to develop collaborations with managed care plans, in which they act as co-managers of care, in order to preserve their funding and maintain continuity of care. They were supported in this effort through their work with the School Health Policy Initiative, sponsored by Montefiore Medical Center in New York, a national program that was studying issues related to structuring relationships between managed care plans and school-based health centers.

Of course, the collaboration would not have worked if it did not make sense from managed care plans' perspective as well. For plans, partnerships with school-based health clinics allow them to take advantage of existing care patterns, minimize their costs, and provide an increased opportunity for health promotion and for attaining certain performance measures (Zimmerman, 1996).

Still, a number of sensitive issues concerning scope of services and authorization requirements need to be worked out, as Health Start discovered in negotiating with the four Medicaid managed care plans with which it now has contracts. These contracts call for Health Start to provide a full range of services; it does not have to obtain preauthorization for basic services. Health Start assumes responsibility for any services that students need outside of the school health clinic, making sure students who need follow-up or specialty services use the health plan's network and understand how to access services. It has worked out elaborate policies to protect patient confidentiality, while exchanging necessary information with managed care plans about routine primary care visits. Health Start meets all the credentialing and other criteria of the health plans, and cooperates in all of the plans' quality improvement activities (Zimmerman, 1996).

Financing is, not surprisingly, a complex issue. Health Start is currently reimbursed on a fee-for-service basis; the health plans that capitate all of their primary care services must withhold some of their primary care capitation to pay for adolescent services. The bulk of the claims paid to Health Start come from a large risk pool of providers that includes the St. Paul community clinics and a hospital provider. For Health Start, one possibility under consideration is to move from a fee-for-service arrangement to capitation for a portion of primary care services, based on utilization studies. Few school-based health clinics could qualify as full primary care providers or as specialty care providers, because few can accept full primary care risk or are open 365 days a year and have 24-hour on-call capabilities (Health Start has 365-day, 24-hour coverage for prenatal care, but for all other services arranges for call coverage through the health plans and the students' outside primary care site). The ideal arrangement may well be as comanagers of care, an arrangement well suited to the needs of vulnerable populations, who often benefit from having a complementary access point for health care (Zimmerman, 1996).

Health Start also hopes to expand from Medicaid contracts to commercial contracts. The ultimate goal is to move from one-on-one negotiations with plans to more global budgeting for school health, which would amass all the resources for school health (school nursing service, board of education, local health departments, managed care plans) and apply some of those funds toward specific programmatic initiatives. One possibility would be the creation of an umbrella organization or consortium of clinics that would provide the mechanism and opportunity for health plans to contribute to services in schools (e.g., through immunizations or family planning education) (Zimmerman 1996).

In developing such collaborations, agreement about a common set of goals is key. Quality improvement efforts can supply that set of goals. In conjunction with its health plans, Health Start has agreed on the criteria for establishing those goals—they must have an impact on cost and be evidence-based, measurable, within the control of the school-based health center, and important to the health plan. Among the goals it has agreed to with health plans are increasing access; ensuring the provision of risk reduction prevention services, particularly at the adolescent level (e.g., through groups like Tobacco Free Teens or weight-control groups); delivering early and effective interventions; increasing user satisfaction; and structuring a full and seamless continuum of care, so that students get some services in the school-based clinics and some in health plan clinics (Zimmerman, 1996).

It is worth noting that the collaboration in Minnesota was not mandated by the state; the state Department of Human Services provided some initial assistance, but the collaboration itself depended on the voluntary cooperative efforts of Health Start and individual managed care plans. Health Start's experience with health plans suggests that the relationship between special needs providers and managed care organizations need not be adversarial, that both have important strengths to bring to a collaboration, and that the crucial first step may be identifying a set of common goals.

Children with Special Health Care Needs

One of the biggest concerns child health professionals and advocates have about managed care is its impact on children with special needs. Managed care promises more coordinated care, which is particularly important for children with chronic conditions, but there are also a number of risks, among them the risk of underutilization, the risk that managed care plans may not have the staff to handle the full range of needs of these children, and the incentives inherent in managed care to limit services. Professionals who have been providing care to children with special needs worry that managed care plans will assume responsibility for the care of these children before they are equipped to provide adequate care. Spurred by these concerns, pediatricians in various parts of the country are working aggressively to develop relationships to promote good care for children with special needs.

In Cleveland, Access Better Care (ABC), a comprehensive, interdisciplinary program for children with developmental disabilities, is a joint effort of United HealthCare, a for-profit managed care company, and Metro Health Medical Center, which is under contract to the Ohio Department of Human Services. ABC is modeled on the program developed by Bob Master at the Boston University School of Public Health. ABC gives the pediatrician full authority for care rendered to patients, and there are no preapproval requirements for referrals to specialty or subspecialty providers. Subspecialty providers are reimbursed on a fee-for-service basis. They receive fees that are above average for Medicaid and in addition they receive a care coordination fee. The capitation is paid by the Ohio Department of Human Services to United HealthCare. Financing of the program is through an eight-tiered capitation program (based on actual usage by the enrollee in the previous fiscal year, using Ohio Medicaid data; the managed care fee is 95 percent of the fee-for-service rolled forward with an inflation factor). There is a stop-loss provision in which the state shares the cost of caring for excessively expensive patients. An administrative and case management allowance of 10 percent is paid in addition to the capitation fee; 4.5 percent of that fee goes to United HealthCare for member services, marketing, and enrollment; 4.5 percent goes to the hospital for care coordination services; and the final 1 percent is used for evaluation (Bilenker, 1996).

Physicians, nurses, nurse practitioners, and social workers work together as a care team. ABC also provides 24-hour access to a nurse coordinator, who oversees the care provided by nurse practitioners in the home. ABC has succeeded in changing the location of services from inpatient to outpatient and home-based services. It also seeks to organize care in such a way that the child and parents play a powerful role in care coordination, making the family the focus of the health care delivery system. This is particularly important in the case of children with special needs (Bilenker, 1996). In addition, ABC has developed a series of care plans, some generic, others dealing with specific illnesses, which outline expectations for ordinary screening measures and prevention and frequency of assessments; a copy is sent to a central location, providing a ready audit trail to track compliance with care agreements (Bilenker, 1996). Enrollment is voluntary.

Among the strengths of the program are its ability to deliver coordinated care; team approach; involvement of families; provision of wraparound services (transportation, nonprescription drugs, 24-hour telephone access to primary care provider); and individual care plans mandating family involvement. This approach sharpens the focus on the medical problem but also emphasizes psychological and social issues and needs (Bilenker, 1996).

ABC is currently developing a baseline profile of utilization and measures of quality of care for evaluative purposes. It will compare ABC enrollees with nonenrolled persons with regard to baseline utilization and establish a cross-site enrollee database that will include measures of health and financial status, utilization, selected quality of care measures, reasons for disenrollment, and incidence of voluntary disenrollment (Bilenker, 1996).

One of the chief challenges has been marketing the program. ABC cannot market its services directly, so the success of its efforts to broaden enrollment depends on its ability to explain the program to the benefits educators who in turn explain the program to potential enrollees.

In Arizona, Phoenix Pediatrics has been serving children with special health care needs on a capitated basis for 12 years. Of the 30,000 children in the practice, 2,000 have substantial special health care needs, including children with developmental disabilities, attention deficit disorder, cerebral palsy, and epilepsy, as well as children who require gastrostomy tube feedings or who are tracheostomy- or home-ventilator-dependent. Many of these children are in capitated managed care plans, while others are fee-for-service patients.

The pediatricians in the practice have learned how to manage the care of children outside the hospital and outside the office, resulting in a decline and stabilization in the rate of office visits for children with special needs. The pediatricians in the practice have developed a range of programs to train parents; they also developed the first home ventilator-care programs and tracheostomy home care programs in Arizona and are developing programs for children in foster care, who are currently excluded from managed care in Arizona (Barela, 1996). When hospitalization is necessary, the pediatricians work collaboratively with specialists. Expeditious discharge planning and aggressive case management are also key elements of the program's philosophy. The upshot of this approach is documented decreases in hospital lengths of stay (Barela, 1996).

As others have noted, physicians require special training if they are to take on a case management role for children with special needs; they receive little or no training during medical education for the management of special health care needs children outside the hospital setting (e.g., how to change tracheostomy or gastrostomy tubes in the office or to manage seizures at home). The demands of effective case management range from the simply time-consuming—in a typical month, the practice makes 860 phone calls for medical management—to the more complex—the pediatricians have had to learn how to do gynecological examinations, arrange for formulary exceptions and enteral feeding orders, and complete eligibility applications for nursing home and mental health referrals (Barela, 1996).

Because there are no quality indicators for the outpatient management of children with special needs, the practice collects its own data to document utilization and patterns of care; these data are used to negotiate rates directly with managed care organizations. Reimbursement is based on a tiered program depending on the number of disabilities that a child has (Barela, 1996).

The experience of ABC in Cleveland and Phoenix Pediatrics demonstrates that managed care may indeed be a suitable kind of care for children with special needs, provided adequate attention is paid to issues of case management, coordination, and education of parents and care providers.

Developing the Necessary Information Systems

In order for any of these collaborations to work, there has to be information and the ability to communicate it. Considerable effort and resources are being invested in developing information gathering and sharing systems, yet a host of issues remain to be resolved: technological (software/hardware), professional (whose responsibility is it?), and philosophical (what kinds of information are necessary?). The subject is complicated by the fact that the tools for measuring health status are so rudimentary. The fact that children often see multiple health care providers, and may repeatedly lose and gain insurance coverage, casts into question even the most well designed of information tracking systems.

Some states are further along in this effort than others. For the last 15 years Rhode Island has published 23 health status indicators for each of the state's census tracts. These indicators constitute a set of touch points, allowing public health staff to assess risks and respond to trends in health status. They focus on prepregnancy testing with a prenatal risk assessment, universal newborn screening (which includes information about parents' education, insurance status, and marital status), criteria for in-home assessment and follow-up, and an assessment of social and environmental risks (Hollinshead, 1996).

The state was thus well positioned to do some consolidation in 1991–92, when it discovered that there were at least nine programs in Rhode Island that were in the process of creating tracking and longitudinal follow-up systems. Recognizing that these systems would be highly redundant, the state department of health developed an integrated plan that started from the universal newborn screening system that was already in place. The data from this screening are combined with vital records information to create a single file for each child; a nurse coordinator at the hospitals responsible for maternal and child health generates newborn screen forms to build a locator file. Eventually, many different kinds of screening information get "dropped into" this file (e.g., immunizations, metabolic screening numbers, hearing and vision screening results). All of this information is accessible to all providers who are licensed by the department of health to provide primary care, including providers in hospital outpatient departments, school clinics, and outreach services. Any of these providers can update the record as well and are expected to enter additional information as they provide tracked services (Hollinshead, 1996).

These data have proven extremely useful in developing contracts with managed care plans, and also in justifying the public health messages and investments that the state has made in the past. The data allow precise comparisons between children who are enrolled in managed care and those who are not, and those whose mothers received comprehensive prenatal care services and those whose mothers did not (Hollinshead, 1996).

This system allows the state to track discharges by payers in real time, and has allowed the state to identify some important issues. For example, the newborn screening data revealed that Medicaid patients, even high-risk ones (single mothers, teenage mothers, mothers with limited education), were being discharged as swiftly as privately insured patients. This information was used to inform the debate in the state legislature about 48-hour discharge (Hollinshead, 1996).

The system is also used to track patterns of lead poisoning. The state department of health still provides free lead tests, and all plans are required to do lead testing and submit their results to the department of health. The department of health discovered a 20 percent drop in the number of lead specimens reported following the advent of managed care from all providers except hospital outpatient departments and could analyze this information by provider site, managed care plan, ethnicity, and community. These findings led to intense discussions with providers and plans to improve accountability measures (Hollinshead, 1996).

Conclusion and Implications
These model programs demonstrate that it is possible to improve the coordination and quality of services available to children, even within the constraints of a system that often appears under siege. The key to successful collaborations—whether they are voluntary or mandatory, whether they involve one sector or several, or whether they are proactive or reactive—is effective communication and joint problem solving. Adequate resources (e.g., through enhanced capitation) are also needed to support planning and information gathering. Structuring incentives and standards so that different sectors are at the very least not discouraged from cooperative efforts is also key. Still, there is enough expertise in the system, and enough commitment to the goal of improving conditions for children, to lead to significant—and much needed—improvements in the care available to U.S. children.

References

Barela TD. 1996 March 5. A pediatric practice specializing in chronic illness care. In: Child health care in a managed care environment: Balancing personal and community health needs. Unpublished conference proceedings. New York: United Hospital Fund.

Bilenker RM. 1996 March 5. A capitated program for children with special health care needs. In: Child health care in a managed care environment: Balancing personal and community health needs. Unpublished conference proceedings. New York: United Hospital Fund.

Hollinshead WH. 1996 March 5. Rhode Island's statewide infant tracking and information system. In: Child health care in a managed care environment: Balancing personal and community health needs. Unpublished conference proceedings. New York: United Hospital Fund.

Nannis P. 1996 March 5. A collaborative approach following a measles epidemic by a managed care plan and the Milwaukee Health Department. In: Child health care in a managed care environment: Balancing personal and community health needs. Unpublished conference proceedings. New York: United Hospital Fund.

Walker D. 1996 March 5. Joint planning by the Massachusetts Office of Managed Care and the State Health Department. In: Child health care in a managed care environment: Balancing personal and community health needs. Unpublished conference proceedings. New York: United Hospital Fund.

Zimmerman D. 1996 March 5. School-based services for hard-to-reach adolescents. In: Child health care in a managed care environment: Balancing personal and community health needs, Unpublished conference proceedings. New York: United Hospital Fund.

17

Child Health at a Crossroads: Choices for Policymakers

Ruth E. K. Stein and Anthony Tassi

We are guilty of many errors and many faults, but our
worst crime is abandoning the children, neglecting the
fountain of life. Many of the things we need can wait, the
Child cannot. Right now is the time his bones are being
formed, his blood is being made and his senses are being
developed. To him we cannot answer "Tomorrow."
His name is "Today."

—Gabriela Mistral

THE PRECEDING CHAPTERS underscore the many ways in which the United
States fails to ensure that all children have an opportunity to grow into
healthy adults. At any given time, roughly 10 million children lack health
insurance, and despite its large investment in health care, the United States
far exceeds other nations in rates of infant mortality, adolescent pregnancy,
childhood asthma and asthma-related deaths, and violence-related injuries
and deaths. The time has come to confront the inadequacies of the current
health care system and to demand the public policy leadership necessary to
remedy them.

For all of the challenges discussed, the child health agenda is remarkably
simple; it requires a broad-based commitment to protect and strengthen
the service delivery and financing systems already in place, and to build

from this base toward a more effective and comprehensive system for all children. This agenda is articulated in five imperatives raised repeatedly throughout the book:

- Employing a child-specific standard of care
- Aligning incentives to assure appropriate care, particularly for vulnerable and medically costly children
- Expanding coverage to provide universal access to health care services
- Strengthening community health functions
- Investing in the research, education, and information systems necessary to assure the future quality of child health care

Taken individually, each element contributes to the ability of children to reach their potential to thrive and to become productive adult members of the community. Together, the imperatives form the building blocks of a systematic effort to reshape child health in the United States, an effort that must begin today.

Employing a Child-specific Standard of Care

The establishment of a uniform standard of care for all children, regardless of their insurance status, would be a significant step toward assuring all children access to a decent minimum of care. It is predicated on a recognition of the significant ways in which the health needs of children differ from those of adults, and would require state and federal actions to hold all insurers and providers accountable for such a standard.

A child-specific standard. The dynamic nature of childhood development, the differing epidemiology of childhood diseases, and the enormous long-term benefits of health interventions in the early years of life make the adult standard of care, with its emphasis on acute illness and the management of chronic conditions, inherently unsuitable for children. A child-specific standard should explicitly include activities that promote health in the long term—such as health maintenance, behavioral assessments, anticipatory advice about health and development issues, and disease prevention counseling—as well as allow for sufficient access to pediatric subspecialty evaluations, developmental services, other therapeutic interventions, and wraparound services that are not routinely covered for commercially insured adults. A model may be found in Medicaid's Early and Periodic Screening, Diagnosis and Treatment (EPSDT) program, which stipulates the content and timeliness of a broad range of enabling, preventive, and curative services for children.

Enforcing and extending a child-specific standard. To realize the potential of these standards, states must be held accountable for implementing them and ensuring that they are explicitly retained in Medicaid managed care contracts—something that is unlikely to happen if left to market forces. And until market forces or other pressures provide clear and strong incentives for widespread voluntary adoption of such standards, there is a need for public policy intervention to extend the standards beyond the Medicaid program to commercial insurance contracts. Such a step would require states to exercise their regulatory authority over the health insurance industry as well as federal action to reach plans that are exempt from state regulation under the Employee Retirement Income Security Act (ERISA); such plans cover approximately 50 percent of the population (Liston and Patterson, 1996). Current calls for increased state flexibility in the definition of benefits packages do not bode well for a uniform minimum standard, without which millions of middle-class children of working parents will continue to be short-changed when it comes to prevention, monitoring, and early intervention.

An effective standard of care requires more than just words on a paper, of course. Providers need to be continually educated by the child health community on the importance of screening and early detection and intervention, as do policymakers who may otherwise be tempted by the prospects of short-term savings to curtail benefit packages.

Aligning Incentives to Assure Appropriate Care, Particularly for Vulnerable and Medically Costly Children

The managed care and integrated delivery systems taking shape around the country offer an unprecedented opportunity to realize a child-specific standard of care across a continuum of provider sites. Ideally, links among providers would transcend the confines of traditional medicine to integrate the services and resources of environmental, social, and educational agencies.

Need for change. It would be unrealistic to assume that providers will be able to implement a child-specific standard without a mechanism for recovering the costs of additional services and efforts. This is especially true in a system in which insurance is often transient and where the longer term savings that may accrue as a result of up-front investments are likely to be realized by another party or at a much later date (e.g., special education departments may save money as a result of a health plan's intensive therapies and customized treatment plans).

For all the potential benefits of managed care, capitated payment systems bring their own risks, chief among them the incentive for insurers to avoid enrolling or to limit services to vulnerable and medically costly children, who although few in number account for a high proportion of health care expenditures (Kronick et al., 1996). Such incentives have always existed for insurance companies in the fee-for-service system, but with the spread of managed care, similar incentives are not only reinforced for plans, but increasingly extended to group practices and individual physicians (Dameron et al., 1996), who now bear risk for a broad range of services instead of being reimbursed on a fee-for-service basis.

Multi-Tiered Capitation. To overcome the incentives to enroll only the healthiest children, to disenroll the sickest, and to limit services, a system must be developed that adjusts payments to health care plans and providers based on the intensity of medical need and social risk of the child. Ironically, progress in the development of multi-tiered or risk-adjusted capitation may be most feasible for children with disabilities (often so poorly served in today's non-system), because the expenses related to chronic care are more predictable and the "pay-off" from preventive and primary care (in terms of avoiding acute episodes) is more immediate than for the general child population (Kronick et al., 1996; Fowler and Anderson, 1996).

However, a healthy dose of realism is essential. In examining the growth of integrated delivery systems, some observers have noted a gap between the rhetoric of accountability and integration and the reality of price-based competition among loosely affiliated networks of providers (see chapter 14). Furthermore, until providers and plans face either penalties or explicit financial rewards related to their provision of comprehensive care for vulnerable children, it is unrealistic to expect that adverse selection and risk avoidance activities will be replaced with quality-based competition.

These risk aversion issues must also receive attention in the fee-for-service sector, since many children with complex social and medical needs will continue to be treated outside of managed care systems in the near term.

Expanding Coverage to Provide Universal Access to Health Care Services

Aligning financial incentives among providers, plans, government agencies, and families is a complex puzzle, which cannot be solved perfectly in light of the extraordinary discontinuities in coverage and care that characterize the experience of so many children. Until continuous insurance coverage is guaranteed that provides every child with genuine access to the broad range of services discussed throughout this volume, the economics of prevention and early interventions for children will never be realized on a large scale.

Enrolling all children eligible for Medicaid. An obvious starting point would be to optimize current sources of health care coverage and financing. Important opportunities exist within the current Medicaid program by "simply" enrolling all those children actually eligible. For example, in 1994 approximately 4.8 million children under age 11 eligible for Medicaid were not enrolled (Sumner et al., 1996). Of these, 2.7 million children had no other source of coverage. Thus, the number of uninsured children under age 11 (currently near 6 million) could be reduced by as much as 45 percent without any change in law. The remaining 2.1 million children who had some other form of coverage for at least part of the year could also benefit from Medicaid (or, at a minimum, better coordination of coverage with Medicaid), given the notorious limitations and burdensome cost of private health insurance available to poor and near-poor families.

A variety of approaches could be used to maximize enrollment among Medicaid-eligible children. School-based efforts merit serious attention, especially in light of the large number of successful school-based clinics throughout the country. Additionally, given the growing reliance on managed care in Medicaid, health plans could play a central role in identifying and enrolling children, perhaps under a framework of presumptive eligibility. In those states where an independent enrollment broker is used, enrollment of children eligible for Medicaid but not currently covered could be made a specific performance standard. Another option would be to give health care providers financial incentives to enroll children in the plans they are affiliated with or into primary care management programs. Minimum standards for initial visits would be necessary in any strategy that relies on plans or providers, and could serve to improve the timeliness of care for hundreds of thousands of children. The federal government could also play a role: to the extent that federal approval will continue to be required for mandatory managed care initiatives, the federal government could make approval conditional on the state's development of a strategy for enrolling all Medicaid-eligible children. Lastly, an outreach effort might be built around the extraordinary network and reach of religious institutions, which have proved so effective a platform for previous advocacy efforts.

As with many of the initiatives mentioned in this volume, the current political climate may well work against the effort to enroll all eligible children. For example, the 1996 welfare law (the "Personal Responsibility and Work Opportunity Reconciliation Act of 1996") severed the automatic link between eligibility for cash assistance (Aid to Families with Dependent Children [AFDC] and Supplemental Security Income [SSI]) and Medicaid enrollment and gave individual states the option of redefining eligibility rules. This provision is cause for great concern since only 38 percent of children under age 11 who were eligible for Medicaid but not eligible for cash assistance under AFDC or SSI were actually enrolled in Medicaid in 1994 (Sumner et al., 1996). Thus, the first step toward optimizing Medicaid enrollment under current law is to prevent a wholesale retrenchment in the program likely to stem from increased state flexibility in the eligibility determination process.

Accelerated expansions in coverage. Another possibility for providing more children with access to care would be to accelerate the expansions of coverage stipulated by current law, whereby all children up to age 19 living under the poverty line will qualify for coverage by 2002 (Davis, 1996). In addition, the income threshold could be raised to a higher percentage of poverty. Because of its limited scope and incremental nature, this approach could garner wide support even among traditional opponents of larger efforts to guarantee coverage. For example, a recent survey showed 38 percent of businesses would be willing to support Medicaid expansions to cover uninsured children, as compared to only 14 percent who would support a requirement that all employers contribute at least half the cost of covering the children of their employees (Meyer et al., 1996).

Establishing a minimum period of Medicaid eligibility. Currently, discontinuities in coverage, as families lose and gain Medicaid eligibility, pose almost as much of a problem as lack of coverage. A minimum period of eligibility and continuous enrollment (e.g., one year for children and two years for infants) would be of great benefit to families relying on Medicaid coverage by enhancing the ability of managed care organizations to serve as a medical home. Plans would be more likely to pay closer attention to required screenings, early interventions, and general member services if they knew that their enrollees would remain in the plan for a year or more.

Private insurance subsidies. While there is a need (and an opportunity) to rationalize and expand Medicaid coverage to the fullest extent possible, roughly half the states have also implemented a variety of initiatives to subsidize the cost of children's-only private insurance coverage. For example, New York's Child Health Plus, originally enacted in 1990 as a modest program to provide outpatient benefits to children under 13 in low-income families not qualifying for Medicaid, now enrolls more than 100,000 children. The covered benefits were recently expanded to include inpatient hospitalization and other services, while the age and income eligibility thresholds were also increased. Sliding scale premium subsidies are available up to 222 percent of poverty, funded through a combination of provider and payer assessments (assessments originally enacted to fund uncompensated hospital care).

Likewise, Massachusetts has received considerable attention for its Children's Medical Security Plan (CMSP) funded through a tobacco tax. Expanded in 1996 as part of a broader-based health insurance expansion, the CMSP is projected to provide primary care and emergency coverage to 125,000 children under age 18 in 1997. Florida has also been credited with implementing a small (roughly 20,000 enrollees) but successful program of subsidized coverage available to children through grade 12. The Florida model is unique for its use of school districts as a grouping mechanism to lower the costs of insurance for children, while facilitating greater access to preventive care and early interventions.

Individually, the scope of many of the "kids-only" initiatives may seem limited in comparison to the identified needs of uninsured children. Their shortcomings are well documented: they exclude the majority of the uninsured—that is, adults—prohibiting a genuine family-centered approach to health care; they use scarce resources inefficiently due to favorable selection in the programs and by potentially replacing existing coverage rather than adding new children to the rolls (the "crowding out" effect); they leave the fate of millions of uninsured children to the political vagaries of 50 different state legislatures; and they imply that a child living in a state with a weaker economic base or lower level of political commitment to children should not be afforded the same basic protections as a child in a wealthier or more committed state. These faults point unequivocally to the need for a more comprehensive, universal solution to the problems related to insurance: a federal guarantee of coverage for every individual.

However, in the immediate future, the benefit of incremental programs cannot be denied. Taken together, they represent a substantial, politically popular commitment of resources to children's health care. Already, a number of different approaches have been proposed on the federal level to expand on the "success" of these initiatives—including tax credits for working families, state-administered voucher programs, and Medicaid managed care buy-in programs. Making children's-only coverage available to families who do not qualify for Medicaid may form a logical base for additional incremental expansions in eligibility and scope of benefits (e.g., incorporating a child standard of care) necessary to reach all children with comprehensive coverage. Additionally, this approach may be necessary in the coming years as the impact of the recent welfare and immigration legislation becomes felt, very likely increasing the number of children without meaningful access to care (Meyer and Silow-Caroll, 1996).

There are a variety of approaches to cover all children: voluntary or mandatory; federal or state-level; private or public; tax credit or subsidies; "kids-only" or universal. These options and the trade-offs that accompany them have tended to divide (and conquer) numerous earlier attempts at meaningful expansion of health care coverage. With an unrelenting focus on the goal of a rationalized health care system where no members of society are singled out for exclusion, pragmatic steps must be taken and agreements reached in order to sustain (and in some areas, create) momentum in the political arena. With each uninsured or underinsured child remaining, the challenges in developing an effective child health system become more difficult.

Strengthening Community Health Functions

Even when children are universally insured, there will continue to be a need for a strong independent community health function. As noted in chapter 15, the community health function is essential to monitor health status and identify health problems in the community, as opposed to a covered population.

Public Health Infrastructure. For the immediate future, most managed care organizations are unlikely to extend their focus beyond personal health care. Therefore, a public health infrastructure is needed to diagnose and investigate health problems and health hazards in the community. Furthermore, the need continues—as strong today as ever—for public vigilance and enforcement of laws and regulations that protect health and ensure safety. Infectious disease control and regulation of toxic materials are but two concrete examples of functions that can never be left to the market. A host of more mundane functions—like pest and rodent control—are also crucial to a healthy environment.

The benefits of such a function are all around us. A dramatic reduction in poisoning accompanied the regulation of packaging of medications and other toxic substances. Likewise, in other countries, the number of injuries, the leading cause of death and morbidity throughout the childhood years, was dramatically reduced as a result of standards and regulations designed to make the environment safer for children, ranging from the placement of electrical sockets out of toddlers' reach to the creation of bicycle pathways that are separate from vehicular traffic to regulating the size of unprotected window openings. Similar results occurred in several large U.S. cities when regulations were enforced regarding window guards in high-rise apartment buildings, markedly decreasing the number of children who suffered severe injuries or death from falls. Such environmental manipulations reduce the hazards associated with childhood morbidity more effectively than one-to-one counseling by the pediatrician.

However, many of the cross-subsidies that have supported public health agencies are being squeezed, just as a revitalized infrastructure is badly needed. The maintenance of governmental responsibility for this function is key: to preserve its independence and public accountability and assure national uniformity of basic services and environmental protections that are so important in this age of high population mobility. This is not to argue that implementation of all public health policies should be performed by governmental agencies; it is the policy setting and monitoring responsibility that should occur at that level. Personal and public health providers must continue to work collaboratively and use the levers of government to protect the citizenry—experimenting with a mix of incentives, penalties, subsidies, and prohibitions to meet new challenges as they are identified.

In their role as monitor, public health agencies must hold providers accountable for their progress not only in meeting service standards for children's preventive and primary care, but also for their progress in meeting the full range of articulated community health goals such as those outlined in *Healthy People 2000* or *Healthy Children 2000*. Advocates must hold the states accountable, whether care is delivered through fee-for-service or managed care delivery systems. States and localities must require health plans to participate more actively in public health planning and interventions and need to reward them for their contributions. This is a complicated task because the benefits of such investments are not always easily quantifiable and may accrue to other programs (such as education). Likewise, plans must be held accountable for their lack of initiative or effectiveness. As health plans and provider systems speak of community and of population-based medicine, we cannot rely entirely on their good will in living up to their rhetoric; they need to be held accountable both by public health agencies and through the force of informed public opinion.

Involving the Community in Community Health. Strengthening communities is an important piece of the child heath care agenda, whether by providing meaningful support to families in childrearing (e.g., through such measures as the 1993 Family and Medical Leave Act) or by using the power of taxation to discourage economic activity that poisons the child's environment. U.S. businesses must be held accountable for the impact of wage, benefit, and child care policies on the health and welfare of children. It is important to highlight the impact of corporate downsizing and employment policies on children and their rates of health care coverage. Moreover, communities have a variety of tools at their disposal to send a clear message to U.S. corporations that they will be held accountable for the systemic impacts of boardroom decisions on families and communities, their natural resources, and their economic bases. Consumer buying guides, social investment screens, and child health impact statements (especially with increased media attention) could be used to reward companies that adopt children-friendly and community-building policies.

Investing in Research, Education, and Information Systems to Assure the Future Quality of Child Health Care

The continued development of quality-based care is unlikely to occur without a continuing investment in research, education, and integrated information systems. These are elements that are essential to the field and cannot be expected to be supported by the marketplace on its own; they are areas requiring managed cooperation, rather than unmanaged competition focused on the bottom line.

Research. A strong research infrastructure is needed to continue advances in medical sciences that improve the treatment and quality of life of children who experience health conditions. The United States has been a leader in discovering cures and preventive techniques for conditions that were previously fatal or caused significant morbidity (e.g., leukemia, poliomyelitis). Such a leadership role depends on sustained investment in scientific research both at the level of the basic science laboratory and in the translation of bench findings to the clinical setting.

In addition, the current research agenda must include a commitment to develop better methodologies for the improvement of child health measures and technologies for risk adjustment, and for health services evaluation to determine the optimal ways of providing child health care services. While there has been an increase in the funding of health services research generally, a very small portion of this effort has focused on child health issues, in large part because much of the current agenda is driven by high-cost items in adult care.

Education. Education of health care professionals with expertise in child health issues is another critical public good. The dynamic needs of children and the special forms their health problems take require that a steady supply of individuals with expertise in their care be maintained and cultivated, both through the primary education of child health professionals and through the retraining of existing providers for new and expanded responsibilities and roles. The latter is especially necessary as providers are being asked to assume new responsibilities under managed care. In some places, attempts to form and implement progressive systems of care for children with special needs have floundered as a result of a lack of appropriately trained health professionals able to fulfill the challenges of the new paradigm.

Information Systems. Finally, much of the data needed for research and monitoring are currently unavailable. The power of information systems and emerging software technologies must be harnessed. Beyond developing basic (but, as of yet, unrealized) functions such as immunization registries, information systems visionaries are needed to provide the data and record-keeping infrastructure necessary for true coordination of care among providers. Flexibility, adaptability, and useability are driving forces in commercial software development; these attributes are sorely needed in children's health care as well. Here again, many needs are specific to child health issues and systems designed for adults are not easily adapted.

A Broader Vision of Health

The five steps outlined above would take us a long way toward assuring that each child in the United States has access to a basic level of health care, but none of them will happen on their own. There is a pressing need for public policy leadership and for active efforts on the part of concerned citizens to pressure their elected officials into assuming this leadership role.

As many of the book's authors remind us, however, we cannot restrict our efforts to the health care system alone; we need to address the broader economic and social factors that influence children's well-being. The negative impacts of poverty, racism, and environmental degradation—inextricably tied to the structure of our economy—cannot be denied and must be addressed. Stitching together a broad coalition active in each of these areas and committed to action to improve the conditions of U.S. children will be necessary if we are to make significant progress.

Finally, although we cannot escape the political reality that the United States has always tended to act in an incrementalist mode in altering its health care policies, it seems self-evident that our best chance for a better tomorrow lies in a complete overhaul of the child health care delivery system. A system that is really designed to address the needs of children would assure that every child was covered for a broad package of care defined by a child-specific standard of medical necessity, had access to a primary care provider, and was protected by a set of strong public health elements that would assure that all children grow up in safer communities. Realizing even a portion of the child health agenda articulated in this book will make a tangible difference in the lives of millions of children throughout the country. Change requires a sustained focus on these issues, and a long-term commitment to our children and the future of society. It is our hope that this volume will mobilize a pragmatism rooted in today's reality and guided by a vision of tomorrow's equity that will bring us closer to these goals.

References

Cantor JC, Miles EL, Baker LC, Barker DC. 1996. Physician service to the underserved: Implications for affirmative action in medical education. Inquiry 33:167–80.

Dameron TH, Fessler JC. 1996. Underwriting: A key to healthy capitation agreements. Healthcare Financial Management 50(9):43-5.

Davis K. 1996. Incremental coverage of the uninsured. Journal of the American Medical Association 276:831–2.

Fowler EJ, Anderson GF. 1996. Capitation adjustment for pediatric populations. Pediatrics 98(1):10–6.

Heyman SJ, Earler A, Egleston B. 1996. Parental availability for the care of sick children. Pediatrics 98:226–30.

Kronick R, Dreyfus T, Lee L, et al. 1996. Diagnostic risk adjustment for Medicaid: The disability payment system. Health Care Financing Review 17(3):7–33.

Liston D, Patterson MP. 1996. Analysis of the number of workers covered by self-insured health plans under the Employee Retirement Income Security Act of 1974—1993 and 1995. A Report to the Henry J. Kaiser Family Foundation.

Meyer JA, Silow-Carroll S. 1996. Options to assure access to health care for people leaving welfare for work. A report prepared for the Annie E. Casey Foundation.

Meyer JA, Naughton DH, Perry MJ. 1996. Assessing business attitudes on health care.

Sumner L, Parrott S, Mann C. 1996. Millions of uninsured and underinsured children are eligible for Medicaid. Center on Budget and Policy Priorities.

About the Editor and Authors

Ruth E. K. Stein, MD, is professor and vice chairman of the department of pediatrics and director of the division of general pediatrics at the Albert Einstein College of Medicine. She is also pediatrician-in-chief at the Jacobi Medical Center. For the past two years she has been a scholar-in-residence at the United Hospital Fund.

Amy B. Bernstein, ScD, is a senior associate at the Alpha Center in Washington, DC, where she is part of the national program office for The Robert Wood Johnson Foundation's Changes in Health Care Financing and Organization program.

Jeffrey Blustein, PhD, is associate professor of bioethics at Albert Einstein College of Medicine and adjunct associate professor of philosophy at Barnard College of Columbia University. Dr. Blustein also serves as clinical bioethicist at Montefiore Medical Center, where he is cochair of the bioethics committee and a member of the bioethics consultation service.

Phyllis Brooks is director of communications at the United Hospital Fund.

Carol Gentry is a freelance writer and a commentator on the public radio show *Marketplace*. She covered the health care system in the 1980s and early 1990s for the *St. Petersburg Times*.

Holly Grason, MA, is director of the Women's and Children's Health Policy Center and a faculty member in the department of maternal and child health at the Johns Hopkins School of Hygiene and Public Health.

Neal Halfon, MD, MPH, is associate professor of pediatrics in the School of Medicine of the University of California at Los Angeles (UCLA), associate professor of community health sciences in the UCLA School of Public Health, and consultant in the social policy department at the RAND Corporation.

Maxine Hayes, MD, MPH, is assistant secretary of the Washington State Department of Health. She is clinical associate professor of pediatrics at the University of Washington School of Medicine and on the MCH faculty in its School of Public Health. She is president of the Association of Maternal and Child Health Programs and national program director for The Robert Wood Johnson Child Health Initiative.

Miles Hochstein, PhD, is the assistant director for the National Center for Infancy and Early Childhood Health Policy at the University of California at Los Angeles (UCLA).

Dana C. Hughes, DrPH, is a senior policy analyst with the Institute for Health Policy Studies at the University of California at San Francisco. She teaches health policy and public health at the University of California at San Francisco and at the University of California at Berkeley School of Public Health.

Vince L. Hutchins, MD, MPH, is Distinguished Research Professor at Georgetown University's National Center for Education in Maternal and Child Health. After a decade in the private practice of pediatrics, he entered federal service in 1971 with the Maternal and Child Health Program, which he directed from 1977 to 1992.

Lorraine V. Klerman, Dr. Ph, is professor and chairperson of the department of maternal and child health at the School of Public Health, University of Alabama at Birmingham.

Sheila Leatherman is executive vice president for United HealthCare Corporation, where she founded the Center for Health Care Policy and Evaluation. Ms. Leatherman is a senior fellow at the Institute for Health Services Research at the University of Minnesota and senior associate at the Judge Institute of Management Studies at Cambridge University in Great Britain.

Debra J. Lipson, MHSA, is an associate director at the Alpha Center in Washington, DC.

Douglas McCarthy is director of public policy for United HealthCare Corporation, and a Public Policy Fellow at the Humphrey Institute of Public Affairs of the University of Minnesota.

Madlyn Morreale holds faculty appointments in the departments of maternal and child health and health policy and management at the Johns Hopkins University School of Hygiene and Public Health. She also serves as the community planning and policy coordinator for the Johns Hopkins University Center for Adolescent Health Promotion and Disease Prevention.

Paul W. Newacheck, DrPH, is professor of health policy in the department of pediatrics and codirector of the Maternal and Child Health Policy Research Center at the University of California at San Francisco. Dr. Newacheck is a member of the Board on Children, Youth and Families for the National Academy of Sciences.

Judith Palfrey, MD, is chief of the division of general pediatrics at Children's Hospital in Boston and the T. Berry Brazelton Professor of Pediatrics at Harvard University Medical School. She is the immediate past president of the Ambulatory Pediatric Association and chair of the Building Bright Futures initiative.

Michelle Pearl, MPH, is a research analyst with the Institute for Health Policy Studies at the University of California at San Francisco and a doctoral student in epidemiology at the University of California at Berkeley.

Janet D. Perloff, PhD, is associate professor of health and social policy in the School of Social Welfare and the School of Public Health at the University at Albany of the State University of New York.

Robert Restuccia is executive director of Health Care for All. He is an adjunct professor at the Boston University School of Public Health.

Sara Rosenbaum, JD, is director of the Center for Health Policy Research and professor at the George Washington University Medical Center. Ms. Rosenbaum also holds appointments in the university's schools of business and law.

Susan Sherry is director of Community Catalyst, a national support center for community health action serving state and local consumer organizations. She was founding director of Health Care For All, the Massachusetts consumer health organization.

Barbara Starfield, MD, MPH, is University Distinguished Service Professor with appointments in the departments of health policy and management and pediatrics at the Johns Hopkins School of Hygiene and Public Health and School of Medicine.

Jeffrey J. Stoddard, MD, is assistant professor of pediatrics and preventive medicine at the University of Wisconsin Medical School in Madison, Wisconsin. He also teaches medical students and residents in community-based pediatric clinics and has assisted in the development of academic-community partnerships focusing on child health.

James R. Tallon, Jr., is president of the United Hospital Fund. Prior to joining the Fund in 1993, Mr. Tallon served for 19 years in the New York State Assembly. He serves as chair of the Kaiser Commission on the Future of Medicaid and is a member of the Prospective Payment Assessment Commission (ProPAC), and the Joint Commission on the Accreditation of Healthcare Organizations.

Anthony Tassi is a health policy analyst at the United Hospital Fund, where he is researching the continuing evolution of Medicaid managed care in New York City.

Deborah Klein Walker, EdD, is the assistant commissioner for the Bureau of Family and Community Health in the Massachusetts Department of Public Health. Dr. Walker is currently Region I Councillor of the Association of Maternal and Child Health Programs and chair of the Association's Committee on the Health.

Michael Weitzman, MD, is pediatrician in chief at Rochester General Hospital and professor and associate chairman of pediatrics at the University of Rochester School of Medicine and Dentistry, where he is also director of the division of general pediatrics. Dr. Weitzman is chairperson of the American Academy of Pediatrics' Committee on Community Health Services.

Index

Current Publications

Better Jobs, Better Care: Building the
Home Care Work Force *Paper Series*
#7038   56 pages   1994 $10.00

Beyond the Clinic: Redefining Hospital
Ambulatory Care
#7348   48 pages   1997 $20.00

Building Bridges: Community Health
Outreach Worker Programs
A Practical Guide
#7186   40 pages   1994 $10.00

A Clearing in the Crowd: Innovations in
Emergency Services *Paper Series*
#7119   48 pages   1994 $10.00

A Death in the Family: Orphans of the
HIV Epidemic
#7135   178 pages   1993 $10.00

Health Care Annual: Data on Hospitals in
New York City, Long Island, and the
Northern Metropolitan Area, 1997
Update
#7321   72 pages   1997 $20.00

Health Care for Children: What's Right,
What's Wrong, What's Next
#7313   416 pages   1997 $40.00

Hospital Watch: A Quarterly Report on
Hospital Finance and Utilization
No charge

Mediating Bioethical Disputes *A
Practical Guide*
#7194   104 pages   1994 $20.00

Medicaid Managed Care Currents
No charge

Meeting Patients' Needs: Quality Care in
a Changing Environment *Paper Series*
#7275   36 pages   1995 $12.00

Monitoring Medicaid Managed Care:
Developing an Assessment and
Evaluation Program *A Special Report*
#7259   52 pages   1995 $25.00

New York City Community Health
Atlas, 1994
#7003   192 pages   1994 $50.00

Reshaping Inpatient Care: Efficiency and
Quality in New York City Hospitals
Paper Series
#7291   44 pages   1996 $12.00

The State of New York City's Municipal
Hospital System, Fiscal Year 1996
#7305   48 pages   1996 $10.00

An Unfinished Revolution: Women and
Health Care in America
#7178   304 pages   1994 $20.00

Zip Code Area Profiles, 1994
#7208   358 pages   1994 $100.00 (book)
$250 (disk*—*please specify Lotus or SPSS*)

* Includes hard copies of *New York City
Community Health Atlas* and *Zip Code
Area Profiles.*

*To order, please write to the United Hospital Fund, Publications Program, Empire State
Building, 350 Fifth Avenue, 23rd Floor, New York, NY 10118. Checks should be made
payable to the United Hospital Fund and include $3.50 for shipping and handling. For infor-
mation about bulk orders or for a complete list of publications, please call 212-494-0700.*